THE WASHINGTON MANUAL™

Cardiology **Subspecialty Consult**

Second Edition

Editors

Phillip S. Cuculich, MD
Fellow, Cardiovascular Diseases
Washington University School of Medicine
Barnes-Jewish Hospital
St. Louis, Missouri

Andrew M. Kates, MD
Associate Professor of Medicine
Washington University School of Medicine
Barnes-Jewish Hospital
St. Louis, Missouri

Series Editors

Katherine E. Henderson, MD
Instructor in Medicine
Department of Internal Medicine
Division of Medical Education
Washington University School of Medicine
Barnes-Jewish Hospital
St. Louis, Missouri

Thomas M. De Fer, MD
Associate Professor of Internal Medicine
Washington University School of Medicine
St. Louis, Missouri

 Wolters Kluwer | Lippincott Williams & Wilkins
Health
Philadelphia · Baltimore · New York · London
Buenos Aires · Hong Kong · Sydney · Tokyo

Acquisitions Editor: Ave McCracken
Managing Editor: Michelle LaPlante
Project Manager: Bridgett Dougherty
Marketing Manager: Kimberly Schonberger
Manufacturing Manager: Kathleen Brown
Design Coordinator: Risa Clow
Cover Designer: Joseph DePinho
Production Service: Aptara, Inc.®

Second Edition

© **2009 by Department of Medicine, Washington University School of Medicine**

Printed in China

9 8 7 6 5 4 3 2 1

Library of Congress Cataloging-in-Publication Data

The Washington manual cardiology subspecialty consult.— 2nd ed. / editors, Phillip S. Cuculich, Andrew M. Kates.

  p. ; cm.— (Washington manual subspecialty consult series)
  Includes bibliographical references and index.
  ISBN 978-0-7817-9151-9
1. Cardiology—Handbooks, manuals, etc. 2. Heart—Diseases—Handbooks, manuals, etc. I. Cuculich, Phillip S. II. Kates, Andrew M. III. Title: Cardiology subspecialty consult. IV. Series.
  [DNLM: 1. Cardiovascular Diseases—Handbooks. 2. Cardiology—methods—Handbooks. WG 39 W3173 2008]
  RC669.15.W37 2008
  616.1'2—dc22

                                                                      2008018120

To purchase additional copies of this book, call our customer service department at **(800) 638-3030** or fax orders to **(301) 223-2320**. International customers should call **(301) 223-2300**.

Visit Lippincott Williams & Wilkins on the Internet: http://www.lww.com. Lippincott Williams & Wilkins customer service representatives are available from 8:30 am to 6:00 pm, EST.

To our wives and families, who give our hearts reason to beat.
—PSC & AMK

American College of Cardiology/American Heart Association Clinical Practice Guidelines

Rating Scheme for the Strength of the Recommendations

Class I: Conditions for which there is evidence and/or general agreement that a given procedure or treatment is beneficial, useful, and effective.

Class II: Conditions for which there is conflicting evidence and/or a divergence of opinion about the usefulness/efficacy of a procedure or treatment.

> **Class IIa:** Weight of evidence/opinion is in favor of usefulness/efficacy.

> **Class IIb:** Usefulness/efficacy is less well established by evidence/opinion.

Class III: Conditions for which there is evidence and/or general agreement that a procedure/treatment is not useful/effective and in some cases may be harmful.

Rating Scheme for the Strength of the Evidence

Level of Evidence A: Data derived from multiple randomized clinical trials or meta-analyses.

Level of Evidence B: Data derived from a single randomized trial or nonrandomized studies.

Level of Evidence C: Only consensus opinion of experts, case studies, or standard-of-care.

Gibbons RJ, Smith S, Antman E. American College of Cardiology/American Heart Association clinical practice guidelines: Part I: where do they come from? *Circulation* 2003;107:2979–2986.

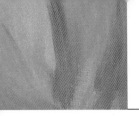

Table of Contents

PART VII. VASCULAR DISEASE

PART VIII. CARDIAC IMAGING AND PROCEDURES

PART IX. SPECIAL POPULATIONS

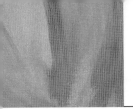

Contributing Authors

Michael O. Barry, MD
Clearwater Cardiovascular &
Interventional Consultants
Clearwater, Florida

Russell M. Canham, MD, MCS
Fellow, Clinical Cardiology
Barnes-Jewish Hospital
St. Louis, Missouri

Daniel H. Cooper, MD
Fellow, Clinical Cardiology
Barnes-Jewish Hospital
St. Louis, Missouri

Phillip S. Cuculich, MD
Fellow, Cardiovascular Diseases
Washington University School of Medicine
Barnes-Jewish Hospital
St. Louis, Missouri

Tillmann Cyrus, MB, MD
Senior Scientist
Washington University School of Medicine
St. Louis, Missouri

Sitaramesh Emani, MD
Resident, Internal Medicine
Washington University School of Medicine
St. Louis, Missouri

Steven M. Ewer, MD
Research Fellow, Cardiology
Washington University School of Medicine
St. Louis, Missouri

Anthony Hart, MD
Resident, Internal Medicine
Washington University School of Medicine
St. Louis, Missouri

Christopher Holley, MD
Chief Medicine Resident
Washington University School of Medicine
St. Louis, Missouri

Raksha Jain, MD
*Clinical Fellow, Pulmonary, Critical Care
and Sleep Medicine*
Barnes-Jewish Hospital
St. Louis, Missouri

Sujith Kalathiveetil, MD
Fellow, Clinical Cardiology
Barnes-Jewish Hospital
St. Louis, Missouri

Andrew M. Kates, MD
Associate Professor of Medicine
Washington University School of Medicine
Barnes-Jewish Hospital
St. Louis, Missouri

Brian R. Lindman, MD
Fellow, Clinical Cardiology
Barnes-Jewish Hospital
St. Louis, Missouri

Kan Liu, MD
Fellow, Clinical Cardiology
Barnes-Jewish Hospital
St. Louis, Missouri

Stacey Mandras, MD
Fellow, Clinical Cardiology
Barnes-Jewish Hospital
St. Louis, Missouri

Santhosh Jay Mathews, MD, MS
Fellow, Clinical Cardiology
Barnes-Jewish Hospital
St. Louis, Missouri

Jennifer L. Peura, MD
Research Fellow, Cardiology,
Washington University School of Medicine
St. Louis, Missouri

John Phillips, MD
Resident, Internal Medicine
Washington University School of Medicine
St. Louis, Missouri

Peter Rao, MD
Research Fellow, Cardiology
Washington University School of Medicine
St. Louis, Missouri

Ibrahim M. Saeed
Assistant Professor of Medicine
Washington University School of Medicine
St. Louis, Missouri

Joel Schilling, MD, PhD
Research Fellow, Cardiology
Washington University School of Medicine
St. Louis, Missouri

Timothy W. Schloss, MD
Fellow, Clinical Cardiology
Barnes-Jewish Hospital
St. Louis, Missouri

Jasvindar Singh, MD
Associate Professor of Medicine
Washington University School of Medicine
St. Louis, Missouri

Sumeet Subherwal, MD
Resident, Internal Medicine
Washington University School of Medicine
St. Louis, Missouri

Courtney Virgilio, MD
Fellow, Clinical Cardiology
Barnes-Jewish Hospital
St. Louis, Missouri

Michael Yeung, MD
Resident, Internal Medicine
Washington University School of Medicine
St. Louis, Missouri

Chairman's Note

Medical knowledge is increasing at an exponential rate, and physicians are being bombarded with new facts at a pace that many find overwhelming. The Washington Manual™ Subspecialty Consult Series was developed in this context for interns, residents, medical students, and other practitioners in need of readily accessible practical clinical information. They, therefore, meet an important unmet need in an era of information overload.

I would like to acknowledge the authors who have contributed to these books. In particular, the series editors, Katherine E. Henderson, MD and Thomas M. De Fer, MD, for their oversight of the project. I'd also like to recognize Melvin Blanchard, MD, Chief of the Division of Medical Education in the Department of Medicine at Washington University for his guidance and advice. The efforts and outstanding skill of the lead authors are evident in the quality of the final product. I am confident that this series will meet its desired goal of providing practical knowledge that can be directly applied to improving patient care.

Kenneth S. Polonsky, MD
Adolphus Busch Professor
Chairman, Department of Medicine
Washington University School of Medicine
St. Louis, Missouri

Preface

We, the editors of the second edition of *The Washington Manual*™ *Cardiology Subspecialty Consult*, extend our gratitude and respect to you, the reader. Gratitude, for choosing our book as worthy of your time to learn about diseases of the heart and blood vessels; and respect, for your desire to care for patients with cardiovascular disease in the most contemporary manner.

We thank the Series Editor, Dr. Katherine Henderson, for her tireless efforts and patience while this book was built one chapter at a time. We acknowledge the thoughtful framework of the first edition provided by the editor, Dr. Peter Crawford. We are most indebted to the marvelous effort of those who contributed to the current edition: house staff, fellows, and attending physicians alike. While we expected excellence from our authors, we were overwhelmed by the high quality of information and clear passion for teaching that is found in each chapter.

The innumerable advances in cardiology as well as our authors' dedication have resulted in the rewriting of nearly every chapter in the second edition. The overriding theme of each chapter is a front-line application of up-to-date guidelines with focus on patient care. We deliberately stress the most useful information as it relates to the patient's diagnosis and treatment. Each chapter is built on a foundation of practical knowledge, buttressed, where appropriate, with mnemonics and easily remembered bullet-point lists, as well as bold-faced clinical pearls and easy-to-read figures. As repetition is essential for learning, chapters conclude with a "Key Points to Remember" section. To keep the text thin enough to be portable, guidelines from the American Heart Association and American College of Cardiology are emphasized with journal and online references at the end of each chapter. We strongly encourage reading these current practice recommendations as well as peer-reviewed journals, review articles, and primary textbooks to supplement the material in this handbook.

We are enormously excited about the quality and scope of this handbook. Seven new chapters have been added to the second edition. The tremendous growth in cardiac imaging is highlighted in its own chapter, which addresses newer imaging tools such as cardiac CT, cardiac MRI, PET, and IVUS. The heightened awareness of the association of coronary and peripheral vascular diseases has necessitated a dedicated chapter as well. The importance of individualization of medicine has helped shape three new chapters on cardiovascular diseases in specific patient populations, including women, the elderly, patients with HIV, and patients with diabetes.

These new chapters are coupled with a logical restructuring of the organization of the book, grouping chapters together by specific disease. At the end of the text, an innovative appendix allows for a quick recall of the most common cardiovascular medications, common doses, and important side effects.

This is a thrilling time to be interested in cardiovascular disease. Ongoing research has led to new discoveries and improvements, and with it new clinical challenges of practicing "evidenced-based" cardiology. This process requires a continuous synthesis and evaluation of the most recent clinical trials into daily practice while maintaining diagnostic skills that are at the center of cardiovascular disease management. It is our hope that both the information and the enthusiasm contained in the chapters that follow provide you with the means to meet these challenges and with it become a better teacher, a better learner, and a better physician.

—PSC & AMK

Approach to the Cardiovascular Consult

Andrew M. Kates

1

he cardiovascular consultant is unique in medicine and cardiology may be considered a most rewarding specialty to pursue. Consultative cardiology affords the opportunity to integrate physiology with physical examination skills in the setting of rapidly developing procedures and techniques, to practice evidence-based medicine in a constantly advancing technological environment, and above all to make a significant difference for the patient and the patient's family.

There are many reasons why physicians are asked to see a patient with presumed cardiac problems, including atrial fibrillation, elevated cardiac enzymes, an abnormal stress test, heart failure, tachy- or bradycardia, and so on. In approaching the patient with potential cardiac issues, it is helpful to understand the role of the consultant in this process—that is, to know what makes a "good," effective consultant. Such a consultant should do the following:

- Define what the referring physician wants from the consultation
- Establish urgency
- Investigate for him- or herself ("trust but verify")
- Address the referring physician's concerns
- Make specific and succinct recommendations
- Include a problem list
- Limit the number of recommendations to fewer than six if possible
- Call the referring physician
- Make a follow-up visit

As an aside, it is understood that not all requests for consultation are expressed in a clear manner. In a teaching hospital, consults may be requested by medical students or junior house officers who are unfamiliar with the patient or the issues regarding the consultation. In a community hospital, it may be a nurse or secretary, with even less information about the patient, who requests the consult. Although there are rules for a "good referral," it is up to the consultant both to determine the reason for the consultation and to assess the patient.

This being said, the aforementioned footprint for effective consultation can be modified to apply specifically to the cardiology consultation. There are several critical questions that should be answered as quickly as possible, especially in assessing a patient who may be critically ill:

- Why is the patient being seen?
- What is the patient's primary problem? (Often distinct from the above.)
- What are his or her vital signs right now?
- Where is the patient right now [home, clinic, patient testing, emergency department, ward, operating room, holding area, intensive care unit (ICU)]?
- How long has the problem been present?
- What are the important exam findings?
- What does the electrocardiogram (ECG) show?

To help answer these questions, consider these issues as the patient is evaluated:

- What diagnostic study, procedure, or therapeutic (medical or surgical) intervention is appropriate for this patient?
- How soon does he or she need it?
- Where does this patient need to be now (e.g., floor, ICU) to best receive care?

After these questions have been answered, workup and management can begin. Obviously, the amount of time it takes to complete this process, including the history and physical exam, will vary depending on the answers to the above questions. The consultant's ability to determine these parameters will develop with knowledge and experience. We hope that this book will serve as a valuable resource for consultant physicians as they care for patients in the myriad of clinical situations likely to be encountered.

Depending upon the complexity of the situation, an opinion regarding management of the patient with cardiac issues can be reasonably rendered by house officers on the medical service or consult service, a cardiology fellow in training, an internist or hospitalist in private practice, or a board-certified cardiologist. Inherent in providing an opinion, however, is an understanding of one's limitations. Although this book may serve as a thorough, useful review of several areas in cardiology—ranging from common clinical presentations (Chapters 3–6), to acute coronary syndromes (Chapters 8–10), to the many faces of heart failure (Chapters 11–14), as well as issues in electrophysiology (Chapters 18–21), valvular disease (Chapters 16 and 17) and many places in between—it is by no means a substitute for reading the primary literature, reviewing published guidelines, amassing clinical experience, or undertaking advanced cardiology training. To quote Hippocrates: "As to diseases, make a habit of two things—to help, or at least to do no harm."

REFERENCES AND SUGGESTED READINGS

Pearson SD. Principles of generalist-specialist relationships. *J Gen Intern Med* 1999;14: S13–S20.

Basic Electrocardiography (ECG 101)

2

Phillip S. Cuculich

INTRODUCTION: "I CAN'T READ AN ECG"

It's 2 A.M. and you are called to see your patient, who is having severe chest pain. He is clearly uncomfortable, sweating, and short of breath. His nurse hands you an ECG and asks you what to do next. In your mind, you say: (1) Wow, this rhythm is fast. (2) Are those ST-segment elevations? (3) Aren't there at least 20 causes of ST elevations?

In general, the electrocardiogram (ECG) may be the single most important and widely used test in the hospital, yet ECG interpretation is usually poorly taught in medical school. There are large gaps in time between each lesson, and ECG basics may never be taught that well in the first place. For example, early in medical school you learn about a guy named Einthoven and his triangle, and several years later you are "pimped" on rounds about the 20 causes of ST elevations. This chapter is not meant to bridge those gaps or to be a complete guide to ECG reading. It is an "in the trenches" practical guide to coming close to a diagnosis, with the ultimate goal of helping you with that 2 A.M. patient mentioned above. Was it a heart attack or just atrial flutter?

Before we dive in, let me mention three very important pieces of advice I was given by my "Jedi masters of cardiology" (influential residents and attendings), which have served me well:

- "Practice, practice, practice"—Invest in a book of unknown ECG tracings with answers. Do online tutorials. Look at ECGs from patients on a cardiology service. Avoid the gaps in time that plagued your learning in med school.
- "Same way every time"—By using the same approach with every ECG, you will become efficient and accurate. More importantly, you will be less likely to miss subtle diagnoses.
- Keep a file of interesting ECGs—By collecting interesting ECGs, you maintain a sense of interest and vigilance. You will begin to recognize certain patterns of disease. Additionally, it will help to have the collection when you must give a conference on short notice.

THE ULTRAPRACTICAL FIVE-STEP METHOD: RATE, RHYTHM, AXIS, INTERVALS, INJURY

Rate: Give a Number

Two useful, easy methods of determining the ventricular rate include these:

- Rely on the computer and look in the upper-left-hand corner of the ECG (risky but often correct).
- Memorize the R-R interval distance chant: "**300, 150, 100 . . . 75, 60, 50 . . . .**" If the distance between two QRS complexes is four big boxes, the ventricular rate is (chant silently: 300, 150, 100) 75 beats per minute.

- Common numbers to know:
  - 60 to 100 bpm: Sinus rhythm
  - 40 to 60 bpm: Junctional escape rhythm
  - 35 bpm: Ventricular escape rhythm
  - 150 bpm: Atrial flutter with 2:1 conduction

Rhythm: Sinus or Otherwise?

- Let's think about the physiology of one normal sinus beat. The impulse starts from the sinus node and depolarizes both atria, then activates the atrioventricular (AV) node, and after some time, the ventricle depolarizes in a coordinated fashion, using the His–Purkinje system. This sentence explains what to look for on an ECG. Here is the same sentence with the ECG findings inserted into the appropriate places: The impulse starts from the sinus node and depolarizes both atria (**P wave**), then activates the AV node, and after some time (**PR interval**), the ventricles depolarize in a coordinated fashion, using the His–Purkinje system (**QRS complex**). When you are determining the rhythm on an ECG, your eyes should follow the same path as the heartbeat: P wave . . . PR interval . . . QRS complex.
- A normal sinus P wave is regularly occurring. There should be one P wave for every QRS ("one for one"). Significant variation in P-wave regularity or shape can imply causes such as an **ectopic atrial tachycardia** (EAT) or **multifocal atrial tachycardia** (MAT). Absence of a P wave usually means **atrial fibrillation**, although atrial standstill can occur with severe hyperkalemia.
- A normal PR interval is less than 200 ms (five small boxes) in duration. It should be the same for every beat. If the PR interval is long, varies between beats, or does not conduct to every QRS complex, some form of **AV block** is to blame. A short PR interval (<40 ms) suggests the presence of an accessory AV connection, known as **Wolff–Parkinson–White (WPW) syndrome**.
- A normal QRS is <120 ms (three small boxes) in duration and should follow every P wave. A wide QRS (>120 ms) can be due to one of four reasons: **left bundle branch block (LBBB); right bundle branch block (RBBB); idioventricular conduction delay** (IVCD, classically due to hyperkalemia), or **ventricular origin**, such as a premature ventricular contraction (PVC) or ventricular tachycardia (VT). Figure 2-1 links these concepts visually with the anatomy of the heart for a better understanding. Determination of the rhythm should rely on the simple concept of the physiology of a heartbeat and *not* on rote memorization.

Axis: Up in Lead I, Up in Lead II

Sorry, but I have to take you back to Einthoven and his triangle briefly. "Axis" is the major direction of the heart's depolarization. Normal direction is inferior and to the patient's left (–30 degrees to +90 degrees; see Fig. 2-2). Determining if an axis is normal requires looking in two leads: lead I and lead II. In Figure 2-2, lead I runs across the top of the diagram, from the patient's right to his or her left. If the QRS is predominantly positive in lead I, the electrical signal is heading in the direction of lead I, or toward the patient's left (anywhere from –90 degrees to +90 degrees). In the same way, we can look at lead II. If it is predominantly positive, we know that the electrical signal is heading in the direction of lead II, or leftward and inferior (anywhere from –30 degrees to 150 degrees). If the QRS is **positive in BOTH lead I and lead II**, the axis must be in the area where the two leads overlap, which is the normal axis between –30 degrees and +90 degrees (light blue in Fig. 2-2).

If the QRS is mostly up in lead I and down in lead II, what is the axis? Well, the signal is moving from the patient's right to his or her left, but now in the opposite direction of lead II. This puts the axis between –30 degrees and –90 degrees, so the answer is left axis

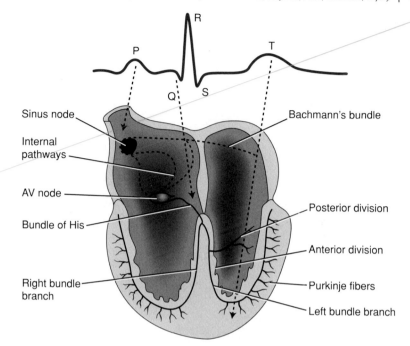

FIGURE 2-1. *Rhythm:* ECG components of the a single sinus beat with anatomic correlation. The P wave reflects atrial activation from the sinus node (green). The PR interval is the time during which the signal is passing through the AV node (purple). The narrow QRS complex represents the coordinated ventricular activation through the His-Purkinje system. The T wave signifies ventricular repolarization.

deviation (LAD). How about if the QRS is down in lead I and up in lead II? Answer: it is between +90 degrees and +150 degrees, or right axis deviation (RAD).

This sounds somewhat confusing, but with practice you should be reading *rate-rhythm-axis* in seconds. It is worth reviewing Figures 2-1 and 2-2 to cement these ideas.

Intervals: Shape and Width

While you are looking at the timing of the intervals (PR interval, QRS interval, QT interval), you should also inspect the shape of the structures (P wave shape, QRS shape). Follow Figure 2-3 as your eyes scan the ECG . . .

- **P waves:** Looking for **left atrial enlargement (LAE)** in V1 (normal is biphasic; abnormal has a large negative component) and **right atrial enlargement (RAE)** in lead II (two little boxes wide by two little boxes tall . . . "2 × 2 in lead II").
- **PR interval:** a normal PR interval is 200 ms (five little boxes). If the PR is longer, it is **AV block**. If the PR is very short, it could be **WPW syndrome**.
- **QRS interval** (width) and **QRS height:**
  - Width—Normally QRS width ranges between 80 and 120 ms. If it is >120 ms, see above (LBBB, RBBB, IVCD, ventricular in origin).

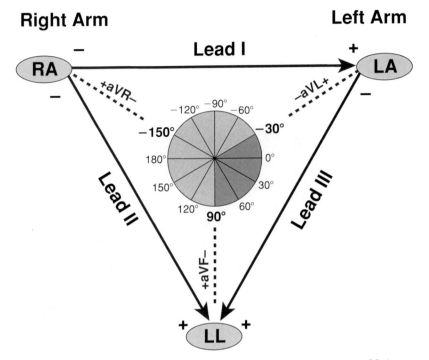

FIGURE 2-2. *Axis:* Einthoven triangle and normal QRS axis (darker screen, −30 degrees to + 90 degrees). (From *Alan E. Lindsay ECG Learning Center in Cyberspace* [http://library.med.utah.edu/kw/ecg], with permission.)

- Height—**Left ventricular hypertrophy (LVH)** can give large voltages. There are many criteria for determining LVH (see Chapter 18), but a commonly used one adds the depth of lead V1 with the height of leads V5 or V6. If >35 mV, then LVH is likely. Small voltages (<5 mV in the limb leads, <10 mV in the precordial leads) can happen when a poorly conductive material gets between the heart and the ECG lead. This is usually due to air [hyperinflated lungs in chronic obstructive pulmonary disease (COPD)], water (pericardial effusion), or fat.
- **QT interval**: the QT interval should be corrected for the underlying heart rate by using the formula QTc = QT (sec)/square root of R-R interval (sec).
  - Normal QTc is 440 ms for men and 460 ms for women. The ECG machine generally does a good job of measuring and calculating this for you. However, especially in situations where prolonged QTc may be a concern, there is no substitute for determing the QT interval yourself.
  - Long QT (LQT) is associated with torsade de pointes, a potentially lethal ventricular rhythm. The five causes of long QT can be grouped into:
    - **Hypos**: hypokalemia, hypocalcemia, hypomagnesemia, hypothermia
    - **Antis**: antibiotics, antiarrhythmics, antihistamines, antipsychotics
    - **Congenital**: LQT syndromes (see Chapter 20)
    - **Intracerebral hemorrhage**: Diffuse, deep, symmetric, large inverted T waves

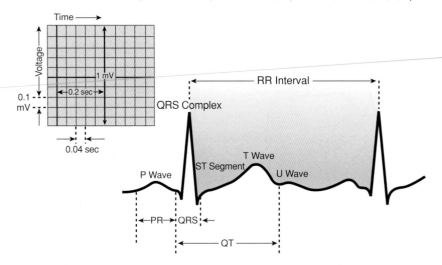

FIGURE 2-3. *Intervals*: Defining the intervals and segments on the ECG and identifying specific pathology to look for in each interval or segment. (From *Alan E. Lindsay ECG Learning Center in Cyberspace* [http://library.med.utah.edu/kw/ecg], with permission.)

P wave size: Look for atrial enlargement (LAE in V1, RAE in lead II).
PR interval: Look for AV block (PR >200 ms) or ventricular preexcitation (PR <40 ms).
QRS size: Large voltage suggests LVH; small voltage suggests pericardial effusion.
QRS interval: Wide QRS (>120 ms) signifies a poorly coordinated beat due to LBBB, RBBB, IVCD, or ventricular beats.
QT interval: Long QT intervals can be due to many causes, including "hypos," "antis," congenital syndromes, intracerebral hemorrhage, or cardiac ischemia (see text).

- **Cardiac ischemia**: In the form of "Wellen's waves" which are deep, symmetric, large inverted T waves particularly seen in V1 to V3, classically associated with proximal left anterior descending (LAD) disease.

Injury (Ischemia/Infarction): The Most Common Reason to Order an ECG

The following are ECG signs of myocardial damage:

- **ST-segment elevation**—classically described in acute myocardial infarction, although it can be seen in LVH, pericarditis, and ventricular aneurysms. Note that ST elevation is best termed an "acute injury pattern" until Q waves (see below) have developed.
- **ST-segment depression**—classically described with myocardial ischemia, although it can be seen in LVH, digoxin toxicity, and WPW syndrome as well as posterior wall injury/infarction.
- **T-wave inversions**—very nonspecific, although Wellen's waves are more suspicious for ischemia.
- **Q waves**—signify a prior infarct that has subsequently developed scar.

The distribution of the particular findings should be noted, as changes consistent throughout a specific coronary artery territory are more likely to indicate a true ischemic finding (Fig. 2-4).

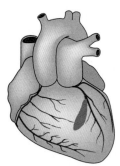

V1, V2 septal infarct

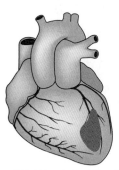

V3, V4 anterior infarct

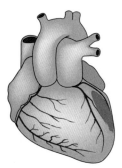

I. aVL, V5, V6 lateral infarct

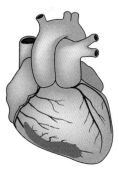

II, III aVF inferior infarct

FIGURE 2-4. *Injury:* ECG leads and coronary artery distributions. ST-segment elevations in specific leads reflect a myocardial injury (infarction or ischemia) in certain anatomic locations, as shown.

- Inferior (usually right coronary artery territory)—leads II, III, aVF
- Anterior (usually LAD territory)—leads V2 to V4
- Lateral (usually left circumflex artery territory)—leads V5 to V6, I, aVL

Put It All Together

When you are initially learning how to read an ECG, talk out loud and say what you see.

- *Rate/Rhythm/Axis:* "The rate is (300, 150, 100) about 75 and the rhythm is sinus. Axis is up in I and down in II, so left axis deviation."
- *Intervals:* "P waves are normal in shape, so there's no atrial enlargement. PR interval is 220 milliseconds, so it's a first-degree AV block. QRS is 100 milliseconds, which is normal. No LVH. QTc interval is 410 ms, which is normal."
- *Injury:* "I don't see any ST elevation or depressions, but there are Q waves in II, III, and aVF, so probably an old inferior myocardial infarct."

Practice will make perfect, so this chapter concludes with several unknown ECG tracing (Figs. 2-5 through 2-8 with answers). Please try out the *rate, rhythm, axis, interval, injury* method.

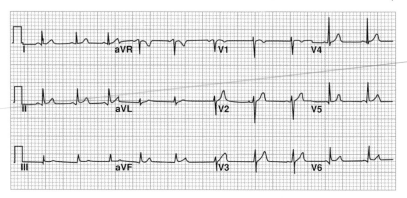

FIGURE 2-5. ECG for interpretation. (From *Alan E. Lindsay ECG Learning Center in Cyberspace* [http://library.med.utah.edu/kw/ecg], with permission.)

Rate: 75 bpm
Rhythm: Sinus (seen best in V1 or lead II).
Axis: Normal (up in lead I and lead II).
Intervals: P waves normal; PR interval normal (<200 ms, five small boxes); QRS normal (<120 ms, three small boxes wide); no LVH; QT interval normal.
Injury: No significant ST elevations or depressions.
Putting it together: Normal ECG.

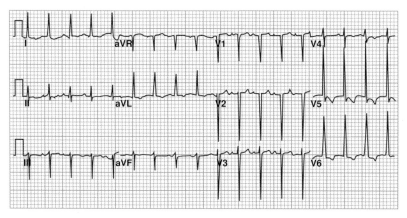

FIGURE 2-6. ECG for interpretation. (From *Alan E. Lindsay ECG Learning Center in Cyberspace* [http://library.med.utah.edu/kw/ecg], with permission.)

Rate: 90 bpm.
Rhythm: Sinus (lead V1).
Axis: Normal (up in lead I, up in lead II).
Intervals: P waves and PR interval normal. QRS narrow but tall. S wave in lead V1 + R wave of lead V5 > 35 mm, so LVH is present. QT interval normal.
Injury: No significant ST elevations or depressions. Inverted T waves in V5 and V6 are from the LVH.
Putting it all together: Left ventricular hypertrophy.

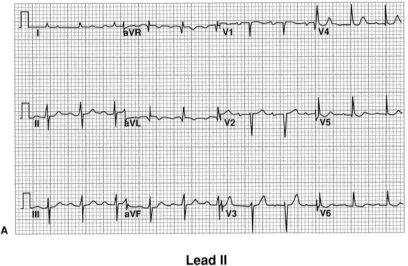

A

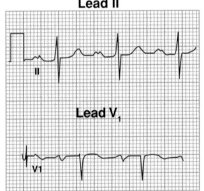

B

FIGURE 2-7. ECG for interpretation. (From *Alan E. Lindsay ECG Learning Center in Cyberspace* [http://library.med.utah.edu/kw/ecg], with permission.)

Rate: 70 bpm.

Rhythm: Sinus.

Axis: Borderline left axis deviation (up in lead I, isoelectric in lead II).

Intervals: Left and right atrial abnormality (see closeup of leads II and V1). PR interval is prolonged (first-degree AV block). Normal QRS size and width. Normal QT interval.

Injury: No significant ST elevation or depression. Q waves in V1 to V2 considered normal septal activation.

Putting it all together: Biatrial enlargement with first-degree AV block.

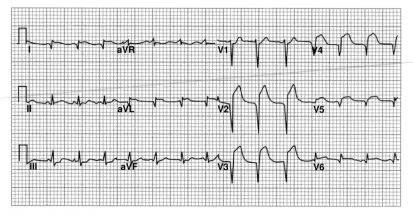

FIGURE 2-8. ECG for interpretation. (From *Alan E. Lindsay ECG Learning Center in Cyberspace* [http://library.med.utah.edu/kw/ecg], with permission.)

Rate: 80 bpm.
Rhythm: Sinus.
Axis: Right axis deviation (down in lead I, up in lead II).
Intervals: Normal P waves and PR interval. QRS normal height and width. QT interval prolonged.
Injury: ST elevations in leads V2 to V6 and leads I and aVL. ST depressions in leads III and aVF. Q waves in leads V2 to V6 and leads I and aVL.
Putting it all together: Anterior–lateral ST-segment myocardial infarction.

KEY POINTS TO REMEMBER

- Interpret ECGs in the same way, every time: *rate, rhythm, axis, intervals and injury.*
- Practice, practice, practice.
- Keep a file of interesting ECGs to stimulate your mind and recognize important ECG patterns.

REFERENCES AND SUGGESTED READINGS

Alan E. Lindsay ECG Learning Center in Cyberspace (http://library.med.utah.edu/kw/ecg)
O'Keefe JH, Hammill S. *The ECG Criteria Book,* 2nd ed. Royal Oak, MI: Physician's Press; 2002.
Rubin D. *Rapid Interpretation of EKGs,* 6th ed. Tampa, FL: Cover Publishing, 2000.
Surawicz B, Knilans T, eds. *Chou's Electrocardiography in Clinical Practice,* 5th ed. Philadelphia: Saunders; 2001.

Evaluation of Chest Pain

Sumeet Subherwal and Christopher Holley

BACKGROUND

Chest pain is the chief complaint for 5% to 10% of all emergency department visits in the United States and represents a wide spectrum of disease, from benign to life-threatening conditions. Consequently the initial evaluation must rapidly focus on ruling out **the five most common life-threatening conditions** that present with chest pain:

- Acute coronary syndrome
- Cardiac tamponade
- Aortic dissection
- Pulmonary embolism (PE)
- Tension pneumothorax

A five-step approach to accurate and rapid triage of patients with chest pain includes **a focused history, a directed physical exam, an electrocardiogram (ECG) performed within 10 minutes of arrival, chest x-ray (CXR), and appropriate laboratory studies.** General appearance should be assessed immediately to identify patients who are critically ill (the "eyeball test"). Patients who are pale, diaphoretic, anxious, and ill-appearing require immediate attention, including hemodynamic assessment, ECG, and CXR. Hemodynamically unstable patients should be evaluated and stabilized per the advanced cardiac life support (ACLS) protocol.

HISTORY

Particular emphasis should be placed on **rapidly and accurately characterizing the current episode of chest pain**. A rapid-fire set of questions following an alphabetical mnemonic (OPQRSTUVW) can provide the framework for a focused, precise history (Table 3-1). This method starts with the most important triaging question of **O**ngoing chest pain and finishes with asking the patient about factors that make the pain **W**orse or better. The remainder of a thorough history can be performed later.

PHYSICAL EXAM

A history-directed physical exam is not a full physical exam. Based on information obtained in the history, the directed exam should confirm a suspected diagnosis or narrow a differential diagnosis list. Much like the focused history, a directed exam should rapidly and accurately characterize the chest pain and screen for life-threatening findings. Most of the few minutes spent examining the patient should be focused on the cardiovascular and pulmonary exams. Clinical pearls for a chest pain–directed exam are listed in Table 3-2.

TABLE 3-1	RAPID AND ACCURATE CHARACTERIZATION OF CHEST PAIN (OPQRSTUVW MNEMONIC)	
	Question	Expected answer
Ongoing	"Are you having ongoing chest pain right now?"	Yes/no; triages high risk patients
Prior	"Have you ever had a heart attack, angiogram, cardiac catheterization or bypass surgery? If so, is this pain like your prior heart attack?"	Yes/no; strongly identifies ACS as a cause
Quality	"What does the pain feel like?"	Sharp, crushing, tearing, tightness, pressure
Radiation	"Can you point to where the pain is?" "Does the pain go anywhere else?"	Epigastric, substernal, scapular, lateral Jaw, shoulder, arms, back, abdomen
Severity	"On a scale from 1 to 10, with 10 being the worst pain you have ever felt, what number would you give this pain?"	Numerical scale from 1 to 10
Timing	"When did it start? How long does it last?"	Abruptness of onset, timing in minutes/hours/days
Underlying disease	For patients without known CAD: "Do you have diabetes, high blood pressure, high cholesterol? Do you smoke? Does anyone in your family have heart disease?"	Risk-stratify for underlying CAD
Various symptoms	"Is your pain related to other new symptoms?"	Diaphoresis, dyspnea, shortness of breath, palpitations, syncope, fatigue, nausea, vomiting, indigestion, hiccups
Worse or better	"What makes your pain worse?" "What makes it better?"	Worse with activity, emotional stress, deep inspiration, food, positional, movement of limbs/trunk, cocaine use Better with rest, nitroglycerin, leaning forward

CAD, coronary artery disease; ACS, acute coronary syndrome.

TABLE 3-2	CHEST PAIN–DIRECTED PHYSICAL EXAM WITH SPECIFIC CLINICAL PEARLS
Blood pressure	• Check both arms, especially if considering aortic dissection • Severe hypertension and hypotension require urgent intervention • Pulsus paradoxus: drop of >10 mm Hg in SBP at end-inspiration (tamponade)
Jugular veins	• Start with patient reclined at 45 degrees. Patients with significantly elevated JVP may need to be sitting up at 90 degrees before the jugular venous pulse can be seen • Hepatojugular reflex: Sustained distention of jugular veins with pressure on abdomen (heart failure) • Kussmaul sign: elevation (or lack of decrease) in JVP with inspiration (constriction)
Carotid arteries	• Palpation for stroke volume: normal carotid upstroke unlikely in severe LV dysfunction or AS • Pulsus parvus et tardus: weak and late pulse (AS)
Palpation	• Laterally displaced PMI (dilated LV) • RV heave (right-sided heart failure)
Heart sounds	• S3 (heart failure) • S4 (HTN and/or heart failure; never heard with atrial fibrillation) • Friction rub (pericarditis)
Murmurs	• Acute AR or MR may not have a murmur • AS: Crescendo–decrescendo systolic murmur, loudest at RUSB, commonly with radiation to the carotids when severe • AR: Diastolic murmur; always pathologic (endocarditis, dissection) • MR: Systolic blowing murmur loudest at apex (ischemia, LV dilation) • VSD: Harsh, loud holosystolic murmur (3–8 days after septal MI)
Pulmonary	• Crackles/rales (atelectasis, pneumonia, pulmonary edema) • Wheezing (usually bronchospasm but sometimes heart failure) • Absent breath sounds with tracheal deviation away from affected side (tension pneumothorax) • Decreased breath sounds, dullness to percussion (pneumonia and/or pleural effusion)
Musculoskeletal	• Pain that is reproducible on exam is rarely cardiac in nature • Dermatomal rash with pain (herpes zoster)
Abdominal	• Hepatomegaly, pulsatile liver, and ascites (heart failure) • Epigastric pain with palpation (PUD or pancreatitis) • RUQ pain (cholecystitis)
Extremities	• Cool extremities (poor cardiac output or occlusive ischemic event if unilateral) • Pitting edema (volume overload)

AR, aortic regurgitation; AS, aortic stenosis; HTN, hypertension; JVP, jugular venous pressure; LV, left ventricular; MI, myocardial infarction; MR, mitral regurgitation; PMI, point of maximum impulse; PUD, peptic ulcer disease; RUQ, right upper quadrant; RUSB, right upper sternal border; RV, right ventricular; SBP, systolic blood pressure; VSD, ventricular septal defect.

TABLE 3-3	ECG FINDINGS RELEVANT TO EVALUATION OF CHEST PAIN
ST-segment elevations	• Any ST elevation in the patient with chest pain is suspicious.
	• Typical ischemic ST elevation has a convex ("tomb-stone") appearance in two or more adjacent leads with reciprocal ST depressions.
	• Diffuse ST elevations with PR depression and/or ST depression in aVR suggests pericarditis in the appropri-ate clinical scenario.
New LBBB	• ST elevation "equivalent" in the appropriate clinical scenario.
ST-segment depression	• Flat or downsloping ST depressions are concerning for ischemia.
	• Specificity of ST depression for ischemia is significantly lower in patients with evidence of prior MI (Q waves) or baseline ST abnormalities.
T-wave inversions	• Not specific but may be first indicator of ischemia.
S1Q3T3	• S wave in I, Q wave and inverted T wave in III: can be seen with PE or right heart strain.

ECG, electrocardiogram; LBBB, left bundle branch block; MI, myocardial infarction; PE, pulmonary embolism.

DIAGNOSTIC TESTING

The **ECG** is critical to the evaluation of chest pain. In fact, for the acutely ill patient, it is prudent to quickly review the ECG prior to completing the history and physical. ECG find-ings that should not be missed are outlined in Table 3-3 and further discussed in Chapters 2 and 18. Prior ECGs for comparison are invaluable. If ischemia is a concern, serial ECGs are useful to look for evolution of the infarct pattern. Suspicion for a right ventricular (RV) infarct should be investigated with right-sided precordial leads, and suspicion for a poste-rior infarct should prompt evaluation with posterior chest leads.

The **CXR** complements the ECG by screening for many of the life-threatening con-ditions that the ECG fails to identify. These include:

- Aortic dissection (widened mediastinum)
- Heart failure (pulmonary edema)
- Pericardial effusion (enlargement of the heart shadow)
- Pneumothorax (free air in the thorax, usually at the apices in an upright patient)
- Pulmonary infiltrates (pneumonia)
- Pulmonary embolism (Hampton's hump: peripherally based, wedge-shaped infarction)
- GI perforation (free air beneath the diaphragm)

Evaluation for myocardial infarction should include measurement of **serial cardiac biomarkers**. Because the levels of these biomarkers rise several hours **after** the onset of infarction, it is important to know that the patient with a myocardial infarction who has sought medical attention without delay may not yet have a positive test. Two negative tests

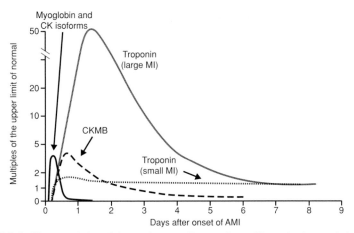

FIGURE 3-1. Characteristics of the various cardiac markers. (From Anderson J. L. et al. *J Am Coll Cardiol* 2007;50:652–726, with permission.)

8 hours apart are usually sufficient to rule out a myocardial infarction. The pattern of elevated biomarker levels can demonstrate the timing and severity of the infarction.

Several assays are available, including troponin I, troponin T, creatine kinase MB fraction (CK-MB), and myoglobin, with specific advantages and disadvantages to each test. Troponin I is the test of choice at our institution (Barnes-Jewish Hospital, St. Louis, MO). Serum levels can rise quickly, and the test is extremely sensitive and specific for myocardial damage. Levels stay elevated for several days after an infarct, which can be a disadvantage in understanding the timing of recurring chest pain in the days after an infarction. CK-MB levels can also rise quickly, and CK-MB is cleared more rapidly than troponin. However, it is significantly less sensitive than troponin. CK-MB levels are useful for diagnosing reinfarction in patients with a recent myocardial infarction who have recurrent symptoms. See Figure 3-1, which describes the characteristics of the various cardiac markers.

Measurement of brain natriuretic peptide (BNP) levels may be helpful to suggest previously undiagnosed heart failure, raising suspicion for an underlying ischemic etiology in patients presenting with chest pain. Lipid profiles are useful for risk stratification for coronary artery disease (CAD) but are of little utility in evaluating acute chest pain. Clinical suspicion may warrant measurement of serum D-dimer pulmonary embolism (PE), amylase/lipase (pancreatitis), or liver function tests (cholecystitis).

TREATMENT

If one of the five most common life-threatening causes of chest pain is identified, an emergent treatment plan should be enacted.

- ST-segment elevation myocardial infarction (STEMI) requires rapid reestablishment of coronary blood flow (IV thrombolytic therapy or percutaneous coronary intervention) (see Chapter 9).
- Cardiac tamponade is managed with urgent pericardiocentesis (see Chapters 6 and 13).
- Suspected aortic dissection should be confirmed with appropriate imaging (transesophageal echocardiography [TEE], computed tomography [CT], or magnetic resonance imaging [MRI]). Type A dissections require emergent surgical consultation (see Chapter 23).

- Tension pneumothorax requires immediate needle decompression followed by chest tube placement.
- Suspected PE can be confirmed by appropriate imaging (CT or $\dot{V}/\dot{Q}$ scan) and treated with anticoagulation. Thrombolytic therapy is considered for patients with significant hemodynamic compromise.

DIFFERENTIAL DIAGNOSIS

When it is clear that the patient is at lower risk and does not have a life-threatening condition, a broader differential diagnosis should include:

- Cardiac: stable angina, non-STEMI, pericarditis, coronary vasospasm
- Pulmonary: pneumonia, pleuritis
- Gastrointestinal: gastroesophageal reflux disease (GERD), peptic ulcer disease, esophagitis, pancreatitis, cholecystitis
- Neuromusculoskeletal: costochondritis, injury of the pectoralis or intercostal muscle, herpes zoster
- Psychiatric: panic attack, anxiety disorder, pain syndromes

KEY POINTS TO REMEMBER

Patients presenting with chest pain deserve a FIVE-STEP rapid and accurate triage response, which consists of:

- A focused history to determine: **O**ngoing pain; **P**rior cardiac history; **Q**uality, **R**adiation, **S**everity, and **T**iming of the pain; **U**nderlying CAD risk factors; **V**arious symptoms associated with the pain; factors that make the pain **W**orse or better (OPQRSTUVW alphabet mnemonic)
- A history-directed physical exam focusing on the cardiovascular and pulmonary systems
- An ECG within 10 minutes of presentation, often prior to the history and exam, specifically screening for evidence of myocardial infarction or ischemia [ST-segment elevations in two consecutive leads or new left bundle branch block (LBBB) signifies infarction; ST-segment depressions or T-wave changes can mean ischemia.]
- A CXR to screen for occult life-threatening conditions
- Appropriate laboratory studies, including serial cardiac biomarkers

REFERENCES AND SUGGESTED READINGS

Boie ET. Initial evaluation of chest pain. *Emerg Med Clin North Am* 2005;23(4):937–957.

Braunwald E, Antman EM, Beasley JW, et al. ACC/AHA guidelines for management of patients with unstable angina: a report of the American College of Cardiology/American Heart Association Task Force on Practice Guidelines (Committee on the Management of Patients with Unstable Angina). *J Am Coll Cardiol* 2000;36:970–1062.

Brown JE, Hamilton GC. Chest pain. *Rosen's Emergency Medicine: Concepts and Clinical Practice,* 6th ed. St. Louis: Mosby, Inc./Elsevier; 2006.

Haro LH, Decker WW, Boie ET, et al. Initial approach to the patient who has chest pain. *Cardiol Clin* 2006;24(1):1–17.

Kelly BS. Evaluation of the elderly patient with acute chest pain. *Clin Geriatr Med* 2007;23(2):327–349.

Lee TH, Cannon CP. Approach to the patient with chest pain. *Braunwald's Heart Disease: A Textbook of Cardiovascular Medicine*, 7th ed. St. Louis: Saunders; 2007.

Winters ME, Katzen SM. Identifying chest pain emergencies in the primary care setting. *Prim Care* 200633(3):625–542.

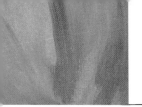

Clinical Presentations
of Heart Failure

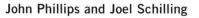

4

John Phillips and Joel Schilling

BACKGROUND

Heart failure (HF) is one of the fastest-growing cardiovascular diagnoses in the United States, where there are over 1 million hospitalizations for HF annually, at a cost exceeding $33 billion. Despite significant advancements in the management of HF, the mortality remains high; once a patient is hospitalized for HF, the 1- and 5-year death rates are ~30% and 50% respectively. In order to improve HF outcomes and reduce hospitalizations, physicians must be able to identify these patients early in their disease and initiate appropriate lifesaving and symptom-reducing therapies.

The clinical presentations of HF can be quite variable. However, patients can be divided into useful subgroups based on the constellation of findings that brings them to medical attention. The purpose of this chapter is to illustrate the manifestations of HF by highlighting different patient presentations.

DEFINITION

HF is a clinical syndrome characterized by dyspnea, exercise intolerance, and fluid retention in the setting of abnormal cardiac function. Most frequently, patients will present with either manifestations of poor cardiac output, such as **fatigue and exercise intolerance**, or volume overload/congestion, such as **pulmonary and peripheral edema**.

ETIOLOGY

There are many causes of myocardial injury that can result in clinically apparent HF. However, in considering the etiology of cardiac dysfunction it is useful to **subdivide patients into those with abnormal systolic function and those with preserved systolic function (PSF)** (Table 4-1). Among patients with abnormal systolic function, defined as ejection fraction ≤40%, approximately two thirds will have an ischemic cardiomyopathy (ICM), usually resulting from prior myocardial infarction (MI). The causes of nonischemic cardiomyopathy (NICM) in patients with systolic dysfunction are more varied and are shown in Table 4-1. Some 80% of patients with reduced left ventricular ejection fraction (LVEF) will have had a prior hospitalization for HF. **The most common presentation for patients with systolic dysfunction is slowly progressive fluid accumulation.**

In HF patients with PSF, the underlying disease processes are distinct. Most disorders leading to HF with PSF affect myocardial relaxation leading to high cardiac filling pressures. The most common causes are hypertension (HTN), diabetes, obesity, and occasionally coronary artery disease (CAD) (~25%). In addition, HF with PSF is more common in females and patients >65 years of age. Atrial fibrillation (AF) and chronic renal insufficiency

TABLE 4-1	COMMON ETIOLOGIES OF HEART FAILURE
Systolic Heart Failure	**Heart Failure with Preserved Systolic Function**
Coronary artery disease	Hypertension
Hypertension	Diabetes
Myocarditis: Infectious Autoimmune	Coronary artery disease
Toxin-induced: Alcohol Cocaine Amphetamines Chemotherapies	Infiltrative: Amyloid Sarcoid Hemochromatosis
Genetic	Hypertrophic cardiomyopathy
Cardiac-specific: Arrhythmogenic right ventricular dysplasia (ARVD) Generalized myopathies: Duchenne or Becker muscular dystrophy	High-output: Arteriovenous malformation Arteriovenous fistula Hyperthyroidism Anemia
Diabetes	Constrictive
Postpartum	Idiopathic cardiac fibrosis
Tachycardia-induced	
Idiopathic	

are frequent comorbidities. Rarer causes of HF with PSF are shown in Table 4-1. Although they can have a more insidious fluid accumulation presentation, **patients with HF and PSF more commonly present with acute pulmonary edema and HTN.**

HISTORY

There are three primary objectives of the history when interviewing a patient with HF:

- Identify etiology of HF
- Assess progression and severity of illness
- Assess volume status

First, it is important to identify factors that may have contributed to the etiology of the HF. For patients with a **first presentation of HF**, questioning should probe the likelihood of ischemic heart disease (history of MI, chest pain, risk factors), myocarditis or viral cardiomyopathy (recent viral illness or upper respiratory symptoms, rheumatologic disease history or symptoms), genetic cardiomyopathy (family history of HF or sudden death), toxic cardiomyopathy (alcohol or drug abuse, history of chemotherapy), and peripartum cardiomyopathy (recent pregnancy). In addition, the presence of HTN and/or diabetes should be elicited. **For patients with a known cardiomyopathy** presenting with an acute decompensation, it is important to **identify the potential triggers of the exacerbation**. A helpful mnemonic is "Patients who are frequently hospitalized for HF eventually VANISH."

- Valvular disease
- Arrhythmia (atrial fibrillation)
- Noncompliance (medications, diet)
- Ischemia or infection
- Substance abuse
- Hypertension

The second critical area to assess in patients with new-onset or established HF is their current functional status and the rate of decline in their activity level. Important questions to ask include what they can do before becoming short of breath currently (How far can they walk? How many flights of stairs can they climb?) and how this compares with what they were able to do 6 to 12 months prior. The answers to these questions allow patients to be categorized into a New York Heart Association (NYHA) functional class and an American Heart Association HF stage (Fig. 4-1), which helps direct therapy and assess prognosis.

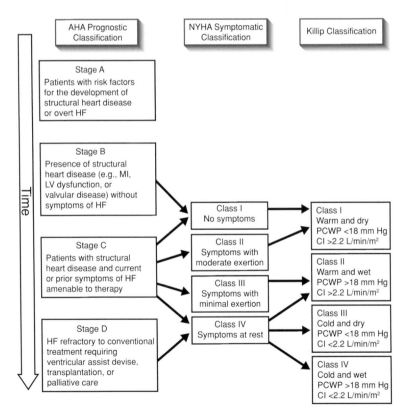

FIGURE 4-1. Classification of heart failure. (Redrawn from McBride BF, White CM. Acute decompensated heart failure: a contemporary approach to pharmacotherapeutic management. *Pharmacotherapy* 2003;(8):997–1020, with permission.)

The third important issue to address with the history is patient volume status. The inability to lie flat (orthopnea) and waking up at night short of breath (paroxysmal nocturnal dyspnea) are very suggestive of volume overload in patients with chronic HF. In addition, changes in body weight should always be discussed with the patient, as increased weight often signifies fluid retention even in the absence of other congestive symptoms. Other manifestations of increased fluid load include abdominal bloating and/or right-upper-quadrant pain and lower extremity edema.

PHYSICAL EXAM

The primary function of the physical exam in patients with HF is to assess volume status. However, the physical exam can also provide important clues as to the etiology of cardiac dysfunction. For example, the presence of a murmur or a pericardial knock may indicate a primary valvular process or pericardial constriction, respectively. In examining a patient, it is important to recognize that the clinical manifestations of HF and volume overload can be highly variable. Common exam findings suggesting systolic dysfunction and volume overload include jugular venous distention, a diffuse and laterally displaced point of maximum impulse (PMI), an S3 gallop, a mitral regurgitation (MR) murmur at the apex, pulmonary crackles, diminished carotid upstrokes, ascites, pulsatile hepatomegaly, and lower extremity edema.

In assessing volume status by physical exam, it is useful to **characterize the patient as hypovolemic, euvolemic, or volume-overloaded.** Jugular venous distention is the most specific and reliable physical exam indicator of volume overload and is best assessed with a penlight and the patient positioned at ~45 degrees. The jugular venous pulse can be distinguished from carotid pulsations by the biphasic appearance of the latter. It is important to remember that elevated neck veins can also be seen with pulmonary hypertension, severe tricuspid regurgitation (TR), and pericardial diseases such as tamponade or constriction. Pulmonary crackles may be present on lung exam and indicate fluid extravasation into the alveoli due to elevated left ventricular end-diastolic pressure (LVEDP). This exam finding is often mistakenly considered mandatory for the diagnosis of decompensated HF. In reality, crackles signify either rapid increases in LVEDP or severe volume overload; they are present in only ~40% to 50% of HF patients with elevated filling pressures. In patients with chronic cardiomyopathy, the gradual increase in LVEDP is compensated for by increased pulmonary lymphatic drainage; thus crackles are a very late sign of decompensation. Lower extremity edema is another marker of fluid overload when present; however, the sensitivity for predicting elevated filling pressures is poor, at ~46%. In addition, some patients can have predominantly abdominal congestive symptoms without any evidence of peripheral or pulmonary edema. In summary, the physical exam is a critical component of volume assessment; however, it is important to know the limitations of common physical exam findings.

CLINICAL PRESENTATION

The clinical presentations of HF are highly variable and range from acute respiratory or circulatory compromise to gradual worsening of dyspnea on exertion. In general, patients with HF can be divided into **three basic presentation phenotypes:**

- "Flash or acute" pulmonary edema with hypertension
- Slowly progressive fluid accumulation
- Low-output state

The most dramatic presentation is acute, or "flash," pulmonary edema. Frequently these patients have a rapid onset of symptoms and elevated blood pressure. The problem is usually not significant volume overload but instead volume redistribution secondary to increased vascular tone and poor left ventricular (LV) relaxation. The slowly progressive HF phenotype most commonly occurs in patients with chronic systolic dysfunction and is typified by normal to mildly elevated blood pressures and signs or symptoms of slowly progressive fluid accumulation. These patients have dyspnea on exertion, paroxysmal nocturnal dyspnea/orthopnea, lower extremity edema, and increased weight. The third and least common presentation type are the patients with a low-output state. These patients are typically hypotensive and have evidence of end-organ hypoperfusion (prerenal azotemia, cold extremities, poor mentation). These patients often require placement of a pulmonary artery (Swan-Ganz) catheter for careful medical management, from which the Killip classification may be determined (Fig. 4-1). Management for each of these clinical presentations is unique and discussed in detail in Chapter 11.

DIFFERENTIAL DIAGNOSIS

It is important to consider other acute diseases that can mimic the presentation of HF with dyspnea, elevated neck veins, and lower extremity edema (i.e. pulmonary hypertension, pulmonary embolism, and pericardial tamponade). Pulmonary inflammatory diseases, progressive pleural effusions, significant anemia, hypothyroidism and some systemic neurologic disorders can present with progressive exertional dyspnea and should remain on the differential diagnosis list if a cardiac cause of the symptoms cannot be found.

KEY POINTS TO REMEMBER

- HF is a common clinical syndrome with significant morbidity and mortality. Early detection can lead to initiation of appropriate lifesaving and symptom-reducing therapies.
- Ischemic cardiomyopathy is the most common cause of HF with reduced LV ejection fraction. Hypertension, diabetes, obesity, and CAD play a contributory role in HF with preserved systolic function.
- The three primary objectives of the history and physical exam are to (1) identify cause of HF, (2) assess the progression and severity of the illness, and (3) assess volume status.
- A mnemonic for the causes of HF decompensation: "Patients who are frequently admitted for heart failure exacerbations often VANISH."
- To guide treatment decisions, the physician's goal is to classify the patient as having one of three common clinical phenotypes: (1) "flash" pulmonary edema with hypertension, (2) slowly progressive fluid accumulation, or (3) a low-output state.

REFERENCES AND SUGGESTED READINGS

Cook DJ, Simel DL. The rational clinical examination: does this patient have abnormal central venous pressure? *JAMA* 1996;275:630–634.
Hunt S, Abraham WT, Chin MH, et al. ACC/AHA 2005 Guideline Update for the Diagnosis and Management of Chronic Heart Failure in the Adult: a Report of the American College of Cardiology/American Heart Association Task Force on Practice Guidelines. *Circulation* 2005;112:e154–e235.

Evaluation of Syncope

Christopher Holley

BACKGROUND

The term "syncope" is reserved for episodes of self-limited, transient loss of consciousness due to global cerebral hypoperfusion. Otherwise, the episode should be referred to as "transient loss of consciousness" (TLOC) so as to include nonsyncopal etiologies in the differential diagnosis.

EPIDEMIOLOGY

Syncope is common, accounting for 3% to 5% of emergency room visits and 1% to 3% of hospital admissions. Many more cases of syncope are not reported. Large population data show at least a 6% incidence over 10 years, with increasing incidence in the elderly. For institutionalized patients over the age of 70, the incidence is as high as 23% over 10 years.

CLASSIFICATION

Syncope first must be differentiated from nonsyncopal events involving real or apparent transient loss of consciousness, such as seizures or falls (Table 5-1). Further subdivision of true syncope is based on specific pathophysiologic etiologies. The four general causes of syncope include **reflex syncope (neurally mediated), orthostatic hypotension, primary cardiac arrhythmias,** and **structural cardiopulmonary diseases** (Table 5-2).

NATURAL HISTORY

Although one-third of patients with syncope will have a recurrent event within 3 years, select subgroups of patients with noncardiac syncope have an excellent prognosis. Young, otherwise healthy individuals with a normal electrocardiogram (ECG) and without identifiable heart disease have essentially no increased risk of death relative to the population at large. Reflex syncope is associated with little or no increase in mortality. Syncope from orthostatic hypotension has an excellent prognosis if the underlying abnormality is easily identified and treated. In contrast, syncope with an identifiable cardiac etiology carries a higher risk of mortality, particularly in patients with advanced heart failure. Mortality approaches 45% at 1 year for patients with syncope and left ventricular (LV) ejection fraction <20%.

EVALUATION

Initial evaluation of syncope utilizes the **history, physical exam,** and **ECG** to classify causes and identify patients who are at high risk for death. There are three key questions that need to be answered with the initial evaluation:

TABLE 5-1	CAUSES OF NONSYNCOPAL TRANSIENT LOSS OF CONSCIOUSNESS	
No Loss of Consciousness	**Partial or Complete Loss of Consciousness**	
Falls	Epilepsy	
Cataplexy/drop attacks	Intoxication	
Psychogenic pseudosyncope	Metabolic disorders (hypoglycemia, hypoxemia)	
TIA, carotid artery disease	TIA, vertebrobasilar disease	

TIA, transient ischemic attack.

- Is loss of consciousness attributable to syncope or not?
- Is heart disease present or not?
- Are there important clinical features in the history that suggest the diagnosis?

HISTORY

Often, the diagnosis of syncope is evident from the history; that is, TLOC occurred and was likely mediated by global cerebral hypoperfusion. Aspects of the history that need to be explored in order to make the diagnosis and further categorize the event include a pro-drome **before** the attack, **eyewitness** accounts during the event, the patient's recollection immediately **after** the attack, **circumstances** that may have played a causative role in the event, and general questions about the patient's medical **history**. A helpful mnemonic is, "I passed out on the BEACH" (Table 5-3).

PHYSICAL EXAM

The **cardiovascular and neurologic exams** are of primary importance. Orthostatic blood pressures are essential to evaluate for orthostatic syncope. Cardiovascular findings that may point to cardiogenic syncope include arrhythmias, murmurs (particularly aortic stenosis or hypertrophic obstructive cardiomyopathy), and evidence for heart failure. Neurologic findings are often absent but might include evidence for autonomic neuropathy (inappropriate sweating, lack of heart rate variability, extreme orthostatic blood pressure changes). A firm massage at the carotid artery bifurcation for 5 to 10 seconds may reproduce symptoms, particularly in the elderly. This maneuver can be performed safely at the bedside with the patient on telemetry monitoring and appropriate bradycardia treatments available. The test is considered positive if it results in a ventricular pause of >3 seconds. Neurologic complications are rare (<0.5%), but the procedure should be avoided in patients with known carotid disease, carotid bruits, or a recent transient ischemic attack/cardiovascular accident (TIA/CVA).

DIAGNOSTIC TESTING

With a focused history, physical exam, and ECG, the cause of syncope is identifiable ~80% of the time (Table 5-2). Specific abnormalities to look for on ECG include:

- Evidence of sinus node dysfunction: sinus bradycardia, sinus pauses >3 seconds, atrial fibrillation (sick sinus syndrome)

TABLE 5-2	CLASSIFICATION AND CLASSIC PRESENTATIONS OF SYNCOPE

Types of Syncope	Classic Presentations
Reflex (neurally mediated)	Combination of reflex bradycardia and/or vasodilation—most common cause of syncope
Vasovagal	Precipitated by emotional stress, prolonged standing association with nausea.
Carotid sinus	Precipitated by carotid artery manipulation.
Situational	Related to micturition, defecation, or coughing.
Orthostatic hypotension	Postural changes resulting in symptoms and/or a drop in SBP >20 mm Hg
Volume depletion	Heat exposure, poor intake, diuretic use
Autonomic failure	Parkinson's disease, diabetes
Drug-induced	Nitrates, alpha blockers, clonidine, other antihypertensives
Cardiac arrhythmia	Insufficient cardiac output to meet systemic demands due to either bradycardia or tachycardia; often preceded by palpitations
Sinus node dysfunction	Symptomatic bradycardia, sick sinus syndrome with atrial fibrillation
AV conduction disease	Beta blockers, calcium channel blockers, Lenègre's disease
Tachycardias	Supraventricular or ventricular tachycardias
Long-QT syndrome	Congenital and/or drug-induced. Current use of certain antiarrhythmic, antihistamine, antibiotic, antipsychotic, or antidepressant medications.
Cardiopulmonary disease	Insufficient cardiac output to meet systemic demands due to abnormalities in the structure or function of the heart. Clues include known cardiac disease, exertional syncope, family history of sudden death, syncope while supine.
Valvular heart disease	Severe aortic stenosis
Acute ischemia/infarction	Particularly RV infarct
Hypertrophic cardiomyopathy	Often exercise-induced syncope
Pulmonary hypertension or embolism	Acute decrease in left ventricular filling
Vascular steal	Subclavian steal syndrome, with increased arterial blood flow to upper extremity causing a reversal of blood flow in the circle of Willis.

AV, atrioventricular; RV, right ventricular; SBP, systolic blood pressure.

TABLE 5-3	ESSENTIAL QUESTIONS TO EVALUATE HISTORY OF SYNCOPE
Before	Nausea, vomiting, feeling cold, sweating, dizziness, visual changes
Eyewitness	Duration of transient loss of consciousness, movements (tonic, clonic, other), description of patient falling
After	Confusion, muscle aches, incontinence, nausea, vomiting, sweating, pallor
Circumstances	Position (supine, standing), activity (rest, exercise, rising to stand, cough, urination), possible precipitants (fear, pain, prolonged standing)
History	Prior syncopal episodes; known cardiac, neurologic, or metabolic disease; medications, family history of sudden cardiac death

- Evidence of AV node dysfunction: AV block (more advanced block is more likely the cause of syncope), ventricular preexcitation, supraventricular tachycardias
- Evidence of cardiomyopathy: Prolonged QT interval, ventricular tachycardia, wide QRS (>120 ms), bifascicular block, Q waves suggestive of prior MI, precordial left ventricular hypertrophy (LVH) with abnormal T waves [hypertrophic cardiomyopathy (HCM)]; right bundle branch block (RBBB) with ST-segment elevation in V1 to V3 (Brugada pattern); RSR' pattern in V1 with abnormal T wave V1 to V3 [arrhythmogenic right ventricular (RV) dysplasia].

For patients with recognizable reflex or orthostatic syncope that occurs infrequently or as an isolated episode, no further workup is necessary. These patients generally have a good prognosis and can be managed as outpatients with treatments listed below.

For patients with a suspected cardiac etiology, an inpatient cardiac evaluation is warranted. This should include patients with exertional syncope, syncope with serious injury, and those with a family history of sudden death. The 2006 American Heart Association/American College of Cardiology (AHA/ACC) algorithm for cardiac evaluation of syncope is shown in Figure 5-1. In addition to the initial history, physical, and ECG, the expanded cardiac evaluation includes an **echocardiogram, exercise testing, and an ischemic evaluation**. In appropriate patients, an exercise stress echo would be sufficient to complete all three aspects of testing (baseline imaging followed by exercise protocol and stress imaging). The echocardiogram alone may be diagnostic in cases of valvular heart disease, cardiomyopathy, or congenital heart disease. Exercise testing should be symptom-limited. Noninvasive testing for ischemia should be followed by cardiac catheterization if there is evidence of ischemia or previously unrecognized infarction. Cardiac magnetic resonance imaging (MRI) or computed tomography (CT) may be helpful in the evaluation for structural heart disease including HCM, arrhythmogenic right ventricular dysplasia (ARVD), or coronary anomalies. Patients should be on continuous telemetry while hospitalized until a cardiac etiology is ruled out. If an arrhythmic cause is suspected but not evident on the initial workup or on expanded cardiac evaluation, **ambulatory cardiac rhythm monitoring** can be achieved through the use of a Holter monitor (24–48 hours of continuous recording), event recorder (1 month of patient-activated recordings to correlate with symptoms), or implantable loop recorder (several months of continuous recording). The choice of monitoring is dependent on the frequency of symptoms and type of suspected arrhythmia. In a highly selected population, the diagnostic yield of ambulatory cardiac monitoring is ~30%.

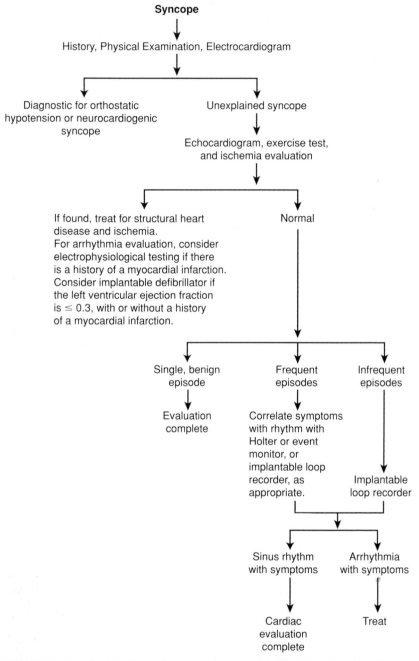

FIGURE 5-1. Algorithm for the evaluation of syncope. (Modified from American Heart Association/American College of Cardiology Foundation. AHA/ACCF scientific statement on the evaluation of syncope. *Circulation* 2006;113:316, with permission.)

If the cardiac evaluation is negative and patients have frequent syncope or recurrent syncope with injury, a reevaluation for reflex syncope may be warranted. In particular, these patients may be treated empirically for reflex syncope (see below) or evaluated with tilt testing. **Tilt testing** can be used to evaluate a patient's hemodynamic response during the transition from a supine to upright state. Physiologically, there is a large volume shift during this everyday repositioning, with 500 to 1000 mL of blood moving from the thorax to the distensible venous system below the diaphragm within the first 10 seconds. Furthermore, the hydrostatic pressures created by the upright position result in a similar volume of fluid moving to the interstitial space within 10 minutes. Autonomic vasoconstriction is the key reflex to counter this orthostatic stress, and failure of the vasoconstriction mechanism at any point may result in syncope. There are numerous protocols for head-up tilt testing, usually with tilt angles of 60 to 70 degrees and a passive testing phase of 20 to 45 minutes. Certain protocols include drug provocation if there is no syncope during the passive phase. Results are classified as primarily vasodepressor, cardioinhibitory, or mixed. Unfortunately, tilt testing can induce syncope in many "normal" individuals who have never had syncope, particularly with more aggressive protocols. Thus, in an unselected population, the predictive value of this test is low. Invasive electrophysiologic testing is potentially useful in selected patients, and appropriate EP consultation should be obtained.

TREATMENT

Treatment of syncope can be broadly defined as **preventing recurrences** and **reducing the risk of injury or death**. In general, this is tailored to treat the individual's underlying etiology of the syncope. For reflex syncope, this may be as simple as avoiding syncopal precipitants. When such precipitants cannot be avoided, coping strategies can be helpful. For example, isometric muscle contractions can improve venous return and abort potential episodes in patients with a recognizable prodrome. Various approaches to treating the four etiologies of syncope are shown in Table 5-4.

TABLE 5-4	TAILORED TREATMENT OF SYNCOPE
Reflex	Avoid precipitants (prolonged standing, overheating); ensure adequate hydration; employ isometric muscle contraction during prodrome to abort episodes; cardiac pacing for carotid sinus syncope with bradycardia
Orthostatic	Adequate hydration; eliminate offending drugs; stand slowly; use support stockings; consider salt supplementation, fludrocortisone, or midodrine
Arrhythmia	Cardiac pacing for sinus node dysfunction or high-degree AV block; discontinue QT-prolonging drugs; ICD for documented VT without correctable cause; endocardial ablation procedure in select patients
Cardiopulmonary	Correction of underlying disorder (valve replacement, revascularization); ICD for syncope with EF <35% even in absence of documented arrhythmia (presumed VT)

AV, atrioventricular; EF, ejection fraction; ICD, implantable cardioverter/defibrillator; VT, ventricular tachycardia.

KEY POINTS TO REMEMBER

- In cases of TLOC, first determine whether or not there was true syncope.
- In cases of true syncope, the initial evaluation is the history, physical exam, and ECG.
- If a cardiac etiology is suspected but not immediately identified, further evaluation should include an echocardiogram, exercise testing, and ischemia testing. Ambulatory cardiac monitoring may be warranted in selected patients.
- For patients with frequent or high-risk syncope and no identifiable cardiac etiology, testing for reflex syncope with a tilt table may be useful.
- Many cases of reflex or orthostatic syncope can be definitively diagnosed with the initial evaluation and do not require further workup. Treatment of these common conditions includes avoiding precipitants, maintaining adequate hydration, and isometric muscle contraction during the prodrome to abort episodes.

REFERENCES AND SUGGESTED READINGS

American Heart Association/American College of Cardiology Foundation. AHA/ACCF Scientific statement on the evaluation of syncope. *Circulation* 2006;113:316.

Grubb BP. Neurocardiogenic syncope. *N Engl J Med* 2005;352:1004.

The Task Force on Syncope, European Society of Cardiology. Guidelines on management (diagnosis and treatment) of syncope—update 2004. *Europace* 2004;6:467.

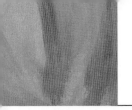

Cardiovascular Emergencies

Phillip S. Cuculich

INTRODUCTION

This chapter highlights the myriad exciting clinical scenarios that require immediate and definitive action from the cardiovascular care team: symptomatic bradycardia, symptomatic tachycardia, ST-segment elevation myocardial infarction (STEMI), late complications of a myocardial infarction, cardiac tamponade, hypertensive emergencies, and cardiogenic shock. After an initial stabilization, patients with these conditions should be cared for in an intensive care setting. This chapter is meant as a hands-on, rapid checklist to help manage patients with the above cardiovascular emergencies. Detailed discussion of each disease can be found elsewhere in this book.

SYMPTOMATIC BRADYCARDIA

Figure 6-1 provides Advanced Cardiac Life Support (ACLS) guidelines for symptomatic bradycardia. As discussed in Chapter 19, a modified version of the "five S" approach to a SSSSSlow heart rate can quickly help organize your thoughts.

- **STABLE:** Is the patient hemodynamically unstable?
- **SYMPTOMS:** Does the patient have symptoms related to the bradycardia? If a patient is hypotensive or having symptoms of bradycardia at rest, particularly syncope, immediate action must be taken:
  - Assess airway, breathing, and circulation (ABCs).
  - Place a monitor/defibrillator on the patient, ideally with transcutaneous pacing pads.
  - Ensure adequate IV access and oxygenation. Call for the crash cart.
- **SOURCE:** Where in the conduction system is the dysfunction?
  - A brief review of the rhythm strip or ECG is important.
  - Advanced atrioventricular (AV) block (second-degree type II or third-degree AV block) is unlikely to respond to the increased atrial heart rates that atropine provides and will likely need urgent pacing.
- **SPEED UP THE HEART:** Medical therapy: atropine then dopamine or epinephrine if necessary.
  - Atropine, 0.5 to 1.0 mg IV. Doses can be repeated every 3 to 5 minutes. The exception to using atropine is type II second-degree AV block, which may be worsened by atropine. Atropine may be given through an endotracheal tube (1–2 mg diluted to a total not to exceed 10 mL of sterile water or normal saline) if IV access is not available.
  - Dopamine, 2 to 10 µg/kg per minute IV. To keep systolic BP >90 mm Hg
  - Epinephrine, 2 to 10 µg/minute IV. To keep systolic BP >90 mm Hg

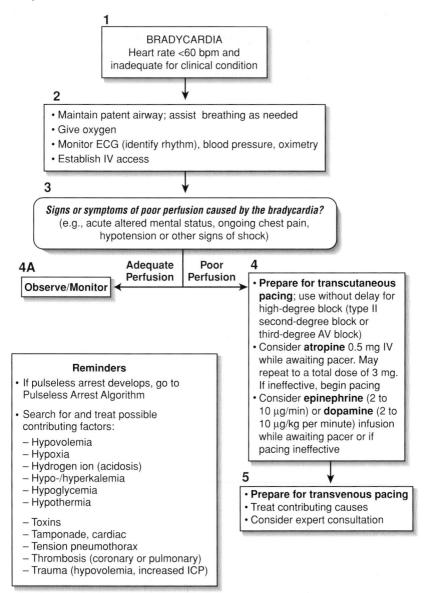

1

BRADYCARDIA
Heart rate <60 bpm and
inadequate for clinical condition

2
- Maintain patent airway; assist breathing as needed
- Give oxygen
- Monitor ECG (identify rhythm), blood pressure, oximetry
- Establish IV access

3

Signs or symptoms of poor perfusion caused by the bradycardia?
(e.g., acute altered mental status, ongoing chest pain,
hypotension or other signs of shock)

4A   Adequate   Poor   **4**
Perfusion   Perfusion

Observe/Monitor

4
- **Prepare for transcutaneous pacing;** use without delay for high-degree block (type II second-degree block or third-degree AV block)
- Consider **atropine** 0.5 mg IV while awaiting pacer. May repeat to a total dose of 3 mg. If ineffective, begin pacing
- Consider **epinephrine** (2 to 10 µg/min) or **dopamine** (2 to 10 µg/kg per minute) infusion while awaiting pacer or if pacing ineffective

Reminders
- If pulseless arrest develops, go to Pulseless Arrest Algorithm

- Search for and treat possible contributing factors:
  - Hypovolemia
  - Hypoxia
  - Hydrogen ion (acidosis)
  - Hypo-/hyperkalemia
  - Hypoglycemia
  - Hypothermia

  - Toxins
  - Tamponade, cardiac
  - Tension pneumothorax
  - Thrombosis (coronary or pulmonary)
  - Trauma (hypovolemia, increased ICP)

5
- **Prepare for transvenous pacing**
- Treat contributing causes
- Consider expert consultation

FIGURE 6-1. ACLS Algorithm for management of bradycardia. [From AHA. American Heart Association guidelines for cardiopulmonary resuscitation and emergency cardiovascular care. *Circulation* 2005;112(IV):1–203, with permission.]

- SET UP FOR PACEMAKER: Get transcutaneous and/or transvenous pacemaker system ready.
- Transcutaneous pacing. Place pads on the anterior and posterior chest walls. Initially begin pacing at the highest output. Rapidly reduce the output until ventricular capture is lost and then increase output until regular capture is seen. If hypotension is not severe, sedate the patient.
- Prepare for transvenous pacing. See Chapter 27.

SYMPTOMATIC TACHYCARDIA

Figure 6-2 provides ACLS guidelines for tachycardia. **Patients who are pulseless or clinically unstable with the tachycardia require immediate defibrillation with unsynchronized high-energy shocks** (200J, 300J, 360J) followed by appropriate ABC attention of ACLS. The cardiac rhythm is briefly assessed between shocks. Administer epinephrine (1 mg IV every 3–5 minutes) or vasopressin (Pitressin, 40 U IV once). Amiodarone (Cordarone, Pacerone, 300 mg IV once, repeat at 150 mg IV once) or lidocaine (1.0–1.5 mg/kg IV, repeat in 3–5 minutes to maximum dose, 3 mg/kg) should be given for continued pulseless ventricular tachycardia (VT). 360J shocks should continue every 30 to 60 seconds if the VT/ventricular fibrillation (VF) continues. Procainamide (Procan, Pronestyl, 20–30 mg/min) can also be considered. If hyperkalemia is suspected, calcium and bicarbonate should be administered.

If the patient has a pulse and is clinically stable, analysis of the ECG dictates the next management steps:

- Narrow-QRS-complex (supraventricular tachycardia, or SVT) tachycardias (QRS <0.12 second) in order of frequency
- Sinus tachycardia
- Atrial fibrillation
- Atrial flutter
- AV nodal reentry (AVNRT)
- Accessory pathway–mediated tachycardia (AVRT)
- Atrial tachycardia (ectopic and reentrant)
- Multifocal atrial tachycardia (MAT)
- Junctional tachycardia
- Wide-QRS-complex tachycardias (QRS ≥0.12 second)
- Ventricular tachycardia (VT)
- SVT with aberrancy
- Preexcited tachycardias (Wolff-Parkinson-White)

Narrow-QRS-complex arrhythmias are further diagnosed (and often treated) by slowing the conduction through the AV node. Essentially, AV nodal blockade will either (1) demonstrate the underlying atrial rhythm without large ventricular QRS complexes obscuring the rhythm (atrial fibrillation, flutter, ectopic atrial tachycardia) or (2) stop the tachycardia if it is dependent on the AV node as part of the tachycardia circuit (AVNRT, AVRT). AV node slowing can be accomplished by increasing vagal tone (carotid sinus massage) or by administering adenosine (6–12 mg IV rapid push with flush).

Wide-QRS-complex arrhythmias present more of a challenge by requiring a working diagnosis **before** the treatment plan is enacted. Treatment of VT is very different than treatment of SVT with aberrancy or a preexcited tachycardia. Clues suggesting VT as the cause:

- In patients with **known structural heart disease**, especially coronary disease, VT is a more likely cause of wide-complex tachycardia.

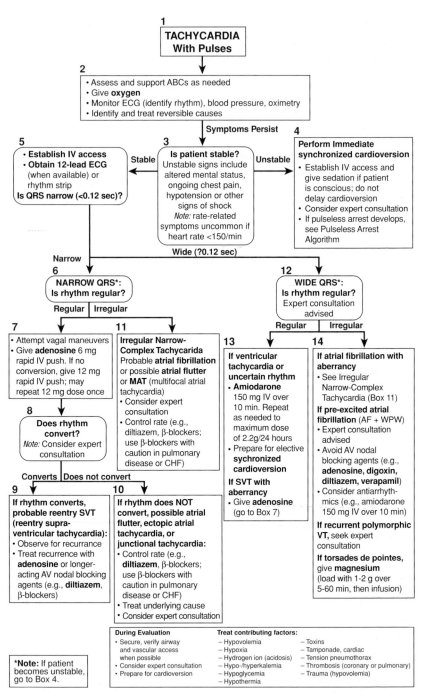

FIGURE 6-2. ACLS Algorithm for management of tachycardia. [From AHA. American Heart Association guidelines for cardiopulmonary resuscitation and emergency cardiovascular care. *Circulation* 2005;112(IV):1–203, with permission.]

- Comparison to the ECG during sinus rhythm is helpful, as a **significant change in the QRS morphology and/or a shift in axis are more suggestive of VT.**
- Other specific findings suggestive of VT include (1) AV dissociation, (2) fusion/capture beats, (3) left bundle-branch block with right-axis deviation, and (4) positive or negative concordance of QRS in ECG leads V1 to V6.
- Should question remain, the Brugada criteria can be used to further determine VT versus SVT (see Chapter 18).

For patients with monomorphic VT, amiodarone (150 mg IV over 10 minutes, followed by 1 mg/min continuous infusion for 6 hours and 0.5 mg/min continuous infusion for the next 18 hours) should be used. Alternative options are procainamide or sotalol. If the patient becomes unstable, or the VT persists, a synchronized defibrillation shock should be delivered.

Polymorphic VT requires immediate attention, as it can become unstable quickly. A prolonged QT interval in sinus rhythm should raise concern of torsades de pointes. Immediate treatment should include administering 4 g IV magnesium, overdrive pacing, or IV isoproterenol (Isuprel) at 5 μg/minute IV infusion. Amiodarone (150 mg IV over 10 minutes) may be helpful, particularly if the QT interval is normal at baseline. Underlying medications or overdoses should be investigated. Persistent torsades de pointes requires defibrillation.

Because coronary artery disease is the most common cause of ventricular tachycardia, an urgent coronary catheterization is warranted, particularly with VT refractory to antiarrhythmic medication.

ST-SEGMENT ELEVATION MYOCARDIAL INFARCTION (STEMI)

The single overriding theme of the countless clinical studies regarding STEMI is that **"time is muscle,"** meaning that early successful coronary reperfusion strategies lead to improved short- and long-term outcomes. In appropriate patients, this is achieved through the use of either IV thrombolytic medication ("lytic") and/or percutaneous coronary intervention ("lab"). Figure 6-3 outlines benchmark goals and a treatment algorithm for STEMI, including medication doses and contraindications. A detailed discussion can be found in Chapter 9.

LATE COMPLICATIONS OF MYOCARDIAL INFARCTION

Postinfarction complication rates have fallen dramatically since the advent of early reperfusion strategies. Nevertheless, many patients (large infarction, silent infarction, late presentation, delayed or incomplete reperfusion) remain at high-risk for life-threatening late complications of myocardial infarction. The role of an **urgent bedside echocardiogram** for a rapid diagnosis cannot be overemphasized. The mnemonic **"FEAR A MI"** is a logical way to remember and respect these potentially life-threatening complications while caring for a patient in the ICU, as demonstrated below:

- **FAILURE:** LV dysfunction is the single most powerful predictor of survival following a myocardial infarction. Clinical symptoms of heart failure are more likely in patients with large infarcts, advanced age, and/or diabetes. Treatment for post-MI heart failure can be found in Chapter 11.
- **EFFUSION AND TAMPONADE:** Post-MI effusions are rarely life-threatening. However, if tamponade physiology is present, consider hemorrhagic effusion from a ventricular rupture (see "Cardiac Tamponade," below).

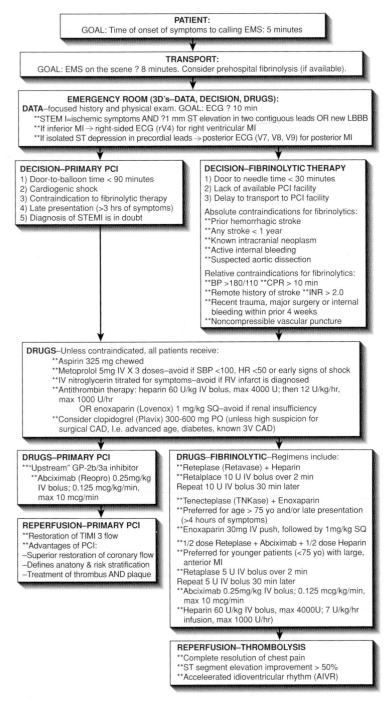

FIGURE 6-3. Benchmark goals and treatment algorithm for ST-segment elevation acute coronary syndrome.

- **ARRHYTHMIA:** Infarction-specific arrhythmias include the following:
  - Accelerated idioventricular rhythm (AIVR) is considered a "reperfusion rhythm," as it is often seen immediately after a successful reperfusion. No treatment is warranted for this arrhythmia when it is combined with a clinical scenario of reperfusion.
  - Ventricular tachycardia (VT) is often the terminal rhythm in the peri-infarct time period and is associated with increased mortality when it occurs in the first 48 hours of hospitalization. Aggressive restoration of sinus rhythm is achieved through the use of antiarrhythmic medications (amiodarone, lidocaine) and/or synchronized DC cardioversion. Because hypokalemia and hypomagnesemia have been associated with the development of sustained ventricular tachycardia, it is reasonable to correct electrolyte levels in the setting of an infarction. In contrast, nonsustained ventricular tachycardia (NSVT) is not associated with an increased risk of death during the index hospitalization or over the first year after infarction.
  - Myocardial infarction can cause a block at any level of the conduction system. In general, proximal (AV nodal) conduction disease is associated with an infarct of the right coronary artery (RCA). This causes a transient AV block and often does not warrant immediate temporary pacemaker placement. One exception is AV block in the setting of right ventricular (RV) infarction, where restoration of AV synchrony can improve RV filling and thus cardiac output. Distal (infranodal) conduction disease is frequently associated with a left anterior descending (LAD)/septal infarct and is longer lasting and life-threatening. Immediate pacing efforts should be pursued.
- **RUPTURE:** The clinical presentation of a ventricular rupture is often striking and life-threatening. The rupture can be in the ventricular free wall, ventricular septum, or papillary muscle. A clinical suspicion and the timely use of echocardiography and a pulmonary artery (PA) catheter are essential for prompt diagnosis of this serious complication, which generally requires emergent surgical consultation.
- **ANEURYSM:** True LV aneurysms complicate less than 5% of acute infarctions but are associated with a considerably lower survival rate. The characteristic ECG findings of LV aneurysm are q-waves with persistent ST elevations, though the diagnosis is best confirmed with a noninvasive imaging study. A pseudoaneurysm, distinct from an aneurysm, can be thought of as a "contained rupture." It is most often seen with an inferior infarction and treatment is emergent surgery. Both surgical and medical treatments carry a very high mortality.
- **MYOCARDIAL INFARCTION:** The complaint of chest pain after a myocardial infarction may represent recurrent ischemia from incomplete revascularization. Ischemia recurs in 20%–30% of patients receiving thrombolytic therapy and up to 10% of patients after percutaneous revascularization. Serial cardiac biomarkers and ECG can help identify at-risk patients. Normally, antianginal medications (nitrates, beta blockers) can control symptoms. Reinfarction due to stent thrombosis usually has a dramatic presentation with severe anginal pain refractory to medical therapy and evolving ST elevations on ECG. These findings warrant additional prompt revascularization efforts.

CARDIAC TAMPONADE

Cardiac tamponade occurs with an increase in intrapericardial pressure due to a pericardial effusion, which is characterized by (1) elevation of intrapericardial pressure, (2) limitation of RV diastolic filling, and (3) reduction of stroke volume and cardiac output. The presence of a pericardial effusion does not necessarily mean tamponade physiology is present.

Cardiac tamponade is a clinical diagnosis, taking into account the history (potential cause, rate of fluid accumulation), physical exam findings (altered mental status, hypotension, jugular venous distention, pulsus paradoxus) and supporting diagnostic information.

- ECG: low voltage, electrical alternans
- CXR: water-bottle-shaped heart
- Echocardiography: pericardial effusion; RV diastolic collapse; right atrial (RA) notching; tricuspid valve (TV) and mitral valve (MV) inflow variation in Doppler velocities of >40% and >25%, respectively; dilated inferior vena cava (IVC).

Initial management consists of **volume expansion** with IV fluids to increase preload. Maintain blood pressure with norepinephrine (Levophed) and dobutamine (Dobutrex) as needed. Avoid vasodilators and diuretics. The decision to drain the pericardial fluid, as well as the method (surgical or percutaneous) and timing (emergent or elective) of the procedure, should be individualized to each patient taking into account the acuity of the patient's condition, availability of trained personnel, and etiology of the effusion.

Percutaneous **pericardiocentesis** is a potentially life-threatening procedure and should be performed by trained personnel with hemodynamic monitoring and echocardiographic guidance whenever possible. Complications of pericardiocentesis include cardiac puncture with hemopericardium or myocardial infarction, pneumothorax, VT, cardiac arrest, coronary artery laceration, bradycardia, trauma to abdominal organs, infection, fistula formation, and pulmonary edema.

In life-threatening emergent situations, a "blind" percutaneous pericardiocentesis may be needed to stabilize a hemodynamically unstable patient. Ideally, a pericardiocentesis kit can be used, which allows for a rapid procedure with appropriate supplies. The 8-cm, 18-gauge blunt-tipped needle should be attached to a syringe and inserted through the subxiphoid region (Fig. 6-4). The tip of the needle is directed posteriorly toward the patient's left shoulder and slowly advanced at a 30-degree angle to the body with gentle aspiration. One suggested way to avoid myocardial puncture is by attaching an ECG electrode to the pericardiocentesis needle. Electrical activity will be seen on the monitor when the needle comes into contact with ventricular myocardium. Aspiration of clear, serous fluid may be from the pericardium or pleural effusion. On the other hand, aspiration of bloody fluid may be from the pericardium or the right ventricle. In general, removal of 50 to 100 mL of pericardial fluid should cause a hemodynamic improvement if tamponade is the cause

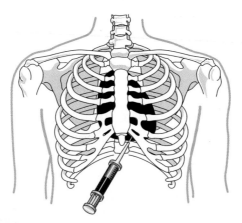

FIGURE 6-4. Approach for percutaneous pericardiocentesis.

of the hypotension. See Chapter 13 for detailed discussion on the etiology, pathophysiology, and management of pericardial effusion.

HYPERTENSIVE EMERGENCY

Hypertensive crises should be differentiated into hypertensive emergency or urgency, based on evidence of end-organ damage. Severe hypertension specifically affects the renal (elevated serum creatinine, hematuria), cardiovascular (angina, heart failure, aortic dissection), and neurologic (headache, mental status changes, vision alterations from retinal damage and papilledema) systems. The presence of end-organ damage (hypertensive emergency) generally means a goal of rapid blood pressure reduction by using IV medications. In contrast, hypertensive urgency can be treated with oral medications with the goal of blood pressure reduction over the course of days.

In general, a reasonable and safe goal for hypertensive emergency is to reduce **the mean arterial pressure by 20% to 25% or to reduce the diastolic pressure to 100 to110 mm Hg within a few hours**. A larger reduction in blood pressure in the first few hours may worsen end-organ damage, particularly in the brain. Exceptions include aortic dissection, LV failure, and pulmonary edema, in which blood pressure should be reduced quickly and to a lower target blood pressure. Placement of an arterial line should be strongly considered for the most accurate blood pressure measurement. The specific antihypertensive medication should be adjusted for the situation. Commonly used first-line IV agents include:

- Sodium nitroprusside (Nipride)—a rapid arterial and venous dilator. IV dosing starts at 0.25 μg/kg per minute and is titrated q5 minutes to a maximum of 10 μg/kg per minute. Thiocyanate toxicity is an uncommon side effect and occurs with prolonged infusions (days) in patients with hepatic or renal insufficiency.
- Labetalol (Normodyne, Trandate)—An alpha- and nonselective beta-antagonist with partial beta-2 agonist quality. Labetalol can be given as bolus doses of 20 to 40 mg IV every 10 to 15 minutes or with an infusion of 0.5 to 2 mg/minute. Relative contraindications to labetalol include heart failure, bradycardia, AV conduction block, and chronic obstructive pulmonary disease (COPD).
- Esmolol (Brevibloc)—A rapidly acting, beta-1–selective agent with a short half-life. Similar relative contraindications to labetalol.
- Nitroglycerin (Tridil)—A weak systemic arterial dilator but should be considered when managing hypertension associated with CAD. The usual initial dose is 5 to 15 μg/minute and can be titrated every 5 minutes to goal blood pressure or onset of headache (common side effect). Nitroglycerin has a rapid onset and offset of action.
- Hydralazine (Apresoline)—A direct arterial vasodilator. A starting dose of 10 to 20 mg IV may be given. The onset of action is 10 to 30 minutes. Hydralazine causes a reflex tachycardia and is contraindicated in myocardial ischemia and aortic dissection.

Specific hypertensive emergencies may warrant specific therapies:

- Hypertensive encephalopathy—The agents of choice are Nipride or labetalol. CNS depressants, such as clonidine (Catapres), should be avoided. In patients having seizures, the use of antiepileptics may help to lower blood pressure.
- Cerebrovascular injury—The need to maintain cerebral perfusion pressure outweighs the acute need to lower blood pressure. If intracerebral pressure (ICP) monitoring is available, cerebral perfusion pressure (mean arterial pressure − ICP) should be kept >70 mm Hg. For patients who have had an acute stroke or intracranial hemorrhage:
  - BP >230/140 mm Hg—Nitroprusside is agent of choice.

- BP 180–230/140–105 mm Hg—Labetalol, esmolol or other easily titratable IV antihypertensive.
- BP <180/105—Defer hypertensive management.
- Aortic dissection—Patients with type A dissections should be referred for emergent surgical correction and aggressively treated with antihypertensives. Type B dissections should be treated with antihypertensives. Labetalol or esmolol should be started initially to lower heart rate, followed by nitroprusside if necessary. See Chapter 23 for a detailed approach to aortic dissection.
- Left ventricular failure with pulmonary edema—Rapid reduction in blood pressure should be achieved with a nitrate [Nipride or nitroglycerin (NTG)]. Small doses of loop diuretics are often effective.
- Myocardial ischemia—IV NTG will improve coronary blood flow, decrease LV preload, and moderately decrease systemic arterial pressure. Beta blockers should be added to decrease heart rate and blood pressure.
- Preeclampsia and eclampsia—Classically, because of large experience in this setting, the centrally acting alpha blocker methyldopa (Aldomet) is the drug of choice for hypertension in pregnancy. IV labetalol may also be used with appropriate fetal monitoring. Angiotensin converting enzyme (ACE) inhibitors are contraindicated in pregnancy.
- Pheochromocytoma—Pheochromocytoma crisis may present with a markedly elevated blood pressure, profound sweating, marked tachycardia, pallor, and numbness/coldness/tingling in extremities. Phentolamine (Regitine), 5 to 10 mg IV, is the drug of choice and should be repeated as needed. Nipride may be added if necessary. A beta blocker should be added only after phentolamine to avoid unopposed alpha-adrenergic activity. Of note, labetalol (alpha and nonselective beta blocker) and clonidine interfere with catecholamine assays used in the diagnosis of pheochromocytoma, so they should be held before the diagnosis is made.
- Cocaine-related hypertensive emergency—Moderate hypertension can be treated with benzodiazepines. Severe hypertension should be treated with nondihydropyridine calcium channel blockers (e.g., IV diltiazem) nitroglycerin, nitroprusside, or phentolamine. Beta blockers should be avoided given the risk of unopposed alpha-adrenergic activity, although labetalol, which has alpha-antagonist activity, may be used.

CARDIOGENIC SHOCK

A logical algorithm for the management of acute decompensated heart failure (ADHF) is presented in Figure 11-2. Patients with the highest immediate mortality (>50%) are those with cardiogenic shock: a low-output state with signs and symptoms of organ underperfusion. There are multiple etiologies of cardiogenic shock; the most common cause is an extensive myocardial infarction (MI), which severely and acutely compromises LV function. Less common causes include RV infarction and mechanical complications, such as papillary muscle dysfunction or rupture, ventricular septal rupture, or free-wall rupture. Underlying cardiomyopathy is a common cause.

Cardiogenic shock usually develops after the patient has been hospitalized. In the SHOCK trial, 75% of patients developed cardiogenic shock after admission at a median of 7 hours after infarction. Risk factors for developing shock include older age, diabetes, anterior infarct, history of previous MI, peripheral vascular disease, decreased LV ejection fraction, and larger infarct.

Patients with cardiogenic shock are profoundly hypotensive, peripherally vasoconstricted (cool to touch), anuric, and often have altered mental status. Pulses are diminished and rapid. Cardiac exam may reveal distant heart sounds with an S3 or S4. Pay close attention for systolic murmurs indicative of a ventricular septal defect (VSD) or papillary muscle rupture. Jugular venous distention (JVD) and pulmonary rales may also be present.

Laboratory testing may show arterial hypoxia, elevated creatinine, and lactic acidosis. Chest x-ray may reveal evidence of pulmonary congestion. Bedside echocardiography gives rapid information regarding LV systolic function and mechanical complications, including acute VSD, severe mitral regurgitation (MR), free-wall rupture, and tamponade. Placement of a pulmonary artery catheter is appropriate in this setting and allows for differentiation of LV and RV infarction, mechanical complication, and volume depletion. In addition, a pulmonary artery catheter will guide treatment when starting inotropes and/or giving volume repletion (see Table 11-1 for interpretation of PA catheter data).

Assuming the patient has "typical" LV pump failure as the cause of cardiogenic shock (systolic BP <90 mm Hg, cardiac index <2.2 L/minute/m^2), the immediate treatment includes:

- **Oxygenation**—Maintain O_2 saturation above 90% if possible. Intubation may be necessary, but be prepared for the further hypotension that results from the sedation and decreased cardiac filling with positive pressure ventilation.
- **IV fluids**—Goal pulmonary capillary wedge pressure (PCWP) is ~18 mm Hg. Patients with low PCWP will benefit from gentle hydration. Patients with pulmonary edema or elevated PCWP will often benefit from diuresis with IV furosemide (Lasix). Be vigilant for hypotension related to the diuresis.
- **Inotropes and vasopressors**—Vasopressor medications are useful in the management of cardiogenic shock but should be titrated with PA catheter guidance.
  - If systolic blood pressure is <70 mm Hg, start norepinephrine at 2 μg/minute and titrate to 20 μg /minute to achieve a mean arterial pressure of 70 mm Hg.
  - If systolic blood pressure is 70 to 90 mm Hg, start dopamine. At 2 to 5 μg/kg per minute, dopamine increases cardiac output and renal blood flow through beta- and dopamine-specific receptors, respectively. At 5 to 20 μg/kg per minute, dopamine has alpha-adrenergic stimulation leading to vasoconstriction.
  - With systolic blood pressure >90 mm Hg, dobutamine (Dobutrex) is the preferred agent. Dobutamine is started at 2.5 μg/kg per minute and **slowly** titrated to effect (usual maximum dose is 10 μg/kg per minute). The phosphodiesterase inhibitor milrinone (Primacor) acts as an inotrope and vasodilator and may be used if other agents prove ineffective.
- **Mechanical support**—Intraaortic balloon pump (IABP) decreases afterload and augments diastolic perfusion pressure to improve cardiac output and coronary perfusion. In several trials, use of IABP has shown a trend toward lower mortality rates when used as a bridge to revascularization (see Chapter 27). Percutaneous and surgical left ventricular assist devices have been used in certain situations.
- **Coronary Reperfusion**—Several trials have examined the benefit of revascularization (percutaneously or surgically) or medical treatment in patients with cardiogenic shock. The SHOCK trial prospectively examined patients who developed cardiogenic shock within 36 hours of acute MI and compared revascularization to aggressive medical management. Although there was no mortality benefit at 30 days, there were significant mortality benefits at 6 months and 1 year. Younger patients (≤75 years) showed greater benefit with revascularization, whereas older patients had better outcomes with medical management.

In the whirlwind of treating cardiogenic shock, it is essential to have objective markers to judge the effects of your treatment. The clinical markers to observe for improvement are mental status, urine output, and arterial and venous oxygenation. Other secondary markers that can be helpful include blood pressure, heart rate, PA catheter values, serum creatinine, and liver enzymes. Further details can be found in Chapter 11.

KEY POINTS TO REMEMBER

- A simplified approach to bradycardia can be remembered with the mnemonic "SSSSS-low heart rate:" Stable patient? Symptoms? Source of AV block? Speed up the heart? Set up for pacemaker.
- Treatment of ANY type of clinically unstable tachycardia is immediate electrical cardioversion/defibrillation. Stable tachycardias afford time to analyze the ECG for the specific diagnosis.
- For patients with STEMI, time to reperfusion relates directly to clincial outcomes. Patients who were not revascularized are at high risk for late, life-threatening complications that can be remembered by the mnemonic "FEAR A MI": Failure; Effusion; Arrhythmia; Rupture; Aneurysm; Myocardial Infarction.
- Cardiac tamponade is a clinical, not an echocardiographic, diagnosis. The decision to drain the pericardial fluid as well as the method (surgical or percutaneous) and the timing (emergent or elective) of the procedure, should be individualized to each patient, taking into account the acuity of the patient's condition, availability of trained personnel, and etiology of the effusion.
- Hypertensive emergency is defined by the presence of end-organ damage (renal, cardiac, or neurologic) and requires urgent lowering of blood pressure by ~25% with IV medications.
- Cardiogenic shock has a high mortality. Immediate treatment includes oxygenation, PA catheter–directed IV fluids, diuretics, inotropes, vasopressors, coronary revascularization (if appropriate), and mechanical support.

REFERENCES AND SUGGESTED READINGS

AHA. 2005 American Heart Association guidelines for cardiopulmonary resuscitation and emergency cardiovascular care. *Circulation* 2005;112(IV):1–203.

Boden WE, Eagle K, Granger CB. Reperfusion strategies in acute ST-segment elevation myocardial infarction: a comprehensive review of contemporary management options. *J Am Coll Cardiol* 2007;50:917–929.

Mann HJ, Nolan PE Jr. Update on the management of cardiogenic shock. *Curr Opin Crit Care* 2006;12:431–436.

Marik PE, Varon J. Hypertensive crises: challenges and management. *Chest* 2007;131;1949–1962.

Roy CL, Minor MA, Brookhart MA, et al. Does this patient with a pericardial effusion have cardiac tamponade? *JAMA* 2007;297:1810-1818.

Wilansky S, Moreno CA, Lester SJ. Complications of myocardial infarction. *Crit Care Med* 2007;35:S348–354.

Stable Angina

Courtney Virgilio and Andrew M. Kates

BACKGROUND

Chronic stable angina is the initial manifestation of ischemic heart disease in approximately half of patients with coronary artery disease (CAD). Approximately 15 million Americans have CAD. Despite the well-documented decline in cardiovascular mortality, ischemic heart disease remains the leading single cause of death in the United States and is responsible for nearly one of every five deaths.

DEFINITION

Angina is a symptom of myocardial ischemia most commonly caused by coronary artery disease. **Typical angina** (definite) is (1) substernal chest discomfort with a characteristic quality and duration that is (2) precipitated by stress and (3) relieved by rest or nitroglycerin (NTG). **Atypical angina** (probable) meets two of these criteria. **Noncardiac chest pain** meets one or none of these criteria. Anginal equivalents vary from patient to patient but may include dyspnea on exertion, fatigue or weakness, diaphoresis, dizziness, nausea, or syncope. Women (more than men) may complain of epigastric discomfort that otherwise presents like typical angina. Diabetic patients may experience anginal equivalent symptoms (e.g., epigastric distress) that should be suspicious for underlying ischemia.

CLASSIFICATION

The **Canadian Classification of Angina** is commonly employed to stratify patients in terms of severity into the following groups:

   I.   Angina only with strenuous activity
   II. Moderate activity, such as walking more than one flight of stairs, yields angina
   III. Mild activity, such as less than one flight of stairs, yields angina
   IV. Any activity, and even rest, yield angina

Keep in mind that in the Canadian Classification, severity of angina is not directly related to the severity of angiographic stenosis. Higher-severity of angina correlates with an increased short-term risk of death or nonfatal myocardial infarction (MI).

CAUSES

Pathophysiology
Stable angina most often results from fixed coronary lesions that produce a mismatch of myocardial oxygen supply and demand with increasing cardiac workload. Determinants of

myocardial oxygen demand include heart rate, afterload or systemic vascular resistance, myocardial wall stress (measured by preload), and myocardial contractility. A fixed stenosis of an epicardial coronary artery, usually >70% of the original luminal diameter of the vessel, is sufficient to limit blood flow distal to the lesion. When myocardial workload (oxygen demand) exceeds the capacity of myocardial blood supply (oxygen delivery), angina may ensue. The presence of ischemic heart disease can predispose patients to additional problems, including heart failure, cardiac arrhythmias, and sudden cardiac death.

Differential Diagnosis

There are other cardiac causes of angina besides coronary artery disease:

- **Congenital anomalies** of the coronary arteries can take many forms. Their prevalence is 1% to 2% of the general population. Anomalous origin of the left or right coronary artery from the contralateral sinus of Valsalva with passage between the aorta and pulmonary artery may produce ischemia and is associated with sudden death.
- **Myocardial bridge** is usually benign but may be associated with ischemic symptoms. The bridging occurs most commonly in the left anterior descending artery. Beta-adrenergic antagonists are helpful to increase diastolic filling, but nitrates can exacerbate the angina. A coronary stent may be indicated in the appropriate circumstances.
- **Coronary arteritis** is associated with collagen vascular diseases such as lupus, polyarteritis nodosa, and scleroderma.
- **Coronary artery ectasia** is characterized by irregular, diffuse, fusiform dilatation of the coronary arteries. Thrombus and obstructive lesions may be associated with these fusiform dilatations. This is most commonly due to hypertension.
- **Radiation therapy** may produce coronary arterial fibrosis with intimal proliferation. This evolves at a variable time course and may lead to ischemia.
- **Cocaine** is associated with vasospasm and thrombus formation, which can produce ischemia. Cocaine also causes endothelial dysfunction and hastens the development of atherosclerosis, which can produce angina.
- **Aortic stenosis** causes angina by subendocardial ischemia due to wall stress.
- **Hypertrophic cardiomyopathy** causes subendocardial ischemia by a mechanism similar to aortic stenosis.
- **Prinzmetal's angina,** or vasospastic angina, is a well-recognized syndrome in which patients present with resting angina and ST-segment elevation. Variant angina is usually associated with an underlying noncritical stenosis; however, a substantial percentage of patients have no evidence of underlying stenosis. This may be due to spasm of the artery, particularly around the area of noncritical stenosis. Coronary artery spasm may be provoked by infusion of dopamine, acetylcholine, or ergonovine.
- **Syndrome X** is typical anginal pain in the setting of normal coronary arteries. Patients may have angiographic stenoses, but these are inadequate to alter coronary blood flow with exercise. Abnormalities in coronary vasomotor tone may mediate angina, resulting in "microvascular angina"—that is, defective endothelial-derived dilatation of the coronary microcirculation. Evidence for myocardial ischemia in syndrome X patients manifests as reversible perfusion defects with thallium scintigraphy and magnetic resonance imaging (MRI) or transient impairment of global or regional ventricular function on echocardiography. This condition should not be confused with metabolic syndrome X (see Chapter 10).

Differential diagnosis of chest pain includes:

- Cardiac:
  - Coronary artery disease (supported by ECG abnormalities—changes in the T waves, ST segments, or conduction pattern; not ruled out by a normal ECG), coronary artery embolism or dissection, coronary artery anomalies
  - Valvular disease, especially aortic stenosis
  - Myocardium—chronic heart failure (thought secondary to myocardial stretch), myocarditis, reversible LV dysfunction related to stress (Tako-tsubo)
  - Pericardial—pericarditis
  - Vasculature—aortic dissection
- Pulmonary:
  - Pulmonary embolism or pulmonary hypertension
  - Lung parenchymal—pneumonia, pneumothorax
  - Pleural tissue—pleuritis or pleural effusion
- Gastrointestinal:
  - Gastroesophageal reflux disease (GERD)
  - Esophageal spasm or abnormal motility
  - Achalasia
  - Esophagitis
  - Esophageal rupture (Boerhaave's syndrome)
  - Peptic ulcer disease
  - Pancreatitis
  - Cholecystitis
- Urologic:
  - Nephrolithiasis
  - Pyelonephritis
- Dermatologic:
  - Herpes zoster
- Musculoskeletal:
  - Costochondritis
  - Rib fractures
  - Rheumatoid arthritis
  - Psoriatic arthritis
  - Fibromyalgia
- Psychiatric:
  - Anxiety disorder
  - Panic disorder
  - Somatoform disorders
  - Delusions

PRESENTATION

Risk Factors (See Chapter 10)

Tobacco abuse is associated with a markedly increased risk of coronary artery disease (CAD) and has a synergistic effect with other risk factors. Environmental exposure to smoke (secondhand smoke) may also increase the risk of heart disease. Successful smoking cessation markedly reduces the risk of CAD. **Hypertension** is associated with increased cardiovascular risk. Lifestyle modification and pharmacologic therapy (if needed) should be used to achieve a goal of less than 140/90 mm Hg. More stringent control (<130/80 mm Hg) is appropriate if comorbid disease—including renal insufficiency, diabetes, or heart failure—is present. CAD is the primary cause of death in people with **diabetes**. In addition, most hospitalizations resulting from diabetes-associated complications are a consequence of CAD. The incidence of CAD is two- to fourfold higher in individuals with diabetes than in those without. Moreover, increased insulin resistance, such as that seen with the **metabolic syndrome**, is also associated with increased risk of CAD. **High LDL, low HDL, and elevated triglycerides** are independent risk factors for CAD. A **family history** of CAD is appropriately defined as premature CAD in a first-degree relative (male relative <55 years; female relative <65 years). **Obesity** increases the risk of CAD and is associated with additional cardiac risk factors, including hypertension, diabetes, and lipid abnormalities. A body mass index >25 kg/m^2 is considered overweight.

Additionally, diseases associated with CAD include peripheral vascular disease, prior cerebrovascular event, and end-stage kidney disease.

History

A thorough history (see Chapter 3) can help determine the correct diagnosis in a patient presenting with chest pain. Focusing on the nature of symptoms as well as other information (risk factors, past history) will help to risk stratify the patient and either increase or decrease the pretest probability of coronary artery disease. Pertinent information about the chest pain includes:

- Location
- Character/quality of the pain
- Setting
- Duration
- Severity
- Associated symptoms
- Aggravating/relieving factors

Pertinent **social history** should include questions concerning tobacco use (pay attention to how much and for how long), alcohol use (moderate alcohol use is associated with a decreased risk of coronary heart disease), and drug use (cocaine use, stimulant use).

Other important points to remember are that diabetic patients may not experience any anginal symptoms despite having ischemic cardiac disease. Additionally, it is important to assess a patient's functional status since a patient who is sedentary may not exert themselves enough to experience angina. Alternatively, a patient who is relatively inactive may be limiting their activity due to anginal symptoms.

Physical Exam

As with the history, the **physical exam** is a key component in the evaluation of the patient with suspected coronary disease. A focused exam must include:

- Vital signs (don't forget blood pressure in **both** arms, and look for tachycardia as well).
- Head, ears, eyes, nose, and throat (HEENT): corneal arcus senilis, xanthelasma, diagonal earlobe crease.
- Neck: carotid artery bruits.
- Lungs: rales (if present during an episode of chest pain may suggest pulmonary edema secondary to ischemia).
- Cardiac: murmurs suggestive of stenotic or regurgitant valves, S3 or S4 gallop
- Abdomen: listen for bruits (aortic or renal arteries), feel for pulsatile mass (abdominal aortic aneurysm).
- Extremities: check the strength of the peripheral pulses (femoral, dorsalis pedis, posterior tibialis, etc.), listen for femoral artery bruits, check for peripheral edema or signs of vascular insufficiency.

Evaluation

The initial evaluation of the patient with cardiac disease can be tailored depending upon clinical suspicion for CAD. A **resting** electrocardiogram (**ECG**) should be obtained during pain and when the patient is pain-free. The ECG will be without abnormality in <50% of patients with chronic stable angina. A normal rest ECG does not exclude the presence of severe CAD. However, ECG abnormalities including (1) pathologic Q waves (>0.4 mV) consistent with a prior MI, (2) resting ST-segment depression, (3) T-wave inversion, or (4) LV hypertrophy increase the likelihood that the chest pain is cardiac in origin. **Biochemical markers** including complete blood count (CBC), fasting glucose, troponin, and lipid profile should be obtained in all patients with suspected CAD or acute coronary syndromes (see Chapter 8). Additionally, elevated baseline C-reactive protein (CRP), lipoprotein(a), and homocysteine levels are associated with increased risk of CAD. **Chest x-ray** should be obtained if there is evidence of congestive heart failure (CHF), valvular disease, or aortic disease.

Exercise stress testing without imaging provides functional information and allows risk stratification in patients with suspected angina. Exercise sufficient to increase the heart rate to 85% of maximum predicted heart rate (MPHR = 220 − age) is necessary for optimal sensitivity. Beta blockers, A-V nodal blocking agents, and nitrates should be discontinued in patients prior to performing stress tests in looking for new ischemia. Medications should be continued if the stress test is performed to optimize medical therapy. Exercise ECG has a sensitivity of 75%. The specificity of the test is adversely affected by the presence of resting ECG abnormalities, inability to exercise, or medication use (beta blockers, digoxin).

A **positive stress test** indicative of severe CAD is defined with the presence of any of the following:

- New ST-segment depression at the start of exercise
- New ST-segment depression >2 mm in multiple leads
- Inability to exercise for more than 2 minutes
- Decreased systolic blood pressure with exercise
- Development of heart failure or sustained ventricular arrhythmias
- Prolonged interval after exercise cessation (>5 minutes) before ischemic ST changes return to baseline.

The **Bruce protocol** is most commonly used, consisting of 3-minute stages of increasing treadmill speed and incline. The patient is monitored for an appropriate physiologic response to exercise with blood pressure and heart rate measurements during the walk and into the recovery period. The patient should be questioned for the presence of anginal symptoms. The patient's ECG is monitored throughout the study to evaluate for ischemic changes.

Prior to obtaining a stress test, it is important to remember **Bayes' theorem**: the posttest likelihood of a condition depends on both the pretest likelihood of the condition being present as well as the actual result of the test (Table 7-1). This pretest probability correlates with the positive and negative predictive values of an abnormal stress test. For example, in a patient who has a very low pretest likelihood of CAD, the stress test does not confer additional useful information. Likewise, in a patient with a very high pretest likelihood of CAD, limited sensitivity significantly increases the possibility of missing the diagnosis. Thus, stress testing is best used for those who have an intermediate likelihood of significant CAD.

The Duke treadmill score provides further prognostic information. It incorporates the duration of exercise on the Bruce protocol, maximal ST-segment deviation on the ECG, and anginal symptoms (Duke score = minutes exercise − [5 × mm ST-segment deviation] − [4 × anginal score]). Scores of >+5, −10 to +4, and <−11 are associated with low, moderate, and high risks, respectively, of subsequent cardiovascular events (Table 7-2).

Patients with a markedly positive stress test should undergo cardiac catheterization to be evaluated for coronary revascularization (see below).

TABLE 7-1	PRETEST LIKELIHOOD OF CAD IN SYMPTOMATIC PATIENTS ACCORDING TO AGE AND SEX (COMBINED DIAMOND/FORRESTER AND CASS DATA)					
	Nonanginal Chest Pain		Atypical Angina		Typical Angina	
Age (years)	Men	Women	Men	Women	Men	Women
30–39	4	2	34	12	76	26
40–49	13	3	51	22	87	55
50–59	20	7	65	31	93	73
60–69	27	14	72	51	94	86

Source: From Gibbons RJ, Abrams J, Chatterjee K, et al. ACC/AHA 2002 guideline update for the management of patients with chronic stable angina. A report of the American College of Cardiology/American Heart Association Task Force on Practice Guidelines (Committee on the Management of Patients With Chronic Stable Angina), 2002. Available at http://www.acc.org/clinical/guidelines/stable.pdf.

Cardiac stress testing with imaging (as opposed to exercise ECG) is an appropriate initial diagnostic study in those patients in the following categories (see Chapters 25 and 26):

- Evidence of preexcitation (WPW)
- LVH
- LBBB (not RBBB) or significant intraventricular conduction defects (IVCD)
- Digoxin effects
- Paced rhythm
- Resting ST- and T-wave changes

Stress myocardial perfusion imaging with thallium-201 (^{201}Tl) or technetium-99m (^{99m}Tc) sestamibi has been reported to increase sensitivity for detection of CAD to 80% and specificity to 80% to 90%. Stress perfusion imaging allows the diagnosis and localization of areas of ischemia, determination of ejection fraction, and determination of

TABLE 7-2	SURVIVAL ACCORDING TO RISK GROUPS BASED ON DUKE TREADMILL SCORES		
Risk Group (score)	Percentage of Total	4-Year Survival	Annual Mortality (%)
Low (≥+5)	62	0.99	0.25
Moderate (−10 to +4)	34	0.95	1.25
High (<−10)	4	0.79	5.0

Source: From Gibbons RJ, Abrams J, Chatterjee K, et al. ACC/AHA 2002 guideline update for the management of patients with chronic stable angina. A report of the American College of Cardiology/American Heart Association Task Force on Practice Guidelines (Committee on the Management of Patients With Chronic Stable Angina), 2002. Available at http://www.acc.org/clinical/guidelines/stable.pdf.

myocardial viability. Owing to its higher cost, it should be performed only in the presence of resting ECG abnormalities (see previous section), inability to exercise, or to evaluate for the presence of in-stent restenosis. A markedly positive stress test demonstrating multiple areas of ischemia, transient LV cavity dilatation, or uptake of radiotracer in the lungs should prompt referral for coronary angiography.

Exercise stress echocardiography can be performed to aid in the diagnosis of CAD. Compared with standard exercise treadmill testing, stress echocardiography provides an additional clinical value for detecting and localizing myocardial ischemia.

Exercise stress testing (generally with a treadmill) is preferable to pharmacologic stress testing. However, when the patient cannot exercise to the necessary level or in other specified circumstances (see above), pharmacologic stress testing may be preferable. Three drugs are commonly used as substitutes for exercise stress testing: dipyridamole, adenosine, and dobutamine. Dipyridamole and adenosine are vasodilators that are generally used in conjunction with myocardial perfusion scintigraphy, whereas dobutamine is a positive inotropic (and chronotropic) agent commonly used with echocardiography. Notably, patients whose resting ECG contains ventricular paced rhythms or LBBB should preferentially undergo adenosine perfusion imaging to avoid potential false positive studies.

Newer imaging modalities include **stress testing with cardiac MRI** and **multiple-slice CT angiography**. These techniques are discussed in detail in Chapter 26.

Exercise stress testing is **contraindicated** patients with the following:

- Acute MI within 2 days
- Unstable angina not previously stabilized by medical therapy
- Cardiac arrhythmias causing symptoms or hemodynamic compromise
- Symptomatic severe aortic stenosis
- Symptomatic heart failure
- Acute pulmonary embolus, myocarditis, pericarditis, aortic dissection

Stress Testing in Specific Populations

Patients without known coronary disease can be considered as being at low, intermediate, and high risk. In general, a "screening" exercise test is not warranted **in asymptomatic patients** at low risk for CAD. **Intermediate-risk patients** can be considered for testing if their occupation is such that impairment might have an impact on public safety (e.g., airline pilot), or they plan to begin a vigorous exercise program. **Patients at high risk for CAD** owing to other diseases, such as diabetes and peripheral vascular disease, can also be considered for testing.

For patients with known coronary disease who remain symptom free after their infarction and have not undergone coronary angiography, **stress testing after MI** provides useful prognostic information in patients. A **submaximal** study performed 4 to 7 days after acute MI or a maximal exercise stress test 4 to 6 weeks after MI aids in determining the patient's ischemic burden, which, if present, should prompt consideration for cardiac catheterization to define the coronary anatomy. **A stress test after acute MI**, either with or without revascularization, helps guide recommendations for a cardiac rehabilitation program. The routine use of stress testing in asymptomatic patients after percutaneous or surgical revascularization remains controversial. If testing is done, it should be performed in conjunction with an imaging modality (nuclear or echocardiographic) to increase the sensitivity of the test and to localize any area(s) of ischemia that may exist.

Women. The use of exercise testing in women presents difficulties that are not experienced in men (see Chapter 28). These difficulties reflect the differences between men and women regarding the prevalence of CAD and the sensitivity and specificity of exercise testing. To compensate for the limitations of the test in women, some investigators have developed predictive models that incorporate more information from the test than simply the amount and type of ST-segment change. Although this approach is attractive, its clinical application remains limited.

Elderly. Performance of exercise testing poses additional problems in the elderly, as functional capacity in these patients is often compromised from muscle weakness and deconditioning (see Chapter 28).

Risk Stratification

Risk assessment of patients with stable angina should be used to help guide decisions on referral for noninvasive or invasive cardiac testing in those with an intermediate or high probability of CAD. Using both the Duke treadmill score as well as the principles of Bayes' theorem, as discussed above, can help to determine if stress testing is appropriate or if the patient should have his or her anatomy defined (either with cardiac CT angiography or conventional coronary angiography).

Invasive Diagnosis of CAD

Coronary angiography or cardiac catheterization (see Chapter 25) is considered the "gold standard" technique for diagnosing CAD. As with noninvasive testing, angiography can be used to establish a diagnosis or to characterize the degree of atherosclerosis in patients with known disease. It should be performed in patients with known or suspected angina with a markedly positive stress test or those who have survived sudden cardiac death. It should be considered for patients with a high pretest probability of left main or three-vessel CAD or for those whose occupation requires a definitive diagnosis. Angiography can also be considered for patients if a recent stress test is nondiagnostic and for individuals who are unable to undergo noninvasive testing. In selected patients with recurrent hospitalizations for chest pain or those with an overriding desire for a definite diagnosis and an intermediate or high pretest probability of CAD, invasive testing can be used to document the presence or extent of disease and facilitate long-term management. Coronary angiography may also be useful in patients with angina who are suspected of having a nonatherosclerotic cause of ischemia (e.g., coronary anomaly, coronary dissection, radiation vasculopathy). Coronary angiography is NOT indicated (class III indication) for stable angina responding to medical therapy (see "Treatment," below).

Several new technologies are available to assist in the diagnosis of CAD; these are discussed further in Chapter 26. **Intravascular ultrasound** can be used in selected patients to assess plaque burden, providing more definitive assessment of the coronary vasculature at the time of the cardiac catheterization. **Doppler flow probe** ("wavewire") is used to determine the functional significance of a coronary lesion by measuring fractional flow reserve across the stenosis. **CT angiography and MR angiography** have both shown promise in the noninvasive evaluation of CAD.

TREATMENT

Rationale

The goal of treatment is twofold: (1) to reduce the likelihood of unstable angina, MI, or death occurring (i.e., to increase the quantity of life) and (2) to reduce symptoms with antianginal therapy (i.e., to increase the quality of life). Both pharmacologic methods and revascularization are important options which should be considered in addition to diet and lifestyle modifications.

Medical Treatment

Specific treatment is aimed at reducing myocardial oxygen demand, improving myocardial oxygen supply, treating cardiac risk factors (hypertension, diabetes, obesity), and controlling exacerbating factors (valvular stenosis, anemia) that may precipitate ischemia.

One approach to guide the treatment of patients with ischemic heart disease is the "ABCDE" mnemonic: Aspirin (antiplatelet agents), antianginal therapy and Angiotensin converting enzyme (ACE) inhibitors; Beta-adrenergic antagonists and blood pressure control; Cholesterol-lowering agents and cigarette-smoking cessation; Diet; and Exercise.

Aspirin use in patients with stable angina has been shown to reduce cardiovascular events by 33%. In asymptomatic patients in the Physician's Health Study, aspirin (325 mg every other day) decreased the incidence of MI. **Clopidogrel** (75 mg/day) can be used in patients who are allergic to or intolerant of aspirin. We strongly encourage consultation with an allergist for the patient suspected of having aspirin allergy.

Beta blockers appear to be effective in controlling angina by decreasing heart rate and blood pressure. The dosage can be adjusted to result in a resting heart rate of 50 to 60 bpm. In patients with persistent angina, a target heart rate <50 bpm is warranted provided that no symptoms are associated with the bradycardia and that heart block does not develop. If stress testing is performed as part of the evaluation, beta-blocker therapy in patients with known heart disease should limit the heart rate response with exercise to <75% of the heart rate associated with the onset of ischemia. Use of beta blockers is **contraindicated** in patients with severe bronchospasm, significant atrioventricular (AV) block, marked resting bradycardia, or decompensated heart failure. In those patients for whom excessive beta blockade results in symptomatic bradycardia, a permanent pacemaker may be indicated. In patients with chronic stable angina, beta blockers decrease the onset of angina or the ischemic threshold is delayed or avoided. Beta blockers, in the absence of contraindications, should be considered initial therapy because of evidence demonstrating their ability to reduce cardiovascular mortality, especially among patients with a history of prior MI. Beta-blocking agents with beta-1 selectivity [such as metoprolol (Lopressor, Toprol-XL) and atenolol (Tenormin)] are preferable in patients with asthma, chronic obstructive pulmonary disease (COPD), insulin-dependent diabetes, or peripheral vascular disease. With increasing dosage, some of the beta-1 selectivity is lost. The resting heart rate goal for patients on beta blockers is 45 to 60 bpm, and with moderate exercise (two flights of stairs) the heart rate should be <90 bpm. Upward titration of beta blockers should occur over 6 to 12 weeks. If side effects warrant discontinuation of beta blockers, the drug should be weaned over a 2- to 3-week period to prevent worsening angina or precipitation of an ischemic event. These medications decrease mortality after MI and decrease symptoms of angina in patients who have not had an MI. Beta blockers decrease myocardial oxygen demand by causing a decrease in heart rate, contractility, and blood pressure. The reduction in heart rate also allows for increased diastolic filling time and may increase coronary perfusion.

Calcium channel blockers can be used in lieu of beta blockers if beta blockers are contraindicated or not tolerated owing to significant adverse effects. They can also be used in conjunction with beta blockers if the latter are not fully effective at relieving anginal symptoms. Long-acting dihydropyridines and nondihydropyridine agents can be used. Use of short-acting dihydropyridines (e.g., nifedipine) should be avoided because of their potential to increase the risk of adverse cardiac events. These agents reduce the transmembrane flux of calcium and thereby decrease coronary vascular resistance and increase coronary blood flow, increasing myocardial oxygen supply. This is the principal mechanism of benefit in vasospastic angina. Calcium antagonists decrease systemic vascular resistance and blood pressure, resulting in a decrease in myocardial oxygen demand. Calcium antagonists, depending on the agent, may also decrease contractility (negative inotropic effects), which can decrease myocardial oxygen demand. Some calcium channel blockers (the nondihydropyridines) decrease heart rate (negative chronotropy) or decrease conduction through the AV node, thereby reducing myocardial oxygen demand.

Nitrates, either long-acting formulations for chronic use or sublingual preparations for acute anginal symptoms, can be used as adjuncts to baseline therapy with beta blockers or calcium antagonists or both. These agents are endothelium-independent vasodilators and venodilators. They reduce myocardial oxygen demand by decreasing blood pressure, thereby decreasing afterload; they decrease preload through venodilation and dilate epicardial coronary arteries, thereby increasing myocardial oxygen supply. The patient should take the medication while seated because of possible side effects of hypotension. Sublingual preparations can be used at the first indication of angina or prophylactically before engaging in activities that are known to precipitate angina. Patients should seek prompt medical attention if angina occurs at rest or fails to respond to the third sublingual dose. Nitrate tolerance, resulting in reduced therapeutic response, may occur with all nitrate preparations. The institution of a nitrate-free period of 10 to 12 hours can enhance treatment efficacy.

Ranolazine has antianginal and anti-ischemic effects that do not depend upon reductions in heart rate or blood pressure. Its exact mechanism of action is unknown; however, it appears to have an effect on the function of cardiomyocyte sodium ion channels. It has shown benefit in providing symptomatic relief of angina.

ACE inhibitors have been investigated for treatment of stable angina. A reduction of exercise-induced myocardial ischemia has been reported with the addition of an ACE inhibitor in patients with stable angina with optimal beta blockade and normal LV function. The effects of the ACE inhibitor ramipril on cardiovascular events in high-risk patients was studied in the HOPE trial, which found that high-risk patients with vascular disease or diabetes plus one other cardiovascular risk factor had a lower rate of death, MI, or cerebrovascular accident (CVA) when treated with ramipril 10 mg/day rather than placebo for 5 years. This benefit is thought to be independent of blood pressure effects.

Cholesterol-lowering agents—including statins, fibrates, bile acid sequestrants, and niacin—have been shown to reduce recurrent events and improve overall outcome in patients with established CAD. By far the most studied of these agents are the HMG Co-A reductase inhibitors (statins). Studies including the Scandinavian Simvastatin Survival Study (4S) trial and the Cholesterol and Recurrent Events Trial (CARE) study established the efficacy of statins in these patients, while more recent studies—including the Heart Protection Study (HPS) and Treating to New Targets (TNT)—indicate that aggressive treatment to LDL levels well below 100 mg/dL was beneficial. PROVE-IT-TIMI 22, the first large study of CAD patients in the setting of acute coronary syndrome, also found that an aggressive approach to LDL reduction was more effective than conventional reduction.

Chelation therapy and **acupuncture** have not been found to be effective in relieving symptoms and are not recommended for treatment of chronic stable angina.

The use of **antibiotics** to treat CAD is not recommended.

Revascularization

Medical therapy with at least two and preferably three classes of antianginal agents should be attempted before treatment is considered a failure. Patients who are refractory to medical therapy should be assessed with coronary angiography if the anatomy has not already been defined. Catheter-based revascularization is ideal for candidates for percutaneous coronary intervention (PCI) who have angina, are <75 years old, have single- or two-vessel CAD, have normal LV function, and do not have diabetes. For most lesions in vessels with diameters >2.0 mm, stents are deployed after percutaneous transluminal coronary angioplasty (PTCA), because long-term patency rates and overall outcomes are improved compared with PTCA alone. There are bare metal stents and drug-eluting stents, each with their own advantages and disadvantages.

The three major **complications of PCI** are **stent thrombosis, restenosis**, and **coronary artery dissection**. **Stent thrombosis** occurring within 24 hours of stent placement is termed **acute** stent thrombosis and is usually red clot (fibrin-mediated); thrombosis occurring within 24 hours to 30 days (with a peak incidence at day 11) is **subacute** stent thrombosis and is usually white clot (platelet-mediated); and thrombosis occurring from 30 days to 1 year is **late** stent thrombosis. More recently, the occurrence of stent thrombosis beyond 1 year, called **very late** stent thrombosis, has been recognized. Very late stent thrombosis appears to be limited to drug-eluting stents and has raised the issue of prolonged dual antiplatelet therapy. **Restenosis** is due to neointimal hyperplasia caused by proliferation of smooth muscle and inflammatory cells. It is defined as a >50% loss in the diameter of the vessel. It is much more common with angioplasty alone and less common with the use of bare metal stents. With the advent of drug-eluting stents, which are coated with antineoplastic agents aimed at preventing restenosis, it is a negligible issue. With bare metal stents, the incidence is <20% (more common in diabetics). The peak incidence is between 3 and 6 months after stent placement. **Coronary artery dissection** often can be repaired with multiple stents but may necessitate bypass surgery.

As the decision is made regarding PCI versus medical management, a discussion of data is appropriate. Patients enrolled in the COURAGE trial had stable angina and were randomized to either percutaneous coronary intervention (PCI) with optimal medical therapy or optimal medical therapy alone and followed for a median of 4.6 years. PCI did not reduce the risk of death, MI, or other major cardiovascular events over the course of the trial. It merits mention, however, that less than 10% of screened patients were enrolled, a substantial number of patients crossed over into the PCI arm, and a relatively small percentage of patients received drug-eluting stents. That having been said, the COURAGE trial does support earlier studies showing no survival benefit to PCI in patients **with stable angina**.

Coronary artery bypass grafting (CABG) is optimal for patients at high risk for cardiac mortality, including those with (1) left main disease, (2) two- or three-vessel disease involving the proximal left anterior descending artery and LV dysfunction, and (3) diabetes and multivessel coronary disease with LV dysfunction.

The risk of surgery includes 1%–3% mortality, a 5% to 10% incidence of perioperative MI, a small risk of perioperative stroke or cognitive dysfunction, and a 10% to 20% risk of vein graft failure in the first year. Approximately 75% of patients remain free of recurrent angina or adverse cardiac events at 5 years of follow-up. The risks of elective PCI include <1% mortality, a 2% to 5% rate of nonfatal MI, and <1% need for emergent CABG for an unsuccessful procedure. The use of internal mammary artery grafts is associated with 90% graft patency at 10 years, compared with 40% to 50% for saphenous vein grafts. The long-term patency of radial artery grafts is currently under review. After 10 years of follow-up, 50% of patients develop recurrent angina or other adverse cardiac events related to late vein graft failure or progression of native CAD. Two U.S. trials—the multicenter BARI and the single-center EAST—evaluated PTCA versus CABG in patients with multivessel disease. The results of these trials at approximately 5 years showed that early and late survival rates are equivalent for PTCA and CABG groups. However, subgroup analysis showed a clear survival benefit with CABG for diabetics and for patients with severe multivessel disease. Of note, the BARI and EAST trials studied PTCA without stents; many believe that the addition of stents drastically changes the long-term results of angioplasty, particularly with drug-eluting stents.

Alternate therapies are available for patients with chronic stable angina who are refractory to medical management and are not candidates for percutaneous or surgical revascularization.

Transmyocardial laser revascularization has been delivered by percutaneous technique (YAG [yttrium-aluminum-garnet] laser) and by epicardial surgical techniques (CO_2 or YAG laser). The percutaneous approach has not been approved by the U.S. Food and Drug Administration and should therefore be considered experimental therapy. The goal in either approach is to create a series of transmural endomyocardial channels. Surgical transmyocardial laser revascularization has been shown to improve symptoms in patients with stable angina, although the responsible mechanism is controversial. The data on whether exercise capacity is improved are conflicting, and no benefit has been demonstrated in terms of increasing myocardial perfusion or reducing mortality.

Enhanced external counterpulsation (EECP) is a nonpharmacologic technique for which 35 hours/week of treatment in patients with chronic stable angina and a positive stress test was shown to decrease the frequency of angina and increase the time to exercise-induced ischemia. This treatment improves anginal symptoms in approximately 75% to 80% of patients; however, additional clinical trial data are required before enhanced external counterpulsation can be definitively recommended.

Chelation therapy is not indicated in the treatment of angina.

Follow-Up

Minor changes in the patient's anginal complaints can be treated with titration or adjustment of the antianginal regimen. If the patient has a significant change in anginal complaints (frequency, severity, or time to onset with activity), a reassessment with a stress test (likely in conjunction with an imaging modality) or a cardiac catheterization is warranted. If the anatomy is amenable to revascularization (either percutaneous or surgical), this approach should be considered.

KEY POINTS TO REMEMBER

- Typical angina is a substernal chest discomfort that may signify CAD. It is stable when caused by a similar amount of activity and relieved with rest or NTG. It is unstable when it is new in onset, occurs at rest, occurs with less activity than usual, or does not resolve.
- The workup of angina includes history and physical exam, followed by ECG. Certain patients should undergo stress testing.
- It is imperative to manage modifiable risk factors (smoking, diabetes, hypertension, lipids, weight). Smoking is the most important risk factor to modify.
- Patients should be referred for coronary angiography only in certain settings, such as class III–IV angina refractory to medications.
- ASA, lipid-lowering therapy, beta blockers, and nitrates form the cornerstone of pharmacotherapy for stable angina. Remember that ACE inhibitors provide a mortality benefit, especially in those patients with LV dysfunction and diabetes.
- Surgical revascularization is indicated in patients with high-grade stenoses, particularly of the left main and left anterior descending coronary arteries, especially if such patients are diabetic or if there is concomitant LV dysfunction or a known large territory of ischemia. The choice of method (percutaneous versus surgical) depends on the number and type of lesions, the presence of diabetes and/or LV dysfunction, and operator experience.

REFERENCES AND SUGGESTED READINGS

Abrams J. Chronic stable angina. *N Engl J Med* 2005;352:2524–2533.

Bello N, Mosca L. Epidemiology of coronary heart disease in women. *Prog Cardiovasc Dis* 2004;46:287–295.

Boden WE, et al. Optimal medical therapy with or without PCI for stable coronary disease. *N Engl J Med* 2007;356:1503–1516.

Braunwald E, Domanski M, Fowler S, et al. Angiotensin-converting-enzyme inhibition in stable coronary artery disease. *N Engl J Med* 2004;351:2058–2068.

Bugiardini R, Merz C. Angina with "normal" coronary arteries. *JAMA* 2005;293:477–484.

Cameron A, Davis KB, Green G, et al. Coronary artery bypass surgery with internal thoracic artery grafts: effects on survival over a 15-year period. *N Engl J Med* 1996;334:216–219.

Cannon C, Braunwald E, McCabe C, et al. Intensive versus moderate lipid lowering with statins after acute coronary syndromes (PROVE-IT-TIMI 22). *N Engl J Med* 2004;350:1495–1504.

CAPRIE Steering Committee. A randomized, blinded trial of clopidogrel versus aspirin in patients at risk of ischemic events. *Lancet* 1996;348:1329–1339.

Cupples LA et al. Preexisting cardiovascular conditions and long-term prognosis after initial myocardial infarction: The Framingham Study. *Am Heart J* 1993;125:863–872.

Davis K, Chaitman B, Ryan T, et al. Comparison of 15-year survival for men and women after initial medical or surgical treatment for coronary artery disease: a CASS registry study. *JACC* 1995;25:1000–1009.

Dunselman P, Liem AH, Verdel G, et al. Addition of felodipine to metoprolol vs. replacement of metoprolol by felodipine in patients with angina pectoris despite adequate beta blockade (FEMINA). *Eur Heart J* 1997;18:1755–1764.

Estacio R, Jeffers B, Hiatt W, et al. The effect of nisoldipine as compared with enalapril on cardiovascular outcomes in patients with non-insulin-dependent diabetes and hypertension. *N Engl J Med* 1998;338:645–652.

Fox KM, Bertrand M, Ferrari R, et al. Efficacy of perindopril, in reduction of cardiovascular events among patients with stable coronary artery disease: randomized, double-blind, placebo-controlled, multicentre trial (the EUROPA study). *Lancet* 2003;362: 782–788.

Frank CW, Weinblatt E, Shapiro S. Angina pectoris in men: prognostic significance of selected medical factors. *Circulation* 1973;47:509–517.

Gianrossi R, Detrano R, Mulvihill D, et al. Exercise-induced ST depression the in diagnosis of coronary artery disease: a meta-analysis. *Circulation* 1989;80:87–98.

Gibbons RJ, Abrams J, Chatterjee K, et al. ACC/AHA 2002 guideline update for the management of patients with chronic stable angina: a report of the American College of Cardiology/American Heart Association Task Force on Practice Guidelines (Committee to Update the 1999 Guidelines for the Management of Patients with Chronic Stable Angina). 2002. Available at www.acc.org/clinical/guidelines/stable/stable.pdf.

Gibbons RJ, Abrams J, Chatterjee K, et al. ACC/AHA 2002 guideline update for the management of patients with chronic stable angina—summary article: a report of the American College of Cardiology/American Heart Association Task Force on Practice Guidelines (Committee on the Management of Patients With Chronic Stable Angina). *Circulation* 2003;107(1):149–158.

Gibbons RJ, Abrams J, Chatterjee K, et al. ACC/AHA 2002 guideline update for the management of patients with chronic stable angina. A report of the American College of Cardiology/American Heart Association Task Force on Practice Guidelines (Committee on the Management of Patients With Chronic Stable Angina), 2002. Available at http://www.acc.org/clinical/guidelines/stable.pdf.

Grundy SM, Cleeman JI, Merz CN, et al. Implications of recent clinical trials for the National Cholesterol Education Program Adult Treatment Panel III guidelines. *Circulation* 2004;110:227–239.

Hannan EL, et al. Long-term outcomes of coronary-artery bypass grafting versus stent implantation. *N Engl J Med* 2005;352:2174–2183.

Heart Protection Study Collaborative Group. MRC/BHF Heart Protection Study of cholesterol lowering with simvastatin in 20,536 high-risk individuals: a randomized placebo-controlled trial. *Lancet* 2002;360:7–22.

Hlatky MA et al. Medical care costs and quality of life after randomization to coronary angioplasty or coronary bypass surgery. *N Engl J Med* 1997;336:92–99.

Hoyert DL et al. *National Vital Statistics Reports; Deaths: Final Data for 2003.* Washington, DC: U.S. Government Printing Office; 2003.

LaRosa J, Grundy S, Waters D, et al. Intensive lipid lowering with atorvastatin in patients with stable coronary disease (TNT). *N Engl J Med* 2005;352:1425–1435.

Merz C, Johnson B, Kelsey S, et al. Diagnostic, prognostic, and cost assessment of coronary artery disease in women. *Am J Manag Care* 2001;7:959–965.

Miki T, Suzuki M, Shibasaki T, et al. Mouse model of Prinzmetal angina by disruption of the inward rectifier Kir6.1. *Nat Med* 2002;8:466–472.

Morice MC, Serruys PW, Sousa JE, et al. A randomized comparison of a sirolimus-eluting stent with a standard stent for coronary revascularization. *N Engl J Med* 2002;346: 1773–1780.

NCEP. Executive Summary of The Third Report of The National Cholesterol Education Program (NCEP) Expert Panel on Detection, Evaluation, and Treatment of High Blood Cholesterol in Adults (Adult Treatment Panel III). *JAMA* 2001;285: 2486–2497.

Pepine C, Cohn P, Deedwania P, et al. Effects of treatment on outcome in mildly symptomatic patients with ischemia during daily life: the atenolol silent ischemia study (ASIST). *Circulation* 1994;90:762–768.

Randomised trial of cholesterol lowering in 4444 patients with coronary heart disease: the Scandinavian Simvastatin Survival Study (4S). *Lancet* 1994;344:1383–1389.

Reis S, Holubkov R, Smith AJ, et al. Coronary microvascular dysfunction is highly prevalent in women with chest pain in the absence of coronary artery disease: results from the NHLBI WISE study. *Am Heart J* 2001;141:735–741.

RITA-2 Trial Participants. Coronary angioplasty versus medical therapy for angina: the second Randomized Intervention Treatment of Angina. *Lancet* 1997;350:461–468.

Sacks F, Pfeffer M, Moye L, et al. The effect of pravastatin on coronary events after myocardial infarction in patients with average cholesterol levels (CARE). *N Engl J Med* 1996;335:1001–1009.

Sangareddi V, Chockalingam A, Gnanavelu G, et al. Canadian cardiovascular society classification of effort angina: an angiographic correlation. *Coron Artery Dis* 2004;15: 111–114.

Tatti P, Pahor M, Byington R, et al. Outcome results of the fosinopril versus amlodipine cardiovascular events randomized trial (FACET) in patients with hypertension and NIDDM. *Diabetes Care* 1998;21:597–603.

The Bypass Angioplasty Revascularization Investigators (BARI). Comparison of coronary bypass surgery with angioplasty in patients with multi-vessel disease. *N Engl J Med* 1996;335:217–225.

Topol E. *Textbook of Cardiovascular Medicine*. Philadelphia: Lippincott Williams & Wilkins; 1998.

Younis LT, Chaitman BR. Management of stable angina pectoris. *Cardiology* 1995;1: 61–64.

Yusuf S, Sleight P, Pogue J, et al. Effects of an angiotensin-converting-enzyme inhibitor, ramipril, on cardiovascular events in high-risk patients (HOPE). *N Engl J Med* 2000; 342:145–153.

Yusuf S, Zucker D, Peduzzi P, et al. Effect of coronary artery bypass graft surgery on survival: overview of 10-year results from randomized trials by the Coronary Artery Bypass Graft Surgery Trialists Collaboration. *Lancet* 1994;334:563–570.

Acute Coronary Syndromes (Unstable Angina/Non–ST-Segment Elevation Myocardial Infarction)

Santhosh Jay Mathews

8

BACKGROUND

Acute coronary syndromes (ACS) represent a broad collection of conditions: acute myocardial ischemia or infarction (AMI) manifested by ST-segment elevation or depression, Q-wave or non–Q-wave myocardial infarction, and unstable angina (UA). For simplicity, ACS can be divided into **ST-segment-elevation acute coronary syndromes/myocardial infarction (STEACS/STEMI) and NSTEACS,** which includes both non–ST-segment elevation myocardial infarction (NSTEMI, both Q wave and non-Q wave) and UA. As opposed to STEACS, which usually results from complete and prolonged occlusion of an epicardial blood vessel, NSTEACS usually results from severe narrowing and/or transient occlusion of coronary arteries. If the stenosis is not severe enough or the occlusion does not persist long enough to cause myocardial necrosis, the syndrome is labeled **UA.** Patients who present with STEACS represent a population in whom immediate reperfusion therapy (e.g., thrombolysis or percutaneous coronary intervention [PCI]) is of primary concern (see Chapter 9). Management of NSTEACS is somewhat more complicated and may dictate a more conservative or early invasive therapeutic strategy, depending on the risk profile of the patient. The primary goal of treatment in NSTEACS is to limit ischemia or infarction and improve overall morbidity/mortality.

EPIDEMIOLOGY

ACS represents almost 1.6 million hospitalizations each year. This syndrome requires early diagnosis and aggressive treatment to minimize myocardial damage. Despite maximal medical therapy, at 1 year, patients with NSTEACS are still at risk for death ($\sim$6%), recurrent myocardial infarction ($\sim$11%), and recurrent need for revascularization ($\sim$50–60%). It is important to note that although the short-term mortality of STEMI is greater than that of NSTEMI, the long-term mortality is the same.

DEFINITION

In the absence of ST-segment elevation, ACS with or without myocardial necrosis falls under the grouping of UA/NSTEMI, or more simply, NSTEACS.

UA can be differentiated from stable angina by meeting one of the following criteria:

- New-onset exertional angina of <2 months' duration that limits physical activity
- Angina that was previously stable, but is now occurring with either increased severity, frequency, duration, or after less exertion
- Angina that occurs at rest that lasts >20 minutes
- Chest pain within 2 weeks of previous MI

UA can progress to NSTEMI, in which case the occlusive event results in objective myocardial necrosis.

The ESC/ACCF/AHA/WHF Task Force further defines acute myocardial infarction as myocardial necrosis in a clinical setting consistent with myocardial ischemia meeting one of the following criteria:

- Elevated cardiac biomarkers with one of the following:
  - Ischemic symptoms
  - Ischemic electrocardiogram (ECG) changes
  - New pathologic Q waves
  - Evidence of infarction by cardiac imaging
- Sudden cardiac death associated with ST elevation or new LBBB (STEACS) and/or fresh coronary thrombus
- Post-PCI, greater the 3× normal elevation of cardiac biomarkers signify PCI-related myocardial infarction
- Post-CABG, greater than 5× normal elevation of cardiac biomarkers with new Q waves/LBBB, graft/native coronary artery occlusion, or infarction by cardiac imaging signify CABG-related myocardial infarction.

CAUSES

Pathophysiology

Myocardial ischemia can be the result of either an increase in myocardial oxygen demand or a reduction in its supply. In the case of NSTEACS, the majority of cases are due to a sudden decrease in blood supply via partial occlusion of the affected vessel. The source of this blockage is most commonly luminal thrombosis secondary to **ruptured atherosclerotic plaque** (55%–60%), **plaque erosion** (30%–35%), or a **calcified nodule** (<10%). Collectively, these three types of plaques are known as **vulnerable plaques**, given their role in thrombosis and ACS. These represent the majority of cases of acute myocardial infarction (AMI) in younger patients (<50 years) and often premenopausal women.

Plaques often do not appear to be severe when visualized with standard arteriography, as up to two-thirds responsible for NSTEACS have subcritical stenosis of <50% lumen diameter. As plaque burden increases, the vessel may undergo **positive remodeling**, in which case overall stenosis is decreased by a compensatory focal increase in vessel size. The plaque can rupture as a result of local factors, including inflammation and shear stress. **Triggers for plaque rupture include increased heart rate, contractility, and hypertension.** After plaque rupture, the lipid-rich subendothelial components become exposed to platelets and inflammatory cells in the bloodstream and act as a very potent substrate for thrombus formation. Concurrently, platelet adhesion commences, followed by release of alpha granules containing multiple substances, including thromboxane A_2, thrombin, serotonin, and adenosine diphosphate. The platelets express glycoprotein IIb/IIIa, which binds to fibrinogen and von Willebrand factor and results in cross-linking/platelet aggregation. In addition to the direct mechanical obstruction caused by the thrombus, the damaged endothelium decreases its production of natural vasodilators, such as nitric oxide. Thrombus is further stabilized by thrombin-mediated conversion of fibrinogen to fibrin. The occlusive matter is usually a platelet-rich "white thrombus," unlike the fibrin-rich "red thrombus" of STEACS, which may partially explain the poor response to fibrinolytic therapy (see "Treatment: Thrombolytics," below).

A minority of patients present with UA from causes other than those listed above (see Chapter 7), including:

- **Vasospastic angina** ("Prinzmetal variant angina") is an uncommon type of episodic, nitrate-sensitive UA that classically is seen in the absence of CAD. The mechanism is not well known but is thought to be related to dysfunctional endothelium resulting in local vasoconstriction severe enough to cause ischemia or even infarction.
- **Cardiovascular "syndrome X"** represents the triad of anginal symptoms with exercise, ST-segment depression with exercise stress testing, and nonobstructive CAD on arteriography. It likely results from impaired, endothelial-dependent or microvascular dilatation, increased sympathetic response, or exercise-induced vasoconstriction.
- **Coronary artery inflammation** or **dissection**
- In **secondary angina**, chest pain arises from some other primary process that then results in an imbalance of oxygen supply and demand (see Chapter 7).

DIFFERENTIAL DIAGNOSIS

While it is essential to recognize that patients with the appropriate risk profile may have NSTEACS, other etiologies for chest pain should also be considered, as they may have significant diagnostic and therapeutic impact. Many conditions can cause patients to present with chest pain that is both typical and atypical for NSTEACS:

- Cardiovascular: acute pericarditis, myocarditis, cardiac tamponade, aortic dissection, aortic stenosis, hypertrophic obstructive cardiomyopathy, congestive heart failure exacerbation
- Pulmonary: pulmonary embolism, pneumothorax, pneumonia, asthma or obstructive lung disease exacerbation
- Gastrointestinal: esophageal spasm, esophagitis, reflux disease, peptic ulcer disease, gastritis, cholecystitis
- Psychiatric: anxiety disorders

PRESENTATION

Risk Factors

NSTEACS is a broad continuum of cardiac events with a diverse range of outcomes. Risk stratification allows patients to be triaged to more aggressive treatment modalities based on the likelihood for obstructive CAD and adverse outcomes. The **TIMI risk score** was developed as a method to differentiate patients based on simple criteria that are easily obtainable on arrival in the emergency department (ED). Using the data from the **ESSENCE** and **TIMI 11B** trials (see "Treatment," below), seven criteria were shown to be significant predictors of death, MI, or emergent revascularization (see Table 8-1).

Increasing risk score has been shown to correlate in a linear fashion with poor outcomes (Fig. 8-1). This score is an effective bedside tool to gauge prognosis at presentation with NSTEACS. Studies have shown that it may be a useful way to discriminate those patients who will benefit from an invasive strategy (see "Early Invasive Versus Conservative Therapy," below).

History

UA is a clinical diagnosis based predominantly on patient history and assisted by physical exam, electrocardiogram, and cardiac enzyme evaluation. Rapid identification of these

TABLE 8-1   CALCULATING TIMI RISK SCORE

Risk Factors

Age >65 years (1 point)

Known CAD (>50% stenosis) (1 point)

Severe anginal symptoms (>2 episodes of chest pain in last 24 hours) (1 point)

ST deviation on admission ECG (1 point)

Elevated serum cardiac markers (1 point)

Use of ASA in the 7 days before presentation (1 point)

≥3 risk factors for CAD

- Family history
- Diabetes
- Hypertension
- Dyslipidemia
- Current smoker

TIMI, thrombolysis in myocardial infarction; CAD, coronary artery disease; ECG, electrocardiogram; ASA, aspirin. (Adapted from Antman et al. *JAMA* 2000, with permission.)

Each positive risk factor is worth one point. Points are added together to determine the TIMI risk score (maximum 7).

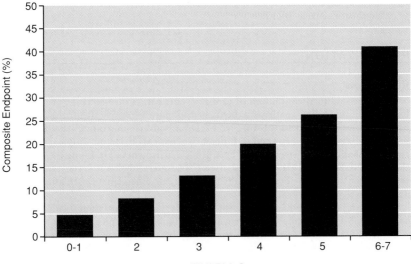

FIGURE 8-1. Fourteen-day rates of death, MI, or urgent revascularization from the TIMI 11B and ESSENCE trials based on increasing TIMI risk score. TIMI, Thrombolysis in Myocardial Infarction; MI, myocardial infarction. (Adapted from Antman et al. *JAMA* 2000, with permission.)

warning symptoms for an ACS allow for initiation of expedited "chest pain protocols" in the Emergency Department (ED).

- Chest pressure or heaviness radiating to the back, shoulders, arms, or jaw
- Indigestion
- "Heartburn," nausea and vomiting with epigastric chest discomfort
- Shortness of breath or dyspnea on exertion
- Weakness, dizziness, light-headedness, or loss of consciousness

Characteristics that can help differentiate UA from chronic stable angina include:

- Chest pain that occurs at rest
- Pain that awakens the patient from sleep
- Episodes lasting >20 minutes
- Pain that develops with less exertion than previously experienced
- Pain that severely limits normal physical activity (i.e., angina with level walking 1–2 blocks or a flight of stairs)

Physical Exam

The physical exam in patients with NSTEACS is rarely specific or sensitive. Often, there are no helpful physical findings. Abnormalities that can support the diagnosis include:

- Extra heart sounds (S3/S4)
- Elevated jugular venous pressure
- Pulmonary rales

MANAGEMENT

Diagnostic Workup and Laboratory Testing

Electrocardiogram
- Approximately 50% of patients with NSTEACS present with significant ECG abnormalities, including:
  - Transient ST-segment elevations and ST depressions as well as T wave inversions
  - ST-segment depression of as little as >0.05 mV (0.5 mm) in two contiguous leads has been shown to be a sensitive indicator of myocardial ischemia, especially when dynamic and associated with symptoms
  - Symmetric T wave inversions of >0.2 mV (2 mm) across the precordium are fairly specific for myocardial ischemia and are particularly worrisome for a critical lesion in the left anterior descending artery (LAD)
  - Less helpful are nonspecific ST-segment changes or T wave inversions (those that do not meet voltage criteria)
- Even in the setting of a normal ECG with chest pain, a least 4% of patients will have UA and up to 6% will go on to have develop NSTEMI

Cardiac Biomarkers
Cardiac markers of myocardial necrosis are of critical importance in the diagnosis of ACS. By definition, NSTEMI occurs when, usually in the setting of UA symptoms, a patient has significant increases in cardiac enzyme assays, confirming myocardial damage. The most common enzyme markers are **creatine kinase/creatine kinase isoenzymes, troponins, and myoglobin** (see Chapter 3).

Creatine kinase/CK-MB is present in both skeletal and myocardial muscle cells. It is no longer considered a sensitive or specific test for diagnosing ACS. However, the CK-MB isoenzyme continues to be an important tool in identifying patients with acute infarction. The isoenzyme is readily detectable in the blood of normal subjects at low levels, but elevated levels can occur with damage to skeletal and cardiac muscle. While it has lower specificity for myocardial necrosis than cardiac troponin, it rises much more quickly. An elevated level is usually present within 4 to 6 hours after injury, with a peak level attained in approximately 10 to18 hours. Serial measurements should be obtained on presentation and repeated in 8 to 12 hours.

- This assay is also very useful for assessing postinfarct ischemia, because a fall and subsequent rise suggests reinfarction.
- It is often checked serially after percutaneous coronary intervention (PCI), as small rises in CK-MB occur with postprocedural distal microembolization but large rises are associated with increased adverse events and cardiac mortality.
- In the acute setting, troponin does not fall rapidly enough for these assessments.

The troponin complex consists of three subunits (troponins C, T, and I), which are responsible for the calcium-mediated contraction of striated muscle. Cardiac troponin components (troponins T and I) present in the peripheral blood are **equally highly specific and sensitive markers of myocardial necrosis**. Serum troponin levels are usually undetectable in normal individuals; therefore any elevation is considered abnormal.

- Levels can usually be detected as early as 2 hours after myocardial damage.
- Peak levels occur 8 to 12 hours after the event and can remain elevated for 10 to 14 days.
- Like CK-MB, troponin levels should be checked serially, with the initial level obtained on arrival and a repeat level obtained in 8 to 12 hours.
- In addition to identifying patients with myocardial necrosis, troponin may be elevated:
  - After direct cardiac injury (e.g., tachyarrhythmias, defibrillator discharges, cardiac surgery or ablation, cardiac contusion, myopericarditis, acute/chronic heart failure exacerbations, and stress induced (Takotsubo cardiomyopathy).
  - Noncardiac conditions (i.e., brain injury, burns, chemotherapy and drug toxicity, sepsis, pulmonary embolism, severe asthma, and renal disease).
  - Elevated troponins have even been found in the circulation of healthy subjects after extreme endurance events.

Myoglobin is a heme-binding protein that is found in myocardium and skeletal muscle that is released into the bloodstream earlier than CK-MB or troponin.

- It can be detected in the serum as early as 2 hours after the event, which explains its appeal among ED clinicians.
- Its low specificity makes myoglobin an inadequate test for the diagnosis of myocardial damage in ACS.

Other biomarkers—such as **lactate dehydrogenase (LDH), alanine transaminase (ALT), and aspartame transaminase (AST)**—are nonspecific markers for NSTEACS and should not be used.

Numerous **inflammatory markers** have been proposed for supplemental use in both diagnosis and risk prediction of ACS and include cytokines, acute-phase reactants, endothelial cell activation and leukocyte adhesion markers, oxidative stress markers, angiogenic growth factors, and matrix metalloproteinases (MMPs). **B-type natriuretic peptide** (BNP), a cardiac myocyte neurohormone released with ventricular stretch, has been well studied among patients with heart failure and shows promise in predicting events in the ACS setting.

Diagnostic Testing: Early Invasive Versus Conservative Therapy
Since the mid-1990s, there has been debate over the usefulness of more aggressive evaluation and treatment of NSTEACS through more liberal use of invasive techniques. This has led to the development of two schemes for patient evaluation.

In the early conservative strategy, the patient is treated with medical therapy at maximally tolerated doses with a "cooling off" period followed by diagnostic testing (usually with stress testing with or without imaging). Coronary angiography is reserved for patients with evidence of recurrent ischemia or a strongly positive stress test despite medical therapy.

- **Low- and intermediate-risk patients** who are free of heart failure and ischemia at rest or during low-level activity for 12 to 24 hours can be further risk-stratified via noninvasive stress testing (class I).
- Ideally, patients should have negative troponins for 24 hours prior to stress testing.
- If a patient has a positive troponin and a noninvasive management plan is undertaken, a patient can have a submaximal or pharmacologic stress test 72 hours after the peak troponin assuming that there are no ongoing symptoms.
- Patients who develop ischemic changes at 6.5 metabolic equivalents (approximately 6 minutes) are considered at high risk and should be referred for cardiac catheterization and possible revascularization.
- If the patient is not able to exercise adequately to obtain the target heart rate due to comorbidities or physical incapacity, a pharmacologic stress test is appropriate (see Chapters 3 and 25).

In the early invasive strategy, patients are routinely recommended for coronary angiography and subsequent revascularization as warranted.

- In general, patients with rest angina, left ventricular dysfunction, or hemodynamic compromise despite maximal medical therapy should be referred for prompt angiography.
- Additionally, high-risk patients, including those with sustained ventricular tachycardia (VT) or prior coronary revascularization (PCI within 6 months or CABG), are best assessed with an early invasive approach.
- An early invasive strategy is also warranted in low- or intermediate-risk patients with repeated ACS presentations despite therapy.
- Coronary angiography is inappropriate for patients in whom percutaneous revascularization is not possible (either for comorbid illness or patient preference).
- Subgroup analyses of three major trials (FRISC II, TACTICS-TIMI 18, and RITA 3) reveal that the benefit of the early invasive strategy is primarily confined to high-risk patients, especially those with refractory angina, dynamic ST-segment changes, elevated cardiac enzymes, and diabetes.

Newer imaging modalities, like cardiac computed tomographic angiography (CCTA) and cardiac magnetic resonance imaging (CMR), are being used to risk-stratify low risk populations (see Chapter 26).

- **CCTA** may prove particularly useful in ruling out obstructive CAD in symptomatic patients who have a low pretest probability for disease, especially with negative ECG and cardiac markers. It is a rapid testing modality that offers good anatomic resolution with the drawback of radiation exposure, contrast dye exposure, poor visualization of small vessels, and need for a regularized heart rhythm.
- **CMR** offers cardiac functional assessment, perfusion imaging (adenosine or dobutamine), and myocardial viability information at the expense of long study times, potential patient claustrophobia, and problems with certain metallic implants (e.g., pacemakers/defibrillators).
- These modalities are still being evaluated and have not been studied in large trials of patients with NSTEACS.

Coronary angiography is useful in providing detailed diagnostic information in patients with symptoms of NSTEACS. Indications for catheterization (and an invasive strategy) include:

- Elevated cardiac biomarkers
- Recurrent symptoms despite medical therapy
- High-risk clinical findings, such as congestive heart failure (CHF), severe mitral regurgitation (MR), hemodynamic instability, and arrhythmias
- Positive results on noninvasive testing, with high-risk findings
- Reduced ejection fraction (<40%)
- New ST-segment depression
- High TIMI risk score
- Prior CABG or PCI within 6 months.

Typical findings of culprit lesions include (1) evidence of new thrombus formation in a location consistent with ECG or imaging studies, (2) eccentric stenoses with uneven edges, and (3) haziness in the area of a subcritical stenosis, indicating possible plaque rupture.

Women and nonwhites (see Chapter 28) are more likely not to have significant epicardial disease. However, it has also been noted that up to one-third of these patients will have evidence of impaired coronary blood flow (i.e., slow washout of dye injection). This may be a result of microvascular disease and warrants continued aggressive medical treatment.

- The ACC/AHA guidelines recommend that women receive similar care to men with NSTEACS. Elderly patients should receive similar care to younger patients with NSTEACS, with appropriate adjustment for medical comorbidities and observation for adverse events.

Treatment

The primary goals of pharmacotherapy in NSTEACS are to **limit clot formation** (by reducing platelet activation/aggregation and subsequent thrombus formation) and **control chest pain** with antianginal medications.

Antithrombotic Therapy (Fig. 8-2)

- **Aspirin** (ASA)
  - ASA (162 mg or 325-mg tablet) is an important initial pharmacotherapy in the management of NSTEACS.
  - Within a few minutes of ingestion, ASA can effectively block platelet aggregation, and should be administered **immediately** by emergency medical services (EMS) or on arrival to the ED.
  - The only **contraindications** to ASA therapy are a history of documented drug allergy and active bleeding. In this situation, consultation with an allergist for possible desensitization is recommended.
- **Adenosine 5′-diphosphate (ADP) antagonists (thienopyridines)**
  - **Clopidogrel** (Plavix) and its predecessor, **ticlopidine** (Ticlid) are selective antagonists of ADP-mediated platelet aggregation. Trials of these medications for secondary prevention of atherosclerotic vascular disease show that they are comparable to ASA in reducing the rates of recurrent MI, stroke, or death.
  - Clopidogrel (given as a loading dose of a bolus dose of 300 to 600 mg followed by 75 mg daily) is preferred to ticlopidine because the latter poses a significant risk of gastrointestinal complications and neutropenia and a small risk of thrombotic thrombocytopenic purpura (TTP).
  - The issue of CABG is of particular concern with regards to clopidogrel administration and timing. It is recommended that clopidogrel be withheld for at least 5 to 7 days if CABG is planned.
  - For patients who are managed noninvasively, clopidogrel should be continued for 1 month and ideally for 1 year.

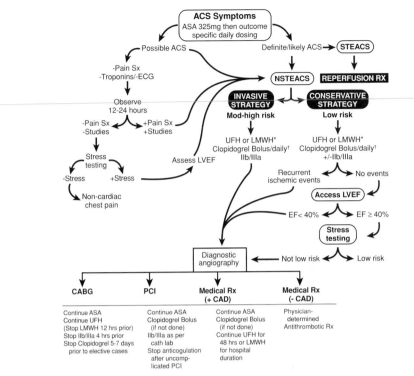

FIGURE 8-2. Strategies for use of antiplatelet/antithrombotic therapy.

*Bivalirudin and fondaparinux are appropriate alternatives to UFH and LMWH.
†Clopidogrel should be given when there is a reasonable certainty that the patient will not require CABG. Otherwise wait until after diagnostic angiography. ACS, acute coronary syndrome; STEACS, ST-elevation acute coronary syndrome; NSTEACS, non–ST-elevation acute coronary syndrome; Rx, treatment; Sx, symptoms; UFH, unfractionated heparin; LMWH, low-molecular-weight heparin; IIb/IIIa, glycoprotein IIb/IIIa inhibitor; LVEF, left ventricular ejection fraction; CAD, coronary artery disease; CABG, coronary artery bypass grafting; PCI, percutaneous coronary intervention. (Adapted from the ACC/AHA 2007 Guidelines for the Management of Patients With Unstable Angina/Non–ST-Elevation Myocardial Infarction.)

- **Heparin**
  - Unfractionated heparin (UFH) acts by binding antithrombin III (ATIII), which in turn inactivates thrombin (factor II), factor IXa, and factor Xa. No trials prove the benefit of heparin administered alone in NSTEACS; however, several trials have shown a trend toward mortality benefit from the combination of UFH with ASA.
  - Therapy should be initiated in all patients with intermediate- or high-risk factors (e.g., TIMI risk score ≥3), especially in the setting of continued chest pain on arrival. IV heparin should be given with a loading bolus of 60 U/kg (maximum 5000 U), then a continuous infusion of 14 U/kg (maximum 1000 U/hour), adjusted to maintain a PTT of 1.5 to 2 times normal (approximately 50–70 seconds).
  - Most studies have continued treatment for 2 to 5 days, and there is no evidence that longer treatment is beneficial.

- In cases of overdosage or refractory, life-threatening bleeding, protamine sulfate can be given (1 mg protamine sulfate IV for every 100 U of active heparin). Prior exposure to protamine-containing insulins, fish allergy, or history of vasectomy may promote adverse reactions via antiprotamine antibodies. Except in rare situations, protamine sulfate should be avoided in patients with NSTEACS.
- **Thrombocytopenia** with heparin therapy can present two ways:
  - **Type I heparin-induced thrombocytopenia** (HIT) is non-immune-mediated, is seen 2 to 3 days after the initiation of therapy, and has a platelet count nadir of approximately 100,000. It resolves with continued use without significant consequence and may be seen in 10% to 20% of patients.
  - **Type II HIT** is much more serious, but much less common (1%–3% of patients) and can occur 4 to 10 days after initiation of therapy or rarely as a delayed manifestation several days after withdrawal of UFH therapy. Patients with known history of type II HIT or active disease potentially with thrombotic complications should be switched to a direct thrombin inhibitor as soon as possible (see below).
- **Low-molecular-weight heparins (LMWHs)**
  - **LMWHs** are obtained by shortening the polysaccharide tail on the heparin molecule. **Advantages** over UFH include better bioavailability, subcutaneous dosing, predictable anticoagulant activity that does not require laboratory monitoring, less heparin-induced thrombocytopenia (approximately 0.2%), and lower overall cost. **Disadvantages** include a long half-life that can make emergent catheterization or PCI more complicated and an inability to effectively reverse its effects in the setting of refractory bleeding (protamine sulfate does not completely bind LMWH).
  - The superiority of LMWH to UFH has been established in several trials including the ESSENCE trial and the TIMI 11b trial (both with enoxaparin) as well as with the FRISC trials using dalteparin (Fragmin).
  - Enoxaparin (Lovenox) should be given at a dose of 1 mg/kg SC every 12 hours. Treatment should be continued through the initial hospitalization.
  - LMWHs require dose adjustment in patients with renal insufficiency, and they should be used with significant caution (and dose reduction by >50%) in patients with a serum creatinine >2 mg/dL or creatinine clearance <30 mL/minute.
- **Fondaparinux** (Arixtra) is a synthetic polysaccharide that contains the same pentasaccharide sequence found in UFH and LMWH. It selectively binds ATIII to predictably inhibit Factor Xa without inhibiting thrombin. Moreover, it lacks the sugar domain necessary to complex with PF4, making HIT unlikely with its use. Fondaparinux (as studied in NSTEACS) is administered 2.5 mg SC daily.
- **Direct thrombin inhibitors (DTI)**
  - Hirudin, lepirudin (recombinant hirudin), and bivalirudin (Angiomax) are examples of DTIs and act by directly binding to thrombin and inactivating it. These agents have been studied in multiple trials as an alternative to treatment with heparin in patients with UA/NSTEMI.
  - **Lepirudin** is delivered as an initial bolus of 0.4 mg/kg IV, followed by continuous infusion at a rate of 0.15 mg/kg per hour. As in the case of heparin, regular monitoring is required, with a goal PTT of 1.5 to 2.5 times normal. **Bivalirudin** is given as a 0.75 mg/kg IV bolus followed by a 1.75 mg/kg per hour IV infusion. It requires dosage adjustment in patients with creatinine clearance <30 mL/minute or those on hemodialysis.
  - The major risk of DTIs is bleeding, which is increased in patients with renal impairment.

- Bivalirudin has taken a dominant role in the management of both cardiac and cardiac surgery patients who have been or are at risk for developing HIT.
- **Glycoprotein IIb/IIIa inhibitors**
  - Glycoprotein IIb/IIIa (GP IIb/IIIa) platelet receptors bind fibrinogen and other ligands, representing the final common pathway for platelet aggregation. GP IIb/IIIa inhibitors work by blocking this receptor. GP IIb/IIIa inhibitors should be considered in the treatment of all high-risk patients with refractory NSTEACS, specifically those with significant ST-T changes or elevated cardiac enzymes.
  - There are three GP IIb/IIIa inhibitors currently available:
    - **Abciximab** (ReoPro) is a murine monoclonal antibody Fab fragment with nonspecific affinity for the human GP IIb/IIIa site. It has been studied predominantly in the setting of percutaneous interventions, where it has been shown to improve outcomes in patients with refractory UA undergoing coronary intervention. Based on the results of GUSTO IV-ACS, abciximab should not be used in patients in whom percutaneous intervention is not planned.
    - **Eptifibatide** (Integrilin) is a peptide sequence similar to one of the fibrinogen-binding sites for GP IIb/IIIa. Tirofiban (Aggrastat) is a nonpeptide mimetic for a similar sequence. Each acts as a competitive inhibitor at the receptor site, and both have been shown to reduce the risk of death or MI in patients with ACS undergoing both invasive and noninvasive treatment.
    - **Tirofiban** (Aggrastat) can be administered with a loading bolus of 0.4 μg/kg per minute over 30 minutes, followed by a maintenance infusion of 0.1 μg/kg per minute. Both doses should be decreased by 50% in patients with a creatinine clearance <30 mL/minute. **Eptifibatide** is given with a loading bolus of 180 μg/kg over 2 minutes, followed by an infusion at 2 μg/kg per minute. The duration of treatment in major studies has been 72 to 96 hours or at least 12 hours after any percutaneous intervention.
    - Eptifibatide and tirofiban are to be used with caution in renal failure and are contraindicated in end-stage renal disease. Abciximab may be used in these settings, as it is not cleared by the kidney. Thrombocytopenia, which can be severe at times, is an uncommon but well-described complication of all these agents and should prompt discontinuation of the drug.
- **Fibrinolytics (thrombolytics)**
  - Thrombolytic therapy has been extensively studied in patients presenting with ACS. The only patients who show a proven benefit from thrombolysis are those who present with persistent ST elevation, posterior MI, or a new left bundle-branch block. Fibrinolytic (thrombolytic) therapy is contraindicated in patients with NSTEACS.
- **Statins**
  - Hydroxymethylglutaryl coenzyme A (HMG-CoA) reductase inhibitors (statins) play a key role in the management of patients with CAD. Initial secondary prevention trials excluded patients with recent or acute MI (see Chapter 10). Several recent trials have demonstrated that statin therapy is useful in this patient population. It is of interest that the effects of statins on risk reduction during the peri-infarct period appears to be independent of the effect of lowering low density lipoprotein (LDL) cholesterol.

Antianginal Treatment

In addition to treatment aimed at preventing or reducing thrombosis, anti-ischemic therapy focuses on improving the balance of oxygen supply to oxygen demand. Antianginal medications mostly work by favorably adjusting this ratio to reduce ischemia and resolve chest pain. The "ABCDE" mnemonic discussed in Chapter 7 is useful here as well.

- Bed/chair rest
  - Patients with active ischemic symptoms should limit activity to bed rest to reduce myocardial oxygen demand. Activity can be increased depending on symptoms and should not be excessively prohibitive. Patients should undergo continuous ECG/telemetry monitoring during this initial phase of hospitalization.
- Oxygen
  - **Supplemental oxygen** is the first step in maintaining adequate myocardial oxygenation supply. Maintenance of a SaO_2 <90% for patients presenting with cyanosis or respiratory distress in the setting of NSTEACS is the goal.
- Nitrates
  - **Nitroglycerin** (NTG) acts as a vasodilator (via nitric oxide) on both the systemic and coronary circulation. By working predominantly as a venodilator, it reduces preload and thereby reduces oxygen demand. At the same time, NTG has an effect on the coronary arteries, leading to increased blood supply through the affected vessel as well as increased collateral flow.
  - NTG can be administered initially via sublingual tablets or spray.
    - Up to three 0.4-mg tablets can be administered 5 minutes apart, with the goal of relieving anginal symptoms.
    - If treatment is successful, the patient can be placed on a standing dose of oral or topical nitrates for the remainder of the observation ("rule out") period to prevent recurrent pain.
    - Dose these medications in such a way as to provide a 6 to 8 hour "nitro-free" period every 24 hours to prevent development of tolerance.
    - If chest pain is **refractory** to the initial treatment, initiate IV NTG at a dose of 10 μg/min; this can be rapidly titrated by 10-μg/min increments every 5 minutes until the patient is free of chest pain or hypotension prevents further increases in dose. There is no maximum dose, but 200 μg/minute should be considered high enough to warrant a change in therapy.
  - Nitrates are generally contraindicated if a patient has severe aortic stenosis, hypertrophic obstructive cardiomyopathy with significant left ventricular outflow tract obstruction, cardiac tamponade, or even restrictive cardiomyopathy, as these patients can be very preload-dependent.
  - Nitrates are contraindicated in patients who have used PDE5 inhibitors (e.g., within 24 hours of sildenafil [Viagra, Revatio] or 48 hours of tadalafil [Cialis]) because of the risk of severe hypotension with the combination. Appropriate timing for vardenafil (Levitra) dosing with nitrates is unknown and should be avoided.
- Beta blockers
  - Beta blockers have a proven benefit on mortality for patients having a myocardial infarction.
  - For patients with active chest pain, initial treatment should be with IV medication, such as **metoprolol** (Lopressor), 5 mg IV every 5 minutes for three doses or IV **esmolol** (Brevibloc) drip started at 0.1 mg/kg per minute. The goals of these measures are to try and reduce the heart rate to 50 to 60 bpm, maintaining a systolic blood pressure greater than 90 to 100 mm Hg. After the IV bolus or in patients without active chest pain, start PO metoprolol, 25 to 50 mg every 6 hours, or atenolol, 50 to 100 mg daily, immediately.
  - These drugs should be held in those patients with evidence of severe congestive heart failure.

- Morphine
  - While no clinical trials show any clinical benefit in the setting of NSTEACS, morphine sulfate is recommended for the relief of chest pain in these patients with NSTEACS due to its analgesic and anxiolytic properties, which reduce sympathetic drive. It is also thought to improve myocardial oxygen demand by reducing preload.
  - When needed, morphine can be dosed in 2 to 4-mg IV boluses with repeated doses as needed to relieve the pain.
  - Morphine causes nausea and vomiting in 20% of patients and also can lead to hypotension and respiratory depression. Naloxone (Narcan) 0.4 to 2 mg IV in 2 to 3 minute intervals (maximum 10 mg) can be given to acutely reverse its effects in the setting of overdosage.
- Calcium Channel Blockers
  - Calcium channel blockers can be used as a third-line agent in patients continuing to have chest pain in the setting of adequate beta blockade and nitrates. These medications have been shown to help with vasospastic angina and among patients in whom beta blockade is contraindicated. Otherwise, no data show significant morbidity or mortality benefit with the use of calcium channel blockers.
  - Short-acting dihydropyridines, such as nifedipine, are associated with an increased risk of death when used without beta blockade in the setting of NSTEACS and are thus contraindicated in this regard.
- Angiotensin converting enzyme (ACE) inhibitors and angiotensin receptor blockers (ARBs)
  - ACE inhibitors and to a lesser extent ARBs have been studied in the setting of acute MI but not in UA.
  - As a majority of the patients presenting with NSTEACS have multiple high-risk features, consider adding an ACE inhibitor to their medical regimens by discharge. ACE inhibitors should be used in patients with LV dysfunction (EF <40%), hypertension, or diabetes presenting with ACS. ARBs are appropriate in patients that are intolerant to ACE inhibitors.
- Other antianginals
  - Blood transfusion
    - Theoretically, increasing blood volume in patients that are anemic should improve oxygen-carrying capacity and improve myocardial oxygen supply. Many clinicians, either as a primary treatment or as a secondary response to bleeding associated with antithrombotic therapy, will transfuse patients with NSTEACS to a hemoglobin >10 mg/dL or hematocrit >30% based on limited data regarding benefit.
  - **Intra-aortic balloon counterpulsation (IABP)** may be useful in patients with refractory ischemic symptoms that persists despite maximal medical therapy or in high-risk patients who are hypotensive with NSTEACS. See Chapter 27 for a discussion of IABP therapy.

Agents to Avoid

- Nonsteroidal antiinflammatory agents
  - Both nonselective cyclooxygenase (COX) inhibitors and COX-2 inhibitors (except ASA) are associated with an increased risk of death, reinfarction, myocardial rupture, hypertension, and heart failure in large meta-analyses.
  - Acetaminophen, low-dose narcotics, and nonacetylated salicylates are acceptable alternatives for treating chronic musculoskeletal pain in patients with NSTEACS.
  - A nonselective COX inhibitor (i.e., naproxen) is reasonable if the above therapies are insufficient.

- Hormone replacement therapy (see Chapter 28)
- Supplements
  - Antioxidant vitamins (e.g., vitamins C, E, and beta-carotene) and folic acid with or without B vitamins have no role in the secondary prevention in patients with NSTEACS.
  - Reduction of homocysteine levels did not significantly impact CAD event rates in the NORVIT (Norwegian Vitamin Trial) or the HOPE-2 trials.

Discharge

After appropriate medical treatment, NSTEACS patients with noninvasive stress testing or coronary angiography/revascularization will be ready for discharge home. The timeline for these events can be as little as 24 hours to several days if CABG is indicated. Important issues to address as the patient is prepared for discharge include:

- Evaluation for aggressive risk-factor control
- Diabetes education and glucose control for diabetic patients
- Smoking cessation
- Improved blood pressure control
- Education on diet, exercise, and weight management
- Lipid-lowering therapy
- Continue patients on medical regimens that have shown benefit in reducing mortality in patients with CAD
  - ASA (81–325 mg/day)
  - Beta blockers
  - ACE inhibitors/ARBs
  - Statin therapy
- All patients with CAD should be discharged with either sublingual or spray versions of NTG for anginal symptom control.
- Refer appropriate patients for cardiac rehabilitation/secondary prevention programs to integrate these lifestyle changes with supervised exercise programs.
- Low-risk patients can be seen in follow-up in 2 to 6 weeks, while high-risk patients should be seen within 14 days after discharge.

SPECIAL TOPICS

Cocaine and Methamphetamine Myocardial Infarction

- An estimated 35 million Americans have used cocaine; it is the most commonly used illicit drug among patients seeking ED care.
- The pathogenesis of cocaine-induced angina is likely secondary to increased myocardial oxygen demand from (1) increased blood pressure, heart rate, and contractility; (2) marked vasoconstriction/vasospasm of epicardial vessels; (3) increased platelet aggregation; and (4) increased coronary thrombosis.
- The risk of infarction in patients otherwise at low risk for cardiac events is increased by a factor of 24 immediately after cocaine use.
- Patients who are at risk of cocaine-induced chest pain should undergo the same diagnostic considerations as other patients with symptoms of NSTEACS.
- However, in patients in whom cocaine-induced chest pain is suspected, the treatment algorithm is modified:
  - All patients should still receive ASA as discussed earlier, owing to increased risk of platelet aggregation.

- Sublingual or intravenous nitrates should also be given, especially in those with ST-segment changes.
- Beta blockers are relatively contraindicated in these patients, as they can lead to unopposed alpha-mediated vasoconstriction and worsening myocardial ischemia (one exception is labetalol, which has both beta- and alpha-blocking properties).
- Calcium channel blockers, such as intravenous diltiazem, can also be used to reduce myocardial oxygen demand, especially in the presence of ST-segment changes.
- Benzodiazepines can be used in this syndrome as an anxiolytic and to reduce ischemia.
- Fibrinolytic therapy can be used in patients presenting with persistent ST-elevation despite NTG and CCB therapy who are not candidates for angiography and have no contraindications. However, immediate angiography is the preferred modality to evaluate these patients, as there are usually comorbid features that preclude use of thrombolytics (e.g., seizures, dissection, and severe hypertension). Patients may often have documented vasospasm on catheterization, but some have luminal thrombosis or plaque rupture, requiring PCI. Given the high risk of stent closure combined with the thrombogenicity of cocaine use and potential for variable antiplatelet drug compliance, bare metal stenting is preferred.

Methamphetamine use is on the rise as are complications associated with its abuse. The incidence of NSTEACS after methamphetamines is unclear, but the pathophysiology is likely similar to that of cocaine abuse. Patients with methamphetamine-induced NSTEACS should therefore be treated as in the case of NSTEACS secondary to cocaine, as data are limited for more specific therapies. Patient education and chemical dependency counseling are important to prevent recurrent events.

KEY POINTS TO REMEMBER

- UA and NSTEMI are treated similarly because they are driven by the same underlying pathophysiology. Together they are known as NSTEACS.
- All patients should receive bed rest, oxygen, ASA, beta blockers, and nitrates for angina suppression **early** in the presentation.
- High-risk patients with NSTEACS (with elevated TIMI risk scores) benefit from a routine, early invasive strategy, including UFH or LMWH, an IV glycoprotein IIb/IIIa inhibitor, clopidogrel, and coronary angiography with revascularization. Carefully tailor therapy plans to individual patients.
- Low-risk patients with NSTEACS can be safely managed with a conservative/selectively invasive strategy where they are medically managed and risk stratified via stress testing prior to discharge.
- The role of LMWH over UFH in NSTEACS is yet to be completely defined, although data are mounting in favor of the former. Bivalirudin and fondaparinux are acceptable alternatives, though evidence for their use is more limited.
- Patients who are unlikely to require CABG within five days of presentation should receive a bolus dose of clopidogrel and daily dosing thereafter. If this issue is unclear, then the bolus dose can be delayed until after angiography.
- Do not forget the importance of secondary prevention. Urge patients to quit smoking, improve their diets, control their diabetes and hypertension, enroll in cardiac rehabilitation, and take a statin (see Chapter 10).

REFERENCES AND SUGGESTED READINGS

Anderson JL, Adams CD, Antman EM, et al. ACC/AHA 2007 guidelines for the management of patients with unstable angina/non–ST-elevation myocardial infarction: a report of the American College of Cardiology/American Heart Association Task Force on Practice Guidelines. *JACC* 2007;50:e1–e157. Available at: http://acc.org/qualityandscience/clinical/statements.htm.

Anderson JL, Adams CD, Antman EM, et al. ACC/AHA 2007 guidelines for the management of patients with unstable angina/non–ST-elevation myocardial infarction: a report of the American College of Cardiology/American Heart Association Task Force on Practice Guidelines (Writing Committee to Revise the 2002 Guidelines for the Management of Patients With Unstable Angina/Non–ST-Elevation Myocardial Infarction) developed in collaboration with the American College of Emergency Physicians, the Society for Cardiovascular Angiography and Interventions, and the Society of Thoracic Surgeons endorsed by the American Association of Cardiovascular and Pulmonary Rehabilitation and the Society for Academic Emergency Medicine. *J Am Coll Cardiol* 2007;50:e1–e157.

Antman EM, Cohen M, Bernink PJ, et al. The TIMI risk score for unstable angina/non–ST-elevation MI: A method for prognostication and therapeutic decision making. *JAMA* 2000;284:835–842.

Antman EM, McCabe CH, Gurfinkel EP, et al. Enoxaparin prevents death and cardiac ischemic events in unstable angina/non–Q-wave myocardial infarction. Results of the thrombolysis in myocardial infarction (TIMI) 11B trial. *Circulation* 1999;100:1593–1601.

Boden WE, O'Rourke RA, Crawford MH, et al. Outcomes in patients with acute non–Q-wave myocardial infarction randomly assigned to an invasive as compared with a conservative management strategy. Veterans Affairs Non–Q-Wave Infarction Strategies in Hospital (VANQWISH) Trial Investigators. *N Engl J Med* 1998;338:1785–1792.

Cannon CP, Weintraub WS, Demopoulos LA, et al. Comparison of early invasive and conservative strategies in patients with unstable coronary syndromes treated with the glycoprotein IIb/IIIa inhibitor tirofiban. *N Engl J Med* 2001;344:1879–1887.

Cohen M, Demers C, Gurfinkel EP, et al. A comparison of low-molecular-weight heparin with unfractionated heparin for unstable coronary artery disease. Efficacy and Safety of Subcutaneous Enoxaparin in Non–Q-Wave Coronary Events Study Group. *N Engl J Med* 1997;337:447–452.

Effects of tissue plasminogen activator and a comparison of early invasive and conservative strategies in unstable angina and non–Q-wave myocardial infarction. Results of the TIMI IIIB Trial. Thrombolysis in Myocardial Ischemia. *Circulation* 1994;89:1545–1556.

Fox KA, Poole-Wilson P, Clayton TC, et al. 5-year outcome of an interventional strategy in non–ST-elevation acute coronary syndrome: the British Heart Foundation RITA 3 randomised trial. *Lancet* 2005;366:914–920.

FRISC II Investigators. Invasive compared with non-invasive treatment in unstable coronary-artery disease: FRISC II prospective randomised multicentre study. Fragmin and Fast Revascularisation during In Stability in Coronary artery disease Investigators. *Lancet* 1999;354:708–715.

Gislason GH, Jacobsen S, Rasmussen JN, et al. Risk of death or reinfarction associated with the use of selective cyclooxygenase-2 inhibitors and nonselective nonsteroidal antiinflammatory drugs after acute myocardial infarction. *Circulation* 2006;113:2906–2913.

Giugliano RP, Braunwald E. The year in non–ST-segment elevation acute coronary syndromes. *J Am Coll Cardiol* 2006;48:386–395.

Kereiakes DJ, Antman EM. Clinical guidelines and practice: in search of the truth. *J Am Coll Cardiol* 2006;48:1129–1135; discussion 1136–1138.

Kleiman NS, Lincoff AM, Flaker GC, et al. Early percutaneous coronary intervention, platelet inhibition with eptifibatide, and clinical outcomes in patients with acute coronary syndromes. PURSUIT Investigators. *Circulation* 2000;101: 751–757.

Lagerqvist B, Husted S, Kontny F, et al. 5-year outcomes in the FRISC-II randomised trial of an invasive versus a non-invasive strategy in non–ST-elevation acute coronary syndrome: a follow-up study. *Lancet* 2006;368:998–1004.

Lange RA, Hillis LD. Cardiovascular complications of cocaine use. *N Engl J Med* 2001;345:351–358.

Lefkovits J, Blankenship JC, Anderson KM, et al. Increased risk of non–Q-wave myocardial infarction after directional atherectomy is platelet dependent: evidence from the EPIC trial. Evaluation of c7E3 for the Prevention of Ischemic Complications. *J Am Coll Cardiol* 1996;28:849–855.

Lefkovits J, Ivanhoe RJ, Califf RM, et al. Effects of platelet glycoprotein IIb/IIIa receptor blockade by a chimeric monoclonal antibody (abciximab) on acute and six-month outcomes after percutaneous transluminal coronary angioplasty for acute myocardial infarction. EPIC investigators. *Am J Cardiol* 1996;77:1045–1051.

Majure DT, Aberegg SK. Fondaparinux versus enoxaparin in acute coronary syndromes. *N Engl J Med* 2006;354:2829; author reply 2830.

Mehta SR, Yusuf S, Peters RJ, et al. Effects of pretreatment with clopidogrel and aspirin followed by long-term therapy in patients undergoing percutaneous coronary intervention: the PCI-CURE study. *Lancet* 2001;358:527–533.

Morrow DA, Antman EM, Tanasijevic M, et al. Cardiac troponin I for stratification of early outcomes and the efficacy of enoxaparin in unstable angina: a TIMI-11B substudy. *J Am Coll Cardiol* 2000;36:1812–1817.

Oler A, Whooley MA, Oler J, Grady D. Adding heparin to aspirin reduces the incidence of myocardial infarction and death in patients with unstable angina. A meta-analysis. *JAMA* 1996;276:811–815.

Patti G, Pasceri V, Colonna G, et al. Atorvastatin pretreatment improves outcomes in patients with acute coronary syndromes undergoing early percutaneous coronary intervention: results of the ARMYDA-ACS randomized trial. *J Am Coll Cardiol* 2007;49:1272–1278.

Platelet glycoprotein IIb/IIIa receptor blockade and low-dose heparin during percutaneous coronary revascularization. The EPILOG Investigators. *N Engl J Med* 1997;336: 1689–1696.

Pursuit Trial Investigators. Inhibition of platelet glycoprotein IIb/IIIa with eptifibatide in patients with acute coronary syndromes. Platelet Glycoprotein IIb/IIIa in Unstable Angina: Receptor Suppression Using Integrilin Therapy. *N Engl J Med* 1998;339: 436–443.

Schwartz GG, Olsson AG, Ezekowitz MD, et al. Effects of atorvastatin on early recurrent ischemic events in acute coronary syndromes: the MIRACL study: a randomized controlled trial. *JAMA* 2001;285:1711–1718.

Steinhubl SR, Berger PB, Brennan DM, et al. Optimal timing for the initiation of pretreatment with 300 mg clopidogrel before percutaneous coronary intervention. *J Am Coll Cardiol* 2006;47:939–943.

Steinhubl SR, Berger PB, Mann JT III, et al. Early and sustained dual oral antiplatelet therapy following percutaneous coronary intervention: a randomized controlled trial. *JAMA* 2002;288:2411–2420.

Stone GW, McLaurin BT, Cox DA, et al. Bivalirudin for patients with acute coronary syndromes. *N Engl J Med* 2006;355:2203–2216.

Stone PH, Thompson B, Anderson HV, et al. Influence of race, sex, and age on management of unstable angina and non–Q-wave myocardial infarction: The TIMI III registry. *JAMA* 1996;275:1104–1112.

Thom T, Haase N, Rosamond W, et al. Heart disease and stroke statistics—2006 update: a report from the American Heart Association Statistics Committee and Stroke Statistics Subcommittee. *Circulation* 2006;113:e85–e151.

Thygensen K, Alpert JS, White HD, et al. Universal definition of myocardial infarction. *Circulation* 2007;116:2634–2653.

Topol EJ, Moliterno DJ, Herrmann HC, et al. Comparison of two platelet glycoprotein IIb/IIIa inhibitors, tirofiban and abciximab, for the prevention of ischemic events with percutaneous coronary revascularization. *N Engl J Med* 2001;344:1888–1894.

Use of a monoclonal antibody directed against the platelet glycoprotein IIb/IIIa receptor in high-risk coronary angioplasty. The EPIC Investigation. *N Engl J Med* 1994; 330(14):956–961.

Virmani R, Burke AP, Farb A, et al. Pathology of the vulnerable plaque. *J Am Coll Cardiol* 2006;47:C13–C18.

Wu WC, Rathore SS, Wang Y, et al. Blood transfusion in elderly patients with acute myocardial infarction. *N Engl J Med* 2001;345:1230–1236.

Yeghiazarians Y, Braunstein JB, Askari A, et al. Unstable angina pectoris. *N Engl J Med* 2000;342:101–114.

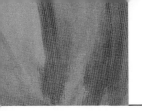

ST-Segment Elevation Myocardial Infarction

9

Peter Rao

INTRODUCTION

Background

ST-segment-elevation myocardial infarction (STEMI) is a clinical entity that merits its own discussion. Compared with unstable angina/non–ST-segment-elevation myocardial infarction (UA/NSTEMI), STEMI is associated with a higher in-hospital and long-term morbidity and mortality. In distinction from UA/NSTEMI (see Chapter 8), the therapeutic paradigm for STEMI mandates a rapid decision regarding reperfusion. This paradigm involves a highly coordinated mobilization of healthcare resources. The success of these efforts, also known as "door-to-balloon" or "door-to-needle" time, has become a major benchmark for the institutional quality of cardiovascular care.

Definition

STEMI, as its name implies, is a form of myocardial infarction. Myocardial infarction has both pathologic and clinical definitions. The pathologic perspective defines myocardial infarction as myocyte cell death, usually due to prolonged myocardial ischemia. A more commonly used clinical definition of myocardial infarction has been established by both the World Health Organization and the American Heart Association/European Society of Cardiology/American College of Cardiology (AHA/ESC/ACC). It requires at least two of the following: **characteristic symptoms, elevation in cardiac biomarkers, or characteristic electrocardiographic (ECG) changes.**

Etiology

Any condition or event that results in interruption of coronary flow sufficient to cause myocardial cell death can lead to STEMI. This usually results from an acute change in a preexisting coronary plaque that leads to activation of thrombotic mediators and subsequent clot formation with obstruction to blood flow. Other conditions that can lead to STEMI include severe coronary vasospasm and embolization. These conditions should be considered in the patient whose clinical findings suggest a process other than acute plaque change (see below, "Differential Diagnosis").

Epidemiology

Despite decades of intensive research and clinical trials, there are still an estimated 500,000 STEMIs annually in the United States. A significant proportion of these patients will die from sudden cardiac death due to ventricular arrhythmia prior to arriving at the hospital. The success of the medical community's concerted effort has led to an impressive 26% reduction in mortality since 1990. Overall survival rates across the majority of U.S. centers is >90%. However, the death rate remains grim among the subgroup of patients who develop cardiogenic shock or other mechanical complications of STEMI, with a mortality approaching 90%. In the United States, there appears to be a falling incidence in STEMI, with a shift towards NSTEMI and UA. This shift is opposed by an increasing incidence of STEMI worldwide, particularly in developing countries.

Classification

The term "acute MI" (AMI) is often used interchangeably with STEMI. The designation of AMI or STEMI includes not only classic ST elevation but also new or presumably new left bundle-branch block (LBBB). The descriptors "Q wave" and "non-Q wave MI," older classifications of AMI, have lost favor, as the majority of STEMI are Q-wave MI.

Pathophysiology

STEMI is most commonly due to coronary artery occlusion by thrombus. The thrombus usually forms in situ at the site of an atheromatous plaque. The mechanisms involved vary by age and gender. In men and older women, the majority of events are due to plaque rupture. In younger women, a more common mechanism is plaque erosion. The setting for this event is believed to involve mild to moderate immature plaques (i.e., those that do not significantly impede coronary flow at baseline) with thin fibrous caps and lipid-rich cores that rupture in the acute setting of inflammation, shear forces, and local rheologic factors. This initiates a sequence of platelet aggregation, fibrin deposition, and vasoconstriction that **completely occludes** the involved artery, predisposing to **transmural MI.** Thus the thrombus formed *in situ* in STEMI is classically the **fibrin-rich red thrombus.** This is why these patients respond to thrombolytics. According to the "open artery theory," rapidly re-establishing blood flow through this occluded artery can limit infarction size and improve survival.

Natural History

Left untreated, the mortality rate of uncomplicated STEMI can exceed 30%. As was seen in the era before thrombolytic and percutaneous catheter–based revascularization, mechanical complications are more common when STEMI is untreated. In addition to the risk of mechanical complications following myocyte cell death, the heart undergoes the detrimental process of remodeling.

PRESENTATION

Patients presenting with a suspected acute coronary syndrome (ACS) should undergo rapid evaluation. A focused history, physical, and ECG interpretation should be performed within 10 minutes of arrival in the emergency department. Each delay of 30 minutes increases the relative risk of 1-year mortality by 8%.

History

The history should be targeted and performed quickly. The goal is to acquire adequate historical information in the setting of diagnostic ECG changes to initiate treatment and mobilize, when appropriate, the team for percutaneous revascularization. Additional details are acquired in parallel with ongoing treatment. Although traditional risk factors such as diabetes, hypertension, hyperlipidemia, tobacco use, and family history of early MI should be reviewed, they are weak predictors of the likelihood of acute infarction as the presenting etiology.

- **Determine the onset of symptoms.** This is important in deciding the appropriate means of reperfusion (see below).
- **Determine the nature of pain.** Chest discomfort, the most common presenting symptom, is typically progressive, substernal to left-sided, and often similar in quality

to typical angina. It is usually intense and prolonged, lasting more than 20 to 30 minutes. Unlike UA/NSTEMI, rest and nitroglycerin usually do not provide significant relief. The discomfort may radiate to the left or right arm, shoulders, neck, jaw, back, and epigastrium.

- **Elicit associated symptoms.** Associated symptoms may include dyspnea, palpitations, diaphoresis, nausea, vomiting, and lightheadedness.
- **Be aware of atypical presentations.** Keep in mind that some patients, particularly women, the elderly, diabetics, and post-operative patients may present with discomfort in a location other than the chest or with an associated symptom without any pain. Acute mental status change may also be the only manifestation.
- **Seek a prior history of CAD or other cardiovascular disease and similarity of previous CAD symptoms to the current presentation.** If the patient has a history of previous cardiac catheterization or revascularization, directing support staff to obtain these records can provide valuable information, particularly in the setting of previous coronary artery bypass in whom urgent percutaneous coronary intervention (PCI) is planned. Obtaining this information, while useful, should not in any way delay definitive therapy.
- **Review absolute and relative contraindications to thrombolytic therapy** if the patient is in a center that provides thrombolytic therapy as a primary treatment option (Table 9-1).
- **Review issues regarding primary PCI.** These include allergy to contrast agents, issues relating to vascular access (peripheral vessel disease or previous peripheral revascularization procedures), previous cardiac catheterizations and complications, history of renal dysfunction, central nervous system disease, pregnancy or bleeding diathesis.
- **Inquire about a history of recent cocaine use, if suspected.** In this setting, a more aggressive approach to medical therapy with nitroglycerin, coronary vasodilators and benzodiazepines should begin prior to initiating reperfusion (see Chapter 8).

Physical Exam

The physical exam, while not contributing significantly to the diagnosis of STEMI, is important in determining other potential sources of chest pain, assessing prognosis, and establishing a baseline that will aid in the early recognition of complications. The goal of a directed physical exam is to determine hemodynamic stability, the presence of cardiogenic pulmonary edema or mechanical complications of MI [papillary muscle dysfunction, free-wall rupture, and ventricular septal defect (VSD)], and exclude other etiologies of acute chest discomfort. As such, the physical exam should include assessment of vital signs and oxygenation with bilateral blood pressures as well as jugular venous pressure; pulmonary exam for pulmonary edema; cardiac exam for arrhythmia, murmurs, gallops friction rub; vascular exam for evidence of peripheral vascular disease and pulse deficits; and neurologic exam (especially prior to administration of thrombolytics).

Differential Diagnosis

The inherent risk of both thrombolytic therapy and primary PCI mandate that alternative diagnoses be considered in patients with chest pain. In particular, administration of thrombolytic agents in certain conditions, such as aortic dissection, may lead to death. In the situation when the diagnosis is uncertain, primary PCI offers a distinct advantage as the initial reperfusion strategy.

Several conditions can mimic the chest pain of acute MI as well as the changes seen on ECG, as shown in the following tables. A brief discussion of a few of these conditions is included.

TABLE 9-1	CONTRAINDICATIONS TO THROMBOLYTIC THERAPY*

Absolute contraindications

    Any prior ICH

    Known structural cerebral vascular lesion (e.g., arteriovenous malformation)

    Known malignant intracranial neoplasm (primary or metastatic)

    Ischemic stroke within 3 months EXCEPT acute ischemic stroke within 3 hours

    Suspected aortic dissection

    Active bleeding or bleeding diathesis (excluding menses)

    Significant closed-head or facial trauma within 3 months

Relative contraindications

    History of chronic, severe, poorly controlled hypertension

    Severe uncontrolled hypertension on presentation (SBP >180 mm Hg or DBP >110 mm Hg)[†]

    History of prior ischemic stroke >3 months, dementia, or known intracranial pathology not covered in contraindications

    Traumatic or prolonged (>10 minutes) CPR or major surgery (<3 weeks)

    Recent (within 2–4 weeks) internal bleeding

    Noncompressible vascular punctures

    For streptokinase/anistreplase: prior exposure (more than 5 days ago) or prior allergic reaction to these agents

    Pregnancy

    Active peptic ulcer

    Current use of anticoagulants: the higher the INR, the higher the risk of bleeding

---

ICH, intracranial hemorrhage; SBP, systolic blood pressure; DBF, diastolic blood pressure; CPR, cardiopulmonary resuscitation; INR, international normalized ratio; MI, myocardial infarction.

*Viewed as advisory for clinical decision making and may not be all-inclusive or definitive.

[†]Could be an absolute contraindication in low-risk patients with MI.

Source: From Antman EM et al. ACC/AHA guidelines for the management of patients with ST-elevation myocardial infarction: a report of the American College of Cardiology/American Heart Association Task Force on Practice Guidelines (Committee to Revise the 1999 Guidelines for the Management of Patients with Acute Myocardial Infarction), 2004; available at www.acc.org.

Differential Diagnosis of Chest Pain

- Life-threatening
  - Aortic dissection
  - Pulmonary embolus
  - Perforating ulcer
  - Tension pneumothorax
  - Boerhaave's syndrome (esophageal rupture with mediastinitis)
- Other cardiac and noncardiac causes
  - Pericarditis

- Myocarditis
- Vasospastic angina
- Gastroesophageal reflux disease (GERD)
- Esophageal spasm
- Costochondritis
- Pleurisy
- Peptic ulcer disease
- Panic attack
- Biliary or pancreatic pain
- Cervical disc or neuropathic pain
- Somatization and psychogenic pain disorder

Differential Diagnosis of ST Elevation on ECG

- Pericarditis
- Pulmonary embolism
- Aortic dissection with coronary artery involvement
- Normal male pattern or normal variant
- Early repolarization
- Left ventricular (LV) hypertrophy with strain
- Brugada syndrome
- Myocarditis
- Hyperkalemia
- Bundle-branch block
- Prinzmetal angina
- Hypertrophic cardiomyopathy
- Aortic dissection

The pain of **acute aortic dissection** is typically a tearing, severe pain that radiates into the back. This condition should be suspected in patients with this type of pain and additional supportive findings on physical exam (bilateral brachial systolic blood pressure differential >20 mm Hg, pulse deficits, aortic regurgitation murmur) and chest x-ray examination (widened mediastinum, calcium sign, pleural effusion, or deviation of the trachea or left mainstem bronchus). The diagnosis should be confirmed with transesophageal echocardiocraphy (TEE), chest computed tomography (CT) or magnetic resonance imaging (MRI), or aortography. Dissections involving the ascending aorta may involve the coronary ostia [particularly the right coronary artery (RCA)], producing an infarction in the compromised territory.

Chest pain associated with **acute pericarditis** (see Chapter 13) is typically worse with recumbency and relieved by sitting upright and leaning forward. The ECG shows diffuse ST-segment elevation, also with PR segment depression and peaked T waves. When the diagnosis is unclear, an urgent echocardiogram can be helpful in differentiating AMI from pericarditis. This is not for assessment of pericardial effusion but for focal wall motion abnormalities accompanying an AMI.

Pulmonary embolism (PE) is very difficult to differentiate from AMI by history and physical exam alone. The onset of chest pain usually involves shortness of breath. A history of conditions that predispose to PE—such as recent surgery, immobilization, malignancy, and hypercoagulable states—may further suggest this diagnosis. Diagnostic evaluation may include V̇/Q̇ nuclear scanning, PE protocol CT, or pulmonary arteriogram.

Risk Stratification
Risk stratification for prognosis should be performed throughout the clinical course of STEMI. Multiple proven risk-assessment tools utilize information obtained during the

TABLE 9-2	KILLIP CLASSIFICATION IN ACUTE MI	
Class	Definition	Mortality (%)
I	No congestive heart failure signs	6
II	+ S^3 and/or basilar rales	17
III	Pulmonary edema	30–40
IV	Cardiogenic shock	60–80

Source: From Killip T III, Kimball JT. Treatment of myocardial infarction in a coronary care unit. A two-year experience with 250 patients. *Am J Cardiol* 1967;20:457, with permission.

history and physical exam as well as the diagnostic evaluation. Examples of risk assessment, which assess 30-day mortality following AMI, include the Killip classification system, the Forrester classification, and the TIMI risk score. The **Killip classification** relies on bedside physical exam findings including an S_3 gallop, pulmonary congestion, and cardiogenic shock (Table 9-2). The **Forrester classification** relies on hemodynamic monitoring of cardiac index and pulmonary capillary wedge pressure (PCWP) (Table 9-3). The **TIMI risk score** (Table 9-4), the most recent prognostic system, combines history and exam findings in patients with STEMI treated with thrombolytics. This is a different risk score than that used for risk stratification in the setting of ACS.

DIAGNOSTIC TESTING

Electrocardiogram (See Chapters 2 and 18)

The ECG, central to the diagnosis of STEMI, should be performed and interpreted within 10 minutes of presentation. If there is clinical suspicion for AMI but the ECG is nondiagnostic, it should be repeated every 20 to 30 minutes for up to 4 hours if the patient has persistent symptoms. Hyperacute T waves, seen as either tall or deeply inverted T waves, may be an early sign of AMI that warrants close monitoring. Recognition of the limitations of the electrocardiogram in AMI is also important as up to 10% of patients with an acute STEMI may have a normal ECG and certain myocardial segments of the left ventricle are not adequately represented, particularly the posterior, lateral, and apical walls.

TABLE 9-3	FORRESTER CLASSIFICATION SYSTEM FOR ACUTE MI		
Class	Cardiac Index (L/min/m²)	PCWP (mm Hg)	Mortality (%)
I	>2.2	<18	3
II	>2.2	>18	9
III	<2.2	<18	23
IV	<2.2	>18	51

Source: From Forrester JS, Diamond G, Chatterjee K, et al. Medical therapy of acute myocardial infarction by application of hemodynamic subsets (first of two parts). *N Engl J Med* 1976;295:1356, with permission.

TABLE 9-4　TIMI RISK SCORE FOR ST-ELEVATION MI

Risk Factor (weight)	Risk Score/30-day Mortality (%)
Age 65–74 years (2 points)	0 (0.8)
Age ≥75 years (3 points)	1 (1.6)
Diabetes mellitus/HTN or angina (1 point)	2 (2.2)
Systolic BP <100 (3 points)	3 (4.4)
Heart rate >100 (2 points)	4 (7.3)
Killip classification II–IV (2 points)	5 (12.4)
Weight <67 kg (1 point)	6 (16.1)
Anterior STE or LBBB (1 point)	7 (23.4)
Time to Rx >4 hours (1 point)	8 (26.8)
Risk score = total points (0–14)	>8 (35.9)

LBBB, left bundle-branch block; STE, ST-segment elevation.

Source: From Morrow DA, Antman EM, Charlesworth A, et al. TIMI risk score for ST-elevation myocardial infarction: a convenient, bedside, clinical score for risk assessment at presentation. *Circulation* 2000;102:2031–2037, with permission.

ECG criteria for diagnosis of STEMI is ≥1 mm (0.1 mV) of ST-segment elevation in two or more contiguous leads. The ECG location (Table 9-5) and degree of ST-segment elevation determines the occluded anatomy and prognosis and can alert the physician to potential complications of MI. Reciprocal changes of ST depressions may be seen in the appropriate leads as well.

Elevated ST segments resulting from occlusion of a coronary artery usually evolve to Q waves over 6 to 12 hours in the absence of spontaneous, medical, or mechanical reperfusion. This manifests as a transmural infarct, with loss of loss of R-wave voltage, as the replacement of cardiac muscle with inflammatory and ultimately scar tissue ensues. It is incorrect to assume that the presence of Q waves implies infarcted myocardium that will not benefit from revascularization, as Q waves can occur early in the presentation of STEMI due to conduction delay in a large area of myocardium.

TABLE 9-5　ANATOMIC DISTRIBUTION BASED ON ECG LEADS

Leads	Myocardium	Coronary Artery
I, aVL	High lateral wall	Diagonal or proximal LCx
V5 to V6	Lateral wall	LCx
V1 to V2	Septal	Proximal LAD
V2 to V4	Anterior wall	LAD
II,III, aVF	Inferior	RCA or LCX

LCx, left circumflex; LAD, left anterior descending; RCA, right coronary artery.

Special Considerations (See Chapter 18)

The presence of a **new left bundle-branch block (LBBB)** in the setting of acute chest symptoms suggests occlusion of the proximal LAD. Patients presenting with this finding should be managed in the same manner as the patient with a classic STEMI. In the setting of **an old LBBB or an RV paced rhythm**, an acute injury pattern may be supported by the following criteria:

- ST-segment elevation ≥ 1 mm in the presence of a positive QRS complex (ST elevation is concordant with QRS)
- ST-segment depression ≥ 1 mm in lead V_1, V_2, or V_3
- ST-segment elevation ≥ 5 mm in the presence of a negative QRS complex (ST elevation is discordant with QRS)

Posterior MI, typically associated with an inferior and/or lateral wall infarct, may be suspected by ST depression in leads V1 to V3. The "reverse-mirror test" is useful to demonstrate this: the ST-segment depression is actually ST elevation of the posterior wall. The prominent R waves in these leads represent posterior Q waves. ST elevation in the inferior leads (II, III, and aVF) and/or the lateral leads (V5 toV6) often accompanies these changes. Typically, inferoposterior and posterolateral MIs involve the right coronary artery (RCA) or obtuse marginal branch of the left coronary artery (LCx), respectively. These changes help distinguish ST depressions in V1 to V3 from the true ST depressions of anteroseptal ischemia, which is treated as an ACS. Posterior leads (V7 to V9) should be placed to help distinguish posterior MI from anterior ischemia or reciprocal depression in all patients presenting with ST depression in leads V1 to V3. Isolated posterior MI is uncommon.

ST elevation in the inferior leads should always prompt a right-sided ECG to assess for **right ventricular (RV) infarction**. ST elevation in leads V3R and V4R suggest right ventricular (RV) involvement. RV infarction should also be suspected on a standard 12-lead ECG when there is ST-segment elevation in V1 along with changes indicating inferior MI. Proximal RCA lesions typically involve the RV, as RV marginal branches arise early from the RCA. Although the principle of revascularization of the RV infarct is the same for other STEMIs, other aspects of treatment are unique, including cautious use of nitrate and beta-blocker therapy.

It is critical to remember the difference between the acute injury pattern of STEMI and ST elevation in **pericarditis**. ST segments normalize before there is T-wave inversion in acute pericarditis, whereas the T waves invert before ST normalization in STEMI. ST-segment elevation in pericarditis is typically diffuse and does not correlate to a particular vascular territory. PR-segment depression in acute pericarditis may also differentiate these two conditions. Pericarditis may, however, complicate AMI.

Cardiac Enzymes

Cardiac enzymes have no role in the initial decision-making process and lead to unnecessary delays in delivering therapy. Initial cardiac enzymes may be normal, depending upon the time in relation to onset of symptoms. Markers used for determining the presence of myocardial necrosis—including CK-MB, troponin, and myoglobin—are discussed in detail in Chapter 8.

Additional Laboratory Evaluation

If available, review of **previous laboratory studies** can aid in decision making but should not delay revascularization. Standard laboratory evaluation should include a basic metabolic profile, magnesium level, liver function, lipid profile, complete blood count, and coagulation studies.

Echocardiography

Echocardiography may be helpful when the diagnosis is in doubt. Segmental wall motion abnormalities suggest myocardial ischemia or infarction (assuming no baseline wall motion abnormality) and can help localize the territory at risk.

Chest Radiography

A standard portable chest x-ray (CXR) should be included in the initial evaluation protocol. The CXR may demonstrate pulmonary edema and/or suggest another cause of chest pain. The CXR should be reviewed for mediastinal widening, suggesting acute aortic dissection, prior to initiating thrombolytic therapy. If clinical suspicion is high, however, normal mediastinal width does not exclude dissection (see Chapter 23).

MANAGEMENT

All medical centers should have in place an easy to follow STEMI protocol that utilizes proven therapies. Centers that do not provide primary PCI as initial therapy should have protocols in place which meet accepted guidelines for time to therapy for either the rapid administration of thrombolytic therapy with subsequent transfer to a PCI center or for initial rapid transport to a center for primary PCI.

Early Adjunctive Therapy

Aspirin

Aspirin should be given immediately to all patients with suspected AMI. The dose is 162 to 325 mg given orally (chewed or crushed) or rectally if necessary. More rapid absorption and earlier drug effect may occur with the non-enteric-coated formulation. **Clopidogrel** should be substituted for patients with a true or suspected aspirin allergy. Subsequent allergy consultation for aspirin desensitization should be obtained. The benefits of aspirin must not be underestimated. The ISIS-2 study demonstrated that the therapeutic benefit of aspirin is equivalent to that of thrombolytic therapy, with a decrease in vascular mortality by 23% and nonfatal infarct by 49%.

Thienopyridines

Clopidogrel (300 mg loading dose followed by 75 mg daily) has been shown to improve survival, decrease reinfarction, and improve vessel patency without an increase in serious bleeding and intracranial hemorrhage when given in conjunction with thrombolytic therapy. As elderly patients were excluded in the CLARITY-TIMI 28 trial and no loading dose was used in the COMMIT/(CSS-2) trial, caution should be exercised with this regimen in those older than 75 years. A similar regimen with an upstream (prior to PCI) dose of 75 to 300 mg should be considered in patients undergoing primary PCI. As mentioned previously, clopidogrel should be given as an alternative to aspirin in the setting of true aspirin allergy.

Beta Blockers

Beta blockers help reduce myocardial O_2 demand, potentially reduce infarct size, and reduce recurrent major adverse cardiac events. Multiple studies have proven that beta blockade reduces mortality, recurrent ischemia, and arrhythmias. Typical regimens include metoprolol, 5 mg IV every 5 minutes, three doses as tolerated, followed by oral metoprolol, up to 50 mg every 6 hours as blood pressure and heart rate permit. Patients with signs of heart failure or cardiogenic shock, such as those in **Killip class II or greater, have increased mortality with early use of beta-blocker therapy**. It is reasonable to withhold beta-blocker therapy in these patients until they have been stabilized. Other **contraindications**

include bradycardia (heart rate <50 bpm); hypotension (SBP <90); first- (PR interval >200 milliseconds) second-, or third-degree AV block; and severe bronchospastic disease.

Supplemental Oxygen

The administration of **supplemental oxygen** increases O_2 supply to ischemic myocytes. The benefit of O_2 is greatest in patients with arterial O_2 desaturation and pulmonary edema. It should be guided by pulse oximetry and is indicated for the first 6 hours following AMI or longer if the oxygen saturation is <92%. Use caution in patients who may be at risk for CO_2 retention.

Nitroglycerin

Nitroglycerin (NTG) causes venodilation and coronary artery dilation. The effect of NTG on survival has not been confirmed by large randomized trials. Sublingual NTG is a first-line agent for relief of angina and should be given unless the patient has hypotension, marked sinus tachycardia or sinus bradycardia, or is suspected of having an RV infarct. It is particularly useful in the setting of AMI and hypertension and/or heart failure. Sublingual NTG 0.4 mg may be given every 5 minutes for three doses if blood pressure permits. In patients who have responded to sublingual NTG, an infusion of IV NTG at 10 μg/minute should be titrated every 5 to 10 minutes to a maximum of 200 to 300 μg/minute as needed for symptom relief and blood pressure control. Nitrates are contraindicated in patients with history of severe aortic stenosis (AS) or hypertrophic obstructive cardiomyopathy. Nitrates are contraindicated in patients who have used PDE5 inhibitors (e.g., within 24 hours of sildenafil [Viagra, Revatio] or 48 hours of tadalafil [Cialis]) because of the risk of severe hypotension with the combination. Appropriate timing for vardenafil (Levitra) dosing with nitrates is unknown and should be avoided. Prolonged continuous use of nitrates >48 hours can lead to reduced drug response due to tachyphylaxis.

Morphine

Morphine acts to provide analgesia for ischemic cardiac pain, produces a favorable hemodynamic effect, and reduces myocardial O_2 consumption. By relieving pain and anxiety, morphine may also exert a beneficial effect by reducing sympathetic activity. When pain is refractory to NTG and beta blockers, morphine can be given as doses of 2 to 4 mg IV and repeated every 10 minutes until pain is relieved or hypotension occurs.

Magnesium

Studies have shown conflicting data regarding administration of empiric **magnesium** on mortality benefit. Use of magnesium presently is indicated when plasma magnesium level is documented to be low or in the setting of torsades de pointes.

Unfractionated Heparin

Although early studies showed no mortality benefit to intravenous heparin, recent meta-analyses have suggested a mortality benefit. The use of heparin with streptokinase (SK) has not been shown to provide any increased survival and had an increased rate of bleeding complications. Therefore patients treated with SK are recommended not to receive heparin until 6 hours after SK infusion (class III indication to give heparin in this setting) and are not recommended to receive a bolus dose. Heparin should be coadministered with newer-generation thrombolytics. The recommended dosing is a bolus of 60 U/kg (maximum 4000 U), followed by an infusion of 12 U/kg per hour (maximum, 1000 U/hour). The infusion rate should be titrated to maintain an aPTT of 50 to 70 seconds.

Low-Molecular-Weight Heparin

Low-molecular-weight heparin (LMWH) is an attractive antithrombotic alternative to heparin because of its more predictable kinetics, easier administration, and absence of monitoring requirement. Enoxaparin (Lovenox) with full-dose tenecteplase (TNKase) significantly improved the composite endpoint of mortality, in-hospital reinfarction, and in-hospital refractory ischemia, with a similar safety profile in the ASSENT-3 trial. In this study, patients received a dose of 1 mg/kg SC of enoxaparin, followed by a 30-mg IV bolus. The SC dose was then repeated every 12 hours to hospital discharge (maximum 7 days). Local preference of the PCI lab should be considered, as many institutions are not equipped to monitor therapeutic effect on factor Xa activity in the catheterization laboratory.

Direct Thrombin Inhibitors

Direct thrombin inhibitors (DTIs) include hirudin (Refludan), lepirudin (Refludan), argatroban, and bivalirudin (Angiomax). They directly inhibit the actions of thrombin and have several potential advantages over other antithrombotic regimens, including the ability to inhibit both clot-bound and circulating thrombin, more predictable plasma levels, and absence of immune thrombocytopenia. Despite these advantages, studies have failed to show significant mortality reduction. At present, use of these agents is reserved primarily for patients who have previously suffered from heparin-induced thrombocytopenia and other operator- and patient-dependent settings.

Glycoprotein IIb/IIIa Inhibitors

Several recent trials have been conducted to evaluate the use of **glycoprotein IIb/IIIa inhibitors** in reducing ischemic complications from STEMI. There appears to be limited benefit when abciximab is used with reduced-dose thrombolytic medications, primarily because of an increased risk of bleeding. However, it is reasonable to start treatment with abciximab, tirofiban, or eptifibatide as early as possible before primary PCI (with or without stenting) in patients with STEMI.

Reperfusion

Reperfusion is most beneficial for patients who are in treated early in the course of their myocardial infarction. The optimal reperfusion strategy should be center-specific, with consideration of available resources. An algorithm to aid in the decision-making process is shown in Figure 9-1.

Briefly, **primary PCI** is the preferred strategy when door-to-balloon time is <90 minutes. Patients who present with MI symptoms >12 hours and <24 hours after pain onset should be considered for reperfusion, particularly in the setting of continued ST-segment elevation, persistent symptoms, recurrent ischemia, LV dysfunction, widespread ECG changes, or prior MI, percutaneous revascularization, or coronary artery bypass grafting (CABG). The administration of thrombolytic therapy to patients greater than 24 hours after symptom onset is contraindicated.

Primary PCI

PCI is the preferred therapy if performed in a timely fashion (door-to-balloon time <90 minutes) by individuals skilled in the procedure (>75 PCIs per year of which 11 are STEMIs) and in high-volume centers (>200 PCIs per year). PCI offers increased early efficacy in opening occluded arteries and improved survival. PCI is also indicated in patients who present with cardiogenic shock, have contraindications to thrombolytics, or whose diagnosis is uncertain. Stenting of the culprit lesion is appropriate, and if significant left-main stenosis is found, consideration of emergent CABG. Percutaneous intervention on the non–infarct-related artery in the setting of an AMI should not be performed unless compelling indications exist.

Rescue PCI

Thrombolytic therapy fails to achieve coronary artery patency in 15% to 50% of patients. Rescue PCI is appropriate for patients who have received thrombolytic therapy but have ongoing symptoms and persistent ST-segment elevation (>50% of original degree of elevation)

STEP 1: Assess Time and Risk
- Time since onset of symptoms
- Risk of STEMI
- Risk of fibrinolysis
- Time required for transport to a skilled PCI lab

STEP 2: Determine if Fibrinolysis or an Invasive Strategy is Preferred
If presentation is less than 3 hours and there is no delay to an invasive strategy, there is no preference for either strategy

Fibrinolysis is generally preferred if:	**An Invasive Strategy is generally preferred if:**
• *Early Presentation (less than or equal to 3 hours from symptom onset and delay to invasive strategy) (see below)*	• *Skilled PCI lab available with surgical backup †‡* Medical Contact-to-Balloon or Door-to-Balloon is less than 90 minutes (Door-to-Balloon) − (Door-to-Needle) is less than 1 hour*
• *Invasive Strategy is not an option* Catheterization lab occupied/not available Vascular access difficulties Lack of access to a skilled PCI lab †‡	• *High Risk from STEMI* Cardiogenic shock Killip class is greater than or equal to 3
• *Delay to Invasive Strategy* Prolonged transport (Door-to-Balloon) − (Door-to -Needle) is greater than 1 hour *§ Medical Contact-to-Balloon or Door-to-Balloon is greater than 90 minutes	• *Contraindications to fibrinolysis including increased risk of bleeding and ICH* • *Late Presentation* The symptom onset was greater than 3 hours ago • *Diagnosis of STEMI is in doubt*

STEMI 5 ST-elevation myocardial infarction; PCI 5 percutaneous coronary intervention; ICH 5 intracranial hemorrhage.
*Applies to fibrin-specific agents (See Figure 15).
†Operator experience greater than a total of 75 Primary PCI cases/year.
‡Team experience greater than a total of 36 Primary PCI cases/year.
§This calculation implies that the estimated delay to the implementation of the invasive strategy is greater than one hour versus initiation of fibrinolytic therapy immediately with a fibrin-specific agent.

FIGURE 9-1. Decision making for reperfusion therapy. (From Antman EM et al. ACC/AHA guidelines for the management of patients with ST-elevation myocardial infarction: a report of the American College of Cardiology/American Heart Association Task Force on Practice Guidelines [Committee to Revise the 1999 Guidelines for the Management of Patients with Acute Myocardial Infarction], 2004; available at www.acc.org.)

90 minutes after administration. Patients with cardiogenic shock, congestive heart failure (CHF), refractory arrhythmias, and particularly with large anterior MIs also should potentially be assessed for mechanical reperfusion. CABG is indicated in the setting of failed percutaneous transluminal coronary angioplasty (PTCA) in patients with ongoing signs and symptoms of ischemia or in similar patients whose coronary anatomy is not suitable for PCI.

Facilitated PCI
Although facilitated PCI using half-dose lytics is attractive in theory, no trial data thus far support its use. In fact, the results of the PACT and ASSENT-4 trials would suggest worse outcomes with this approach.

Thrombolytic/Fibrinolytic Therapy
The benefits of early (<12 hours) thrombolytic therapy are well established in the medical literature, with pooled data from the FTT Collaborative Group displaying an 18% relative reduction in mortality. When given early following onset of symptoms, thrombolytics can be very effective. Thrombolytics have not been shown to be effective in vein grafts. Thus, if a patient post-CABG presents with a STEMI, the preferred mode of reperfusion is PCI. Note that the terms "thrombolytic" and "fibrinolytic" are used somewhat interchangeably.

Fibrinolytic agents are more specific in the coagulation cascade. The absolute and relative contraindications for thrombolytic therapy are shown Table 9-1.

Thrombolytic Agents
Various thrombolytic agents are available and have similar efficacy. These medications vary predominantly by rate of administration. Details are shown in Table 9-6.

Bleeding Risk
Intracranial hemorrhage, the most feared complication of thrombolytic therapy, occurs in 0.7% of cases. Several risk models have determined factors predictive of increased risk. These include age ≥ 65 years, weight below 70 kg, hypertension (SBP >170 or DBP >90 on admission), and use of tissue plasminogen activator (tPA) rather than other agents.

Later Evaluation and Treatment
ICU Monitoring
All patients must be monitored in the ICU for at least 48 hours following STEMI. Patients should have continuous telemetry monitoring, preferably with display of one of the leads involved with ST-segment elevation, to monitor for recurrent ischemia and arrhythmias. Daily evaluation should include assessment for recurrent anginal and heart failure symptoms, physical exam with new murmurs or evidence of heart failure, and a daily ECG. Most patients can safely be transferred to a step-down unit in 24 to 48 hours with telemetry monitoring in the absence of any further problems.

Medical Treatment
ACE Inhibitors
Angiotensin converting enzyme (ACE) inhibitors and angiotensin receptor blockers improve ventricular remodeling and hemodynamics and prevent heart failure. Patients with ejection fractions <40%, large anterior MI, and prior MI derive the most benefit from prompt ACE-inhibitor therapy (within the first 24 hours). Contraindications include hypotension, acute renal failure, allergy, bilateral renal artery stenosis, and hyperkalemia. Care must be taken to avoid hypotension.

HMG-CoA Reductase Inhibitors (Statins)
Several trials have shown the benefit of early and aggressive use of statins following AMI. The goal is at least a 50% reduction in low-density-lipoprotein cholesterol (LDL-C) or LDL-C <70 mg/dL.

Aldosterone Receptor Blockers
Aldosterone receptor blockers, including spironolactone (Aldactone) and eplerenone (Inspra), have shown benefit in patients with symptomatic CHF. In the EPHESUS trial, eplerenone, a selective aldosterone receptor blocker, demonstrated significant benefit compared with placebo in patients with an LV ejection fraction of <40% who also had clinical evidence of heart failure or had diabetes. Caution should be used in patients with hyperkalemia and renal insufficiency (CrCl <30 ml/minute) or severe hepatic impairment.

Complications (See Chapter 6)
Cardiogenic Shock
Cardiogenic shock is an infrequent but serious complication of STEMI. It occurs within the first 48 hours after symptom onset, particularly with large anterior infarcts. An algorithm for managing these complex patients is shown in Figure 9-2.

The SHOCK trial demonstrated a significant benefit of revascularization over medical therapy in patients with cardiogenic shock in whom revascularization could be performed

TABLE 9-6 THROMBOLYTIC AGENTS

	Streptokinase	Alteplase	Reteplase	Tenecteplase-tPA
Dose	1.5 MU over 30–60 min	Up to 100 mg in 90 min (based on weight)*	10 U × 2 each over 2 min	30–50 mg based on weight†
Bolus administration	No	No	Yes	Yes
Antigenic	Yes	No	No	No
Allergic reactions (hypotension most common)	Yes	No	No	No
Systemic fibrinogen depletion	Marked	Mild	Moderate	Minimal
90-min patency rates, approximate %	50	75	81%	75
TIMI grade 3 flow, %	32	54	60	63
Cost per dose (US $)	$613	$2974	$2750	$2833 for 50 mg

MU, mega units.

*Bolus 15 mg, infusion 0.75 mg/kg times 30 minutes (maximum 50 mg), then 0.5 mg/kg not to exceed 35 mg over the next 60 minutes to an overall maximum of 100 mg.

†Thirty milligrams for weight <60 kg; 35 mg for 60–69 kg; 40 mg for 70–79 mg; 45 mg for 80–89 kg; 50 mg for 90 kg or more.

Source: From Antman EM et al. ACC/AHA guidelines for the management of patients with ST-elevation myocardial infarction: a report of the American College of Cardiology/American Heart Association Task Force on Practice Guidelines (Committee to Revise the 1999 Guidelines for the Management of Patients with Acute Myocardial Infarction). 2004; available at www.acc.org.

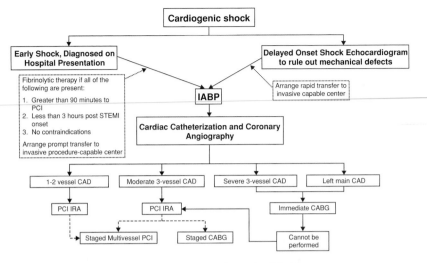

CAD = coronary artery disease; PCI = percutaneous coronary intervention; IRA = infarct related artery; CABG = coronary artery bypass grafting; IABP = intraaortic balloon pump

FIGURE 9-2. Management of Cardiogenic Shock. (From Antman EM et al. ACC/AHA guidelines for the management of patients with ST-elevation myocardial infarction: a report of the American College of Cardiology/American Heart Association Task Force on Practice Guidelines [Committee to Revise the 1999 Guidelines for the Management of Patients with Acute Myocardial Infarction], 2004; available at www.acc.org.)

within 18 hours of onset of shock. Note that the benefit of such therapy did not extend to patients over 75 years of age in this randomized trial.

Free-Wall Rupture
Free-wall rupture occurs 2 to 6 days after MI, more commonly in patients without prior angina or MI and with large infarcts by enzyme criteria. It may present as hypotension, cardiac tamponade, or pulseless electrical activity. Mortality is very high, and management consists of volume resuscitation, inotropes, pericardiocentesis, and surgical repair.

Pseudoaneurysm
A contained rupture sealed by thrombus and pericardium can occur as a complication of an anteroapical MI. It is clinically silent but may be characterized by a to-and-fro murmur. The thrombus may result in systemic emboli. A hemodynamically significant pericardial effusion may result. Diagnosis is by echocardiography, and pseudoaneurysm is often found incidentally. Treatment is surgical in nearly all cases.

Ventricular Septal Defect
VSD typically occurs 2 to 5 days after AMI and is more common in anterior MIs. It presents with a new harsh holosystolic murmur with or without hemodynamic compromise; diagnosis depends on echocardiography with Doppler and/or pulmonary artery (PA) catheterization revealing oxygen step-up. Management involves an intra-aortic balloon pump (IABP), inotropes, vasodilators, and surgical versus catheter-based closure.

Papillary Muscle Rupture

Papillary muscle rupture usually occurs 2 to 7 days after MI and involves the posteromedial papillary muscle due to single blood supply. It is most commonly associated with inferior MI and presents with a new holosystolic murmur (although this may not be present), cardiogenic shock, and pulmonary edema. Diagnosis can be made by echocardiography or PA catheter waveforms with prominent v waves. Treatment involves afterload reduction with IABP or vasodilators, revascularization, and surgical repair.

Right Ventricular Infarct

RV infarct occurs in the setting of inferior MI and is characterized by a triad of hypotension, elevated jugular venous pressure with Kussmaul's sign, and clear lung fields. It is diagnosed by right-sided ECG with ST-segment elevation in V3R and V4R or by witnessed RV wall motion abnormality on echocardiography. Treatment includes volume loading to PCWP of 18 to 20 mm Hg, avoidance of nitrates, and low-dose dobutamine if needed to treat hypotension.

Arrhythmias

Arrhythmias are very common after STEMI. Accelerated idioventricular rhythm should not be treated unless there is hemodynamic disturbance. Prophylactic antiarrhythmic infusion after AMI to suppress ventricular tachycardia/ventricular fibrillation (VT/VF) does not improve mortality and is not indicated. Bradycardias may warrant a temporary transvenous pacer if associated with significant atrioventricular (AV) block. AV block in association with an inferior MI usually portends a good prognosis, as the mechanism is ischemia of the AV node (the AV nodal branch derives from the RCA) and a compensatory Bezold–Jarisch reflex, which stimulates vagal tone. AV block after IMI may persist up to 1 to 2 weeks. AV block in association with an anterior MI usually portends a poor prognosis (permanent pacer likely required), as the mechanism is infarction of part of the distal conduction system.

Post–Myocardial Infarction Pericarditis

Post-MI pericarditis occurs 1 to 4 days after MI and may cause recurrent chest discomfort and widespread ST-segment elevation. PR depression may occur on ECGs but is uncommon; pericardial rub may be found on exam. Treatment consists of high-dose NSAID. Heparin should be avoided owing to risk of hemorrhagic transformation.

Dressler's Syndrome

Dressler's syndrome presents 2 to 10 weeks after MI with fever, malaise, and pleuritic chest discomfort. Often, patients have an elevated erythrocyte sedimentation rate (ESR), and echocardiography may demonstrate pericardial effusion. It is usually managed with high-dose NSAID.

Left Ventricular Thrombus

LV thrombus may occur with large anteroapical MIs that produce akinetic or dyskinetic segments on echocardiogram or left ventriculogram. Treatment consists of anticoagulation with warfarin for 3 to 6 months.

Ventricular Aneurysm

Ventricular aneurysm may occur acutely after an MI and cause significant hemodynamic compromise or develop more insidiously up to 6 weeks after the infarct. Persistent ST elevation more than 4 weeks after AMI is suggestive but not diagnostic of an aneurysm; echocardiography establishes the diagnosis and provides information regarding LV function and presence of thrombus. Treatment involves afterload reduction, preferably with ACE inhibitor to help reduce LV remodeling, with warfarin anticoagulation; and potentially surgical resection in selected cases.

REFERENCES AND SUGGESTED READINGS

Acute Infarction Ramipril Efficacy (AIRE) Study Investigators. Effect of ramipril on mortality and morbidity of survivors of acute myocardial infarction with clinical evidence of heart failure. *Lancet* 1993;342:821–828.

American Heart Association. *2001 Heart and Stroke Statistical Update.* http://www.americanheart.org.

Antman EM, Braunwald E. Acute myocardial infarction. In Braunwald E, ed. *Heart Disease: A Textbook of Cardiovascular Medicine.* Philadelphia: Saunders, 1997.

Antman EM et al. ACC/AHA guidelines for the management of patients with ST-elevation myocardial infarction: a report of the American College of Cardiology/American Heart Association Task Force on Practice Guidelines (Committee to Revise the 1999 Guidelines for the Management of Patients with Acute Myocardial Infarction), 2004; available at www.acc.org.

Assessment of the Safety and Efficacy of a New Treatment Strategy with Percutaneous Coronary Intervention (ASSENT-4 PCI) Investigators. Primary versus tenecteplase-facilitated percutaneous coronary interventions in patients with ST-segment elevation acute myocardial infarction (ASSENT-4 PCI): Randomised trial. *Lancet* 2006;367:569–578.

Boersma, E and the Primary Coronary Angioplasty vs. Thrombolysis Group. Does time matter? A pooled analysis of randomized clinical trials comparing primary percutaneous coronary intervention and in-hospital fibrinolysis in acute myocardial infarction patients. *Eur Heart J* 2006;27(7):779–788. Epub 2006 Mar 2.

Cannon CP, Braunwald E, McCabe CH, et al. The Thrombolysis in Myocardial Infarction (TIMI) trials: the first decade. The TIMI Investigators. *J Interv Cardiol* 1995; 8:117–135.

Cannon CJ, Braunwald E, McCabe CH, for the Pravastatin or Atorvastatin Evaluation and Infection Therapy: Thrombolysis in Myocardial Infarction 22 Investigators.

Comparison of intensive and moderate lipid lowering with statins after acute coronary syndromes. *N Engl J Med* 2004. Published online before print (April 8 issue).

COMMIT (ClOpidogrel and Metoprolol in Myocardial Infarction Trial) collaborative group. Addition of clopidogrel to aspirin in 45 852 patients with acute myocardial infarction: Randomised placebo-controlled trial. *Lancet* 2005;366:1607–1621.

Eikelboom JW, Quinlan DJ, Mehta SR, et al. Unfractionated and low-molecular-weight heparin as adjuncts to thrombolysis in aspirin-treated patients with ST-elevation acute myocardial infarction: a meta-analysis of the randomized trials. *Circulation* 2005;112(25):3855–3867. Epub 2005 Dec 12.

Gershlick AH, Stephens-Lloyd A, Hughes S, et al. Rescue angioplasty after failed thrombolytic therapy for acute myocardial infarction. *N Engl J Med* 2005;353:2758–2768.

Gibson CM. Primary angioplasty compared with thrombolysis: new issues in the era of glycoprotein IIb/IIIa inhibition and intracoronary stenting. *Ann Intern Med* 1999;130:841–847.

Global Utilization of Streptokinase and Tissue Plasminogen Activator for Occluded Coronary Arteries (GUSTO) Investigators. An international randomized trial comparing four thrombolytic strategies for acute myocardial infarction. *N Engl J Med* 1993;329:673–682.

Goldman LE, Eisenberg MJ. Identification and management of patients with failed thrombolysis after acute myocardial infarction. *Ann Intern Med* 2000;132:556–565.

Grines CL, Cox DA, Stone GW, et al. Coronary angioplasty with or without stent implantation for acute myocardial infarction. *N Engl J Med* 1999;341:1949–1956.

Gruppo Italiano Per Lo Studio Della Streptochinasi Nell'Infarct Miocardico (GISSI). Effectiveness of intravenous thrombolytic treatment in acute myocardial infarction. *Lancet* 1987;2:871–874.

Hochman JS, Sleeper LA, Webb JG, et al. Early revascularization in acute myocardial infarction complicated by cardiogenic shock. SHOCK Investigators. Should we emergently revascularize occluded coronaries for cardiogenic shock. *N Engl J Med* 1999; 341:625–634.

International Joint Efficacy Comparison of Thrombolytics. Randomized, double-blind comparison of reteplase double-bolus administration with streptokinase in acute myocardial infarction (INJECT): trial to investigate equivalence. *Lancet* 1995;346:329.

ISIS Collaborative Group. Randomized trial of intravenous streptokinase, oral aspirin, both, or neither among 17,187 cases of suspected acute myocardial infarction. *Lancet* 1988;2:349–360.

Lenderink T, Simoons ML, Van Es GA, et al. Benefits of thrombolytic therapy is sustained throughout five years and is related to TIMI perfusion grade 3 but not grade 2 flow at discharge. *Circulation* 1995;92:1110.

Lincoff AM, Topol EJ, Califf RM, et al. Significance of a coronary artery with thrombolysis in myocardial infarction grade 2 flow "patency" (outcome in the Thrombolysis and Angioplasty in Myocardial Infarction trials). *Am J Cardiol* 1995;75:871–876.

Montalescot G, Barragan P, Wittenberg O, et al. Platelet glycoprotein IIb/IIIa inhibition with coronary stenting for acute myocardial infarction. *N Engl J Med* 2001;344: 1895–1903.

Morrow DA, Antman EM, Charlesworth A, et al. TIMI risk score for ST-elevation myocardial infarction: a convenient, bedside, clinical score for risk assessment at presentation. *Circulation* 2000;102:2031–2037.

Pfeffer MA, McMurray JJV, Velasquez EJ, et al. Valsartan, captopril, or both in myocardial infarction complicated by heart failure, left ventricular dysfunction, or both. *N Engl J Med* 2003;349:1893–1906.

Pfeffer MA, Braunwald E, Moyé LA, et al. Effect of captopril on mortality and morbidity in patients with left ventricular dysfunction after myocardial infarction: results of the Survival and Ventricular Enlargement trial. *N Engl J Med* 1992;327:669–677.

Pitt B, Remme W, Zannad F, et al, for the Eplerenone Post-Acute Myocardial Infarction Heart Failure Efficacy and Survival Study Investigators. Eplerenone, a selective aldosterone blocker, in patients with left ventricular dysfunction after myocardial infarction. *N Engl J Med* 2003;348:1309–1321.

Ross R. Atherosclerosis: an inflammatory disease. *N Engl J Med* 1999;340(2):115–126.

Sabatine MS, Cannon CP, Gibson CM, et al for the CLARITY-TIMI 28 Investigators. Addition of clopidogrel to aspirin and fibrinolytic therapy for myocardial infarction with ST-segment elevation. *N Engl J Med* 2005; available at http://www.nejm.org.

Simoons MI, Maggioni AP, Knatterud G, et al. Individual risk assessment for intracranial hemorrhage during thrombolytic therapy. *Lancet* 1993;342:523–528.

Stone GW, Grines CL, Cox DA, et al. Comparison of angioplasty with stenting, with or without abciximab, in acute myocardial infarction. *N Engl J Med* 2002;346:957–966.

The Assessment of the Safety and Efficacy of a New Thrombolytic Regimen (ASSENT)-3 Investigators. Efficacy and safety of tenecteplase in combination with enoxaparin, abciximab, or unfractionated heparin: the ASSENT-3 randomised trial in acute myocardial infarction. *Lancet* 2001;358:605–613.

The GUSTO Angiographic Investigators. The comparative effects of tissue plasminogen activator, streptokinase, or both on coronary artery patency, ventricular function and survival after acute myocardial infarction. *N Engl J Med* 1993;329:1615–1622.

The GUSTO IIb Angioplasty Substudy Investigators. A clinical trial comparing primary coronary angioplasty with tissue plasminogen activator for acute myocardial infarction. *N Engl J Med* 1997;336:1621–1628.

The GUSTO III Investigators. A comparison of reteplase with alteplase for acute myocardial infarction. *N Engl J Med* 1997;337:1118–1123.

The GUSTO V Investigators. Reperfusion therapy for acute myocardial infarction with thrombolytic therapy or combination reduced thrombolytic therapy and platelet glycoprotein IIb/IIIa inhibition: the GUSTO V randomised trial. *Lancet* 2001;357: 1905–1914.

The International Study Group. In-hospital mortality and clinical course of 20,891 patients with suspected acute myocardial infarction randomised between alteplase and streptokinase with or without heparin. *Lancet* 1990;2:71.

Third International Study of Infarct Survival (ISIS-3) Collaborative Group. ISIS-3: a randomized trial of streptokinase vs tissue plasminogen activator vs. anistreplase and of aspirin plus heparin vs aspirin alone among 41,299 cases of suspected acute myocardial infarction. *Lancet* 1992;339:753.

Thrombolytic Therapy Trialists' (FTT) Collaborative Group. Indications for thrombolytic therapy in suspected acute myocardial infarction: collaborative overview of early mortality and major morbidity results from all randomised trials of more than 1000 patients. *Lancet* 1994;343:311–322.

Weaver WD, Simes RJ, Betriu A, et al. Comparison of primary coronary angioplasty and intravenous thrombolytic therapy for acute myocardial infarction: a quantitative review. *JAMA* 1997;278:2093–2098.

Wu WC, Rathore SS, Wang Y, et al. Blood transfusion in elderly patients with acute myocardial infarction. *N Engl J Med* 2001;345(17):1230–1236.

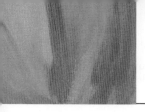

Primary and Secondary Prevention of Cardiovascular Disease

10

Courtney Virgilio and Andrew M. Kates

INTRODUCTION

Background

Cardiovascular disease (CVD) is the leading cause of death among men and women in the United States. In 2004, some 15,800,000 Americans experienced a myocardial infarction (MI), angina, or both. The prevalence of coronary artery disease (CAD) increases with age and is more prevalent in men than in women (Fig. 10-1). CAD is also a major source of morbidity leading to congestive heart failure (CHF), stable and unstable angina, and cardiac arrest. CAD has economic consequences as well. In 2007, it is estimated that the overall cost of CAD will exceed $400 billion. All of these issues highlight the gravity of cardiovascular disease and illustrate the need for prevention. Moreover, there is an inherent association between CAD and other forms of vascular disease, including stroke, transient ischemic attacks (TIAs), and peripheral vascular disease. When combined with CAD, cardiovascular disease accounts for more deaths than the other four leading causes combined.

Definition

Primary prevention is the prevention of disease in a person without prior symptoms of CVD by treating risk factors with lifestyle modifications or drugs. **Secondary prevention** is the prevention of death or recurrence of disease in those patients who are symptomatic or have been diagnosed with CVD.

Primary Prevention

The main target in primary prevention of coronary disease is the prevention of the atherosclerotic process itself. Prevention can be addressed on a large-scale population-wide basis with programs designed to educate and effect change on the population as a whole (e.g., health fairs, smoking seminars, etc.) or on an individual basis with identification of the high-risk patient. This section first focuses on the identification of the at-risk patient and then discusses specific recommendations.

Risk Factors
Key to understanding who is at risk for CAD is in the identification of risk factors. These can be divided into nonmodifiable, modifiable (behavioral), and clinical (physiologic) (Fig. 10-2).

Risk Assessment
The goal of risk assessment is to identify patients without established CAD who may benefit from aggressive medical therapies and lifestyle changes. It is recommended that asymptomatic patients undergo routine risk-factor screening by their primary care provider beginning at age 20. Blood pressure, body mass index, waist circumference, and pulse (to screen for atrial fibrillation) should be recorded at each visit (at least every 2 years). Fasting serum

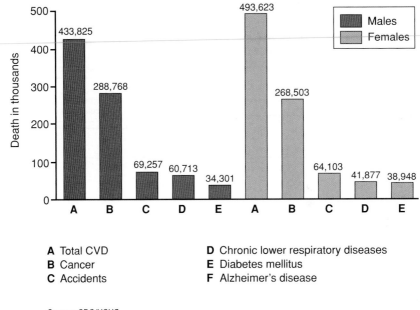

Leading causes of death for all males and females
United States: 2002

A Total CVD
B Cancer
C Accidents
D Chronic lower respiratory diseases
E Diabetes mellitus
F Alzheimer's disease

Source: CDC/HCHS

FIGURE 10-1. Heart Disease and Stroke Statistics, 2005 Update, American Heart Association.

ning at age 20. Blood pressure, body mass index, waist circumference, and pulse (to screen for atrial fibrillation) should be recorded at each visit (at least every 2 years). Fasting serum lipoprotein profile [or total and high-density-lipoprotein cholesterol (HDL-C) if fasting is unavailable] and fasting blood glucose should be measured according to the patient's risk for hyperlipidemia and diabetes, respectively (at least every 5 years; if risk factors are present, every 2 years). Global risk estimation (see below) should be performed every 5 years (or more frequently if risk factors change) in all adults ≥40 years of age to estimate the risk of developing heart disease.

A common tool is the Framingham risk score, which uses "standard" risk factors (smoking, blood pressure, serum cholesterol, HDL cholesterol, blood glucose, and age). Although this is a well-validated model, it may not be as applicable in some patient populations. The key components of the Framingham equation are shown in Figure 10-3. In addition, there are many web-based and personal digital assistant (PDA)-based models for in-office assessment (http://hp2010.nhlbihin.net/atpiii/calculator.asp?usertype=prof). One advantage of risk scores such as Framingham is the identification of those at risk not from a single markedly elevated risk factor but from several moderately elevated risk factors.

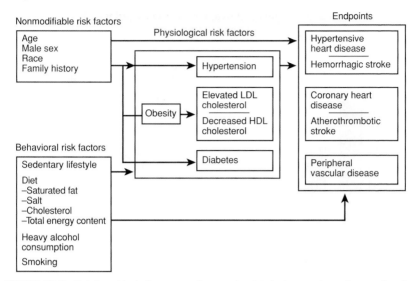

FIGURE 10-2. Relationship between cardiovascular risk factors and cardiovascular disease. (From Wilson, MA, Pearsion, TA. Primary prevention. In Wong ND, Black HR, Gardin JM, eds. *Preventive Cardiology: A Practical Approach.* New York: McGraw-Hill; 2005:493–514, with permission.)

(1) Assess
- CHD history
- Diet
- Body mass index
- Family history of CHD
- Blood pressure
- Physical activity
- Smoking history
- Diabetes

(2) Measure fasting lipids (cholesterol, triglyceride, HDL). Measure glucose, treat if abnormal

(3) Determine absolute risk of future coronary events (using a Framingham risk equation tool)

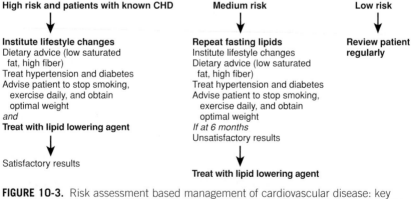

High risk and patients with known CHD

Institute lifestyle changes
Dietary advice (low saturated fat, high fiber)
Treat hypertension and diabetes
Advise patient to stop smoking, exercise daily, and obtain optimal weight
and
Treat with lipid lowering agent

Satisfactory results

Medium risk

Repeat fasting lipids
Institute lifestyle changes
Dietary advice (low saturated fat, high fiber)
Treat hypertension and diabetes
Advise patient to stop smoking, exercise daily, and obtain optimal weight
If at 6 months
Unsatisfactory results

Treat with lipid lowering agent

Low risk

Review patient regularly

FIGURE 10-3. Risk assessment based management of cardiovascular disease: key points. CHD, coronary heart disease; HDL, high-density lipoprotein. (From Hobbs FD. Cardiovascular disease: different strategies for primary and secondary prevention? *Heart* 2004;90(10):1217–1223, with permission.)

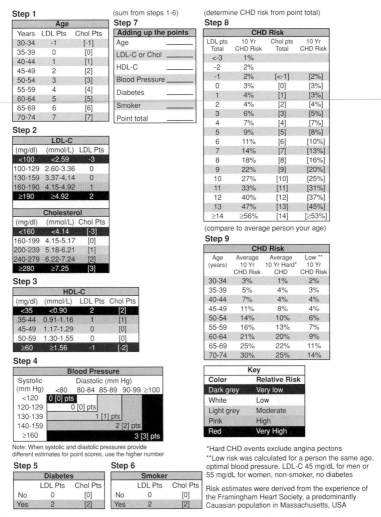

FIGURE 10-4. Components of the Framingham risk score. (From Wilson PW, D'Agostino RB, Levy D, et al. Prediction of coronary heart disease using risk factor categories. *Circulation* 1998;97(18):1837–1847, with permission.)

Using individual risk-assessment methods, asymptomatic individuals can be placed into one of three risk categories: low, intermediate, and high (Fig. 10-4). Intermediate-risk patients may become candidates for further risk stratification through noninvasive procedures that test for the presence of myocardial ischemia or coronary atherosclerotic burden, including high sensitivity C-reactive protein (hs-CRP), coronary calcium screening, and carotid intima–media thickness. Individuals can subsequently be targeted for the recommendations discussed below.

Recommendations

The American Heart Association (AHA) has published guidelines for the primary prevention of cardiovascular disease. Those recommendations as well as more recent ones from the AHA and other societies are incorporated into the section that follows.

BEHAVIORAL RISK FACTORS

Lifestyle Modifications

Diet

Improving diet is a critical component in the prevention of heart disease. Maintaining a healthy diet and lifestyle offers the greatest potential of all known approaches for reducing the risk for CVD. The American Heart Association recently published updated recommendations for a healthy diet and lifestyle for patients both with and without CAD. These recommendations are shown in Table 10-1. Intentionally, no specific diet is recommended; instead, an overall healthy diet is emphasized. Several diets appear to be beneficial. Examples are shown in Table 10-2.

- **Fish Oil.** The AHA recommends regular fish oil consumption, either as n-3 polyunsaturated fatty acids (PUFA), found in fish such as tuna and salmon, or α-linolenic acid, found in flax and rapeseed oil for primary prevention. Data from both the Nurses Health Study and MRFIT provide support for the use of PUFA in primary prevention.

  Patients should limit saturated fat consumption to <7% of total caloric intake and *trans* fats to <1%.

TABLE 10-1	AHA 2006 DIET AND LIFESTYLE RECOMMENDATIONS

- Balance calorie intake and physical activity to achieve or maintain a healthy body weight.
- Consume a diet rich in vegetables and fruits.
- Choose whole-grain high-fiber foods.
- Consume fish, especially oily fish, at least twice a week.
- Limit your intake of saturated fat to <7% of energy, *trans* fat to <1% of energy, and cholesterol to <300 mg per day by
  - choosing lean meats and vegetable alternatives:
  - selecting fat-free (skim), 1%-fat and low-fat dairy products: and
  - Minimizing intake of partially hydrogenated fats.
- Minimize your intake of beverages and foods with added sugars.
- Choose and prepare foods with little or no salt.
- If you consume alcohol, do so in moderation.
- When you eat food that is prepared outside of the home, follow the AHA Diet and Lifestyle Recommendations.

Source: From American Heart Association Nutrition Committee. Diet and lifestyle recommendations revision 2006: a scientific statement from the American Heart Association Nutrition Committee. *Circulation* 2006;114(1):82–96, with permission.

TABLE 10-2 DIET RECOMMENDATIONS

Eating Pattern	DASH*	TLC[†]	Serving Sizes
Grains[‡]	6 to 8 servings per day	7 servings[§] per day	1 slice bread, 1 oz dry cereal,[¶] ½ cup cooked rice, pasta, or cereal
Vegetables	4 to 5 servings per day	5 servings[§] per day	1 cup raw leafy vegetable, ½ cup cut-up raw or cooked vegetable, ½ cup vegetable juice
Fruits	4 to 5 servings per day	4 servings[§] per day	1 medium fruit, ¼ cup dried fruit, ½ cup fresh, frozen, or canned fruit, ½ cup fruit juice
Fat-free or low-fat milk and milk products	2 to 3 servings per day	2 to 3 servings per day	1 cup milk, 1 cup yogurt, 1½ oz cheese
Lean[‖] meats, poultry, and fish	<6 oz per day	≤5 oz per day	
Nuts, Seeds, and legumes	4 to 5 servings per week	Counted in vegetable servings	½ cup (1½ oz), 2 Tbsp peanut butter, 2 Tbsp or ½ oz seeds, ½ cup dry beans or peas
Fats and oils	2 to 3 servings[#] per day	Amount depends on daily calorie level	1 tsp soft margarine, 1 Tbsp mayonnaise, 2 Tbsp salad dressing, 1 tsp vegetable oil
Sweets and added sugars	5 or fewer servings per week	No recommendation	1 Tbsp sugar, 1 Tbsp jelly or jam, ½ cup sorbet and ices, 1 cup lemonade

*Dietary Approaches to stop Hypertension. For more information, please visit http://www.nhlbi.nih.gov/health/public/heart/hbp/dash.

[†]Therapeutic Lifestyle Changes. For more information, please visit http://www.nhlbi.nih.gov/cgi-bin/chel/step2intro.cgi.TLC includes 2 therapeutic diet options: plant stanol/sterol (add 2 g per day) and soluble fiber (add 5 to 10 g per day).

[‡]Whole-grain foods are recommended for most grain servings to meet fiber recommendations.

[§]This number can be less or more depending on other food choices to meet 2000 calories.

[¶]Equals ½ to 1¼ cups. Depending on cereal type. Check the product's Nutrition Facts Label.

[‖]Lean cuts include sirloin tip, round steak, and rump roast; extra lean hamburger; and cold cuts made with lean meat or soy protein. Lean cuts of pork are center-cut ham loin chops, and pork tenderloin.

[#]Fat content changes serving counts for fats and oils: For example, 1 Tbsp of regular salad dressing equals 1 serving: 1 Tbsp of low-fat dressing equals ½ serving: 1Tbsp of fat-free dressing equals 0 servings.

Source: From American Heart Association Nutrition Committee. Diet and lifestyle recommendations revision 2006: a scientific statement from the American Heart Association Nutrition Committee. *Circulation* 2006;114(1):82–96, with permission.

- **Dark Chocolate.** The phenols found in dark chocolate have been postulated to have beneficial cardiovascular effects. There is a recent small randomized controlled trial illustrating that 18 weeks of dark chocolate improved blood pressure measurements in patients with prehypertension. More data are needed on this topic before this intervention can be recommended to patients.

Exercise

Part of a healthy lifestyle and key to the prevention of CAD is exercise. Regular exercise can help prevent CAD by treating many established atherosclerotic risk factors:

- Lowering blood pressure
- Improving insulin resistance and glucose tolerance
- Lowering triglycerides
- Raising high-density-lipoprotein cholesterol (HDL-C)
- Lowering fibrinogen levels and improving fibrinolytic capacity

The AHA and the American College of Sports Medicine have published new recommendations regarding exercise in healthy adults (Table 10-3). These guidelines stress the

TABLE 10-3	PHYSICAL ACTIVITY RECOMMENDATIONS FOR HEALTHY ADULTS

1. To promote and maintain good health, adults aged 18–65 yr should maintain a physically active lifestyle. I (A)
2. They should perform moderate-intensity aerobic (endurance) physical activity for a minimum of 30 min on five days each week or vigorous-intensity aerobic activity minimum of 20 min on three days each week. I (A)
3. Combinations of moderate- and vigorous-intensity activity can be performed to meet this recommendation. For example, a person can meet the recommendation by walking briskly for 30 min twice during the week and then jogging for 20 min on two other days. IIa (B)
4. These moderate- or vigorous intensity activities are in addition to the light intensity activities frequently performed during daily life (e.g., self care, washing dishes, using light tools at a desk) or activities of very short duration (e.g., taking out trash, walking to parking lot at store or office).
5. Moderate-intensity aerobic activity, which is generally equivalent to a brisk walk and noticeably accelerates the heart rate, can be accumulated toward the 30-min minimum by performing bouts each lastng 10 or more minutes. I (B)
6. Vigorous-intensity activity is exemplified by jogging, and causes rapid breathing and a substantial increase in heart rate.
7. In addition, at least twice each week adults will benefit by performing activities using the major muscles of the body that maintain or increase muscular strength and endurance. IIa (A)
8. Because of the dose-response relation between physical activity and health, persons who wish to further improve their personal fitness, reduce their risk for chronic diseases and disabilities, or prevent unhealthy weight gain will likely benefit by exceeding the minimum recommended amount of physical activity. I (A)

Source: From Haskell WL, Lee IM, Pate RR, et al., and the American College of Sports Medicine/American Heart Association. Physical activity and public health: updated recommendation for adults from the American College of Sports Medicine and the American Heart Association. *Circulation* 2007;116(9):1081–1093, with permission.

benefits of **moderate-intensity exercise**. Examples of such exercise include walking at 3 to 4 mph; household or occupational activities such as sweeping, vacuuming, or mowing the lawn; and leisurely sports such as bicycling on a flat surface at 10 to 12 mph or golfing (without a cart!).

Alcohol

Alcohol in moderation has been shown to have beneficial effects on cardiovascular disease. The primary mechanism for alcohol's beneficial effect is by raising HDL. Moderate amounts are considered to be 1 to 3 drinks/day, with women being lower on that range than men. One drink is a 4-oz glass of wine, a 12-oz beer, or 1.5 oz of 80-proof spirit. As for the type of beverage imbibed (wine, beer, or spirits), a meta-analysis of several alcoholic beverage trials showed that the beverage that is drunk in moderation is the one that demonstrates the beneficial effects on cardiovascular disease. Another testament to the importance of moderation is seen in looking at alcohol's effect on cardiovascular disease. There is a J-shaped curve such that, with moderation, there is a decrease in CVD death; but with increasing doses, there is increased death from all causes as well as from cardio-vascular diseases. Remember that increased alcohol consumption can have untoward medical and societal ramifications (i.e., hypertension, alcoholism, cirrhosis, suicide, decreased economic productivity). Therefore there is not enough benefit to recommend that patients increase their alcohol consumption simply to improve their cardiovascular risk profile.

Tobacco Abuse

Smoking is the leading cause of preventable death among older adults. Smoking leads to increases in blood pressure and heart rate as well as platelet activation and coronary plaque destabilization. Recommendations include the following:

- Ask patients about their tobacco use at every visit.
- In a clear, strong, and personalized manner, advise every tobacco user to quit.
- Assess the tobacco user's willingness to quit.
- Assist by counseling and developing a plan for quitting.
- Arrange follow-up, referral to special programs, or pharmacotherapy.
- Urge avoidance of exposure to secondhand smoke at work and at home.
- Consider the use of pharmacotherapy.
- Nicotine patch, nicotine gum, nicotine spray, or nicotine inhalers are available and have been shown to significantly increase the rate of cessation.
- **Bupropion** (Wellbutrin or Zyban), used alone or in combination with replacement therapy, has also been shown to increase cessation rates.
  - The standard regimen is 150 mg PO daily for 3 days, followed by 150 mg PO twice daily for 8 to 12 weeks. The patient is instructed to avoid smoking on day 5 to 7.
  - Bupropion is contraindicated in patients at risk for seizures.
- A newer agent, **varenicline** (Chantix), is used for 12 to 24 weeks and has shown promise in further decreasing the quit rate compared to bupropion or placebo.

CLINICAL/PHYSIOLOGIC RISK FACTORS

Cholesterol

Lowering low-density-lipoprotein cholesterol (LDL-C) is the primary focus in the man-agement of dyslipidemia. Initial attempts should begin with therapeutic lifestyle changes (TLCs) with dietary modifications (see above), increasing physical activity, and reducing weight. Unfortunately, many patients are unable to meet the goal LDL level and will require the addition of pharmacologic therapy. Multiple primary prevention trials have demonstrated the benefit of HMG-CoA reductase inhibitors (statins) in this population.

TABLE 10-4	CLINICAL EVALUATION TO IDENTIFY PERSONS WITH MULTIPLE RISK FACTORS	
Risk Factor	**Definition**	**Comments**
Cigarette smoking	Any cigarette smoking in the past month	
Hypertension	Blood pressure ≥140/90 mm Hg or taking antihypertensive medications	Multiple measures of blood pressure required for diagnosis (see JNC VI for further clinical evaluation)
Low HDL cholesterol	HDL cholesterol <40 mg/dL	
Family history of premature CHD	Clinical CHD or sudden death documented in 1st–degree male relative before age 55 or in	

Source: From the Expert Panel on Detection, Evaluation, and Treatment of High Blood Cholesterol in Adults. Executive Summary of the Third Report of the National Cholesterol Education Program (NCEP) Expert Panel on Detection, Evaluation, and Treatment of High Blood Cholesterol in Adults (Adult Treatment Panel III). *JAMA* 2001;285(19):2486–2497, with permission.

Initiation of lipid-modifying therapy depends upon risk assessment, as discussed above. The guidelines for therapy from the Adult Treatment Panel III (ATP III) are based on a nine-step evaluation process and include consideration for risk factors, baseline cholesterol, and initiation of therapeutic lifestyle changes. Tables 10-4 to 10-6 highlight recommendations from ATP III for cholesterol goals based on the number of risk factors present as well as overall risk as calculated by the Framingham risk score.

Hypertension

Detection of hypertension begins with proper blood pressure measurements, which should be obtained at each health care encounter. To measure blood pressure, the patient should

TABLE 10-5	LDL CHOLESTEROL GOALS FOR THREE RISK LEVELS
Risk Level	**LDL-C Goal**
CHD and CHD Risk Equivalent	<100 mg/dL
Multiple (2+) Risk Factors	<130 mg/dL*
0–1 Risk Factor	<160 mg/dL

*LDL-C Goal for multiple-risk factor persons with 10-year risk >20% = <100 mg/dL

Source: From the Expert Panel on Detection, Evaluation, and Treatment of High Blood Cholesterol in Adults. Executive Summary of the Third Report of the National Cholesterol Education Program (NCEP) Expert Panel on Detection, Evaluation, and Treatment of High Blood Cholesterol in Adults (Adult Treatment Panel III). *JAMA* 2001;285(19):2486–2497, with permission.

TABLE 10-6	MANAGEMENT OF LDL CHOLESTEROL IN PERSONS BEGINNING WITH 10-YEAR RISK ASSESSMENT		
10-Year Risk	LDL Goal	LDL Level at Which to Initiate TLC	LDL Level at Which to Consider Drug Therapy (After TLC)
>20%	<100 mg/dL	≥100 mg/dL	See CHD and CHD risk equivalent
10%–20%	<130 mg/dL	≥130 mg/dL	≥130 mg/dL
<10%:			
Multiple (2+) risk factors	<130 mg/dL	≥130 mg/dL	≥160 mg/dL
0–1 risk factor	<160 mg/dL	≥160 mg/dL	≥190 mg/dL*

*Drug therapy optional for LDL-C 160–189 mg/dL (after dietary therapy).

Source: From the Expert Panel on Detection, Evaluation, and Treatment of High Blood Cholesterol in Adults. Executive Summary of the Third Report of the National Cholesterol Education Program (NCEP) Expert Panel on Detection, Evaluation, and Treatment of High Blood Cholesterol in Adults (Adult Treatment Panel III). *JAMA* 2001;285(19):2486–2497, with permission.

be seated in a chair with the back supported and an arm bared and supported at heart level. Patients should refrain from smoking or ingesting caffeine during the 30 minutes preceding the measurement. Measurement should begin after ≥5 minutes of rest. The appropriate cuff size must be used to ensure accurate measurement. The bladder within the cuff should encircle ≥80% of the arm. Many adults will require a large adult cuff. Record systolic blood pressure, which is the first appearance of sound, and diastolic blood pressure, defined as the disappearance of sound. Two or more readings separated by 2 minutes should be averaged. If the first two readings differ by >5 mm Hg, obtain additional readings and average them. In addition to blood pressure assessment, the physical exam should include a funduscopic exam, vascular exam for bruits, cardiac exam for rhythm and extra heart sounds, lung exam for wheezes or crackles, abdominal exam for bruits or masses, peripheral pulse check, and neurologic exam.

Goal blood pressure is <140/90 mm Hg or <130/80 mm Hg if diabetes, renal insufficiency, or heart failure are present. Recommendations to achieve these goals are reviewed in Table 10-7.

Diabetes Mellitus

The leading cause of death in diabetics is ischemic heart disease. Moreover, the risk of a cardiac event in a diabetic patient is similar to that of a patient who already has symptomatic CAD; hence the ATP III guidelines consider diabetes to be a CAD risk equivalent. Sufficient data from several statin trials, including the diabetic subgroup from the Heart Protection Study and the CARDS trial, suggest that all patients over age 40 with type 2 diabetes benefit from statin therapy regardless of their baseline cholesterol (see Chapter 29).

Obesity

Obesity is associated with hyperlipidemia, hypertension, glucose intolerance, and insulin resistance. Waist-to-hip ratios and body mass index (BMI) have a linear association with CAD, but the waist-to-hip ratio has been found to be a more accurate predictor of CAD. Among obese individuals, those with central adiposity are at particularly high risk of CAD. A combination of diet and exercise is the mainstay of weight loss. Recommendations include:

TABLE 10-7   CLASSIFICATION AND MANAGEMENT OF BLOOD PRESSURE

BP Classification	Systolic BP, mm Hg*		Diastolic BP, mm Hg*	Management* Lifestyle Modification	Initial Drug Therapy Without Compelling Indication	Initial Drug Therapy With Compelling Indications
Normal	<120	and	<80	Encourage		
Prehypertension	120–139	or	80–89	Yes	No antihypertensive drug indicated	Drug(s) for the compelling indications[†]
Stage 1 hypertension	140–159	or	90–99	Yes	Thiazide-type diuretics for most; may consider ACE inhibitor. ARB, β-blocker, CCB, or combination	Drug(s) for the compelling indications Other antihypertensive drugs (duretics. ACE inhibitor, ARB, β-blocker, CCB) as needed
Stage 2 hypertension	≥160	or	≥100	Yes	2-Drug combination for most (usually thiazide-type diuretic and ACE inhibitor or ARB or β-blocker or CCB)[‡]	Drug(s) for the compelling indications Other antihypertensive drugs (diuretics, ACE inhibitor, ARB, β-blocker, CCB) as needed

Abbreviations ACE angiotensin converting enzyme: ARB, angiotensin receptor blocker, BP, blood pressure: CCB, calcium channel blocker.

*Treatment determined highest BP category.

[†]Treat patients with chronic kidney disease or diabetes to BP goal of less than 130/80 mm Hg.

[‡]Initial combined therapy should be used cautiously in those at risk for orthostatic hypotension.

Source: From Chobanian AV, Bakris GL, Black HR, et al., and the National Heart, Lung, and Blood Institute Joint National Committee on Prevention, Detection, Evaluation, and Treatment of High Blood Pressure; National High Blood Pressure Education Program Coordinating Committee. The Seventh Report of the Joint National Committee on Prevention, Detection, Evaluation, and Treatment of High Blood Pressure: the JNC 7 report. JAMA 2003;289(19):2560–2572, with permission.

- Initiation of a weight-management program through caloric restriction and increased caloric expenditure as appropriate.
- For overweight/obese persons, the goal is to reduce body weight by 10% in the first year of therapy.

The Metabolic Syndrome

The metabolic syndrome is characterized by a group of metabolic risk factors that are closely associated with insulin resistance. The underlying causes of this syndrome are overweight/obesity, physical inactivity, and genetic factors. People with the metabolic syndrome are at increased risk of CHD, other diseases related to plaque accumulation in artery walls (e.g., stroke and peripheral vascular disease), and type 2 diabetes.

There are no well-accepted criteria for diagnosing the metabolic syndrome. In fact, there remains some controversy about its very existence. The criteria proposed by the National Cholesterol Education Program (NCEP)/ATP III are the most current and widely used.

According to the ATP III criteria, the metabolic syndrome is identified by the presence of three or more of these components:

- Central obesity as measured by waist circumference:
  - Men ≥40 inches
  - Women ≥35 inches
- Fasting blood triglycerides ≥150 mg/dL
- Blood HDL cholesterol:
  - Men <40 mg/dL
  - Women <50 mg/dL
- Blood pressure ≥130/85 mm Hg
- Fasting glucose ≥100 mg/dL

Secondary Prevention

Recommendations

In 2006, the AHA and the American College of Cardiology (ACC) published a consensus statement on secondary prevention incorporating evidence from clinical trials that emerged since the previous set of guidelines in 2001. It affirmed and broadened the merits of aggressive risk-reduction therapies for patients with established coronary and other atherosclerotic vascular disease, including peripheral arterial disease, aortic disease, and carotid artery disease. This growing body of evidence confirms that aggressive comprehensive risk-factor management improves survival, reduces recurrent events and the need for interventional procedures, and improves quality of life for these patients (Table 10-8).

Aspirin plays an important role in both primary and secondary prevention. It is indicated in patients with a 10-year risk of myocardial infarction (MI) that is >10% and in women over the age of 65. It is not indicated for primary prevention in a patient without risk factors for CVD.

Special Topics in Secondary Prevention

Lipid Management. In 2004 and 2006, updated recommendations were issued that incorporated data on cholesterol management in the high-risk patient. In the **very** high risk patient, an optional goal is treatment to an LDL <70 mg/dL. Very high risk patients are those with established CVD and multiple risk factors (especially diabetes), severe and poorly controlled risk factors (e.g., cigarette smoking), metabolic syndrome (high triglycerides,

TABLE 10-8	SUMMARY OF AHA/ACC RECOMMENDATIONS FOR SECONDARY PREVENTION OF CAD

Risk Factor	Goal
Smoking	Complete cessation. No exposure to environmental smoke.
Blood pressure	<140/80 mm Hg. <130/80 if patient has DM or chronic kidney disease.
Lipid management	LDL-C <100 mg/dL and <70 mg/dL in some very high risk patients (see below).
Physical activity	30 minutes 7 days per week (minimum 5 days).
Weight management	Body mass index 18.5 to 24.9 kg/m^2 Waist circumference: men <40 inches, women <35 inches.
Diabetes management	HbA1C <7%.
Antiplatelet agents/ anticoagulants	ASA 75 to 162 mg/day in all patients unless contraindicated. Clopidogrel 75 mg/day with ASA 162 mg/day in all patients with ACS. Length of therapy and dose of ASA determined by presence and/or type of revascularization (see Chapters 7 and 8).
Renin-angiotensin-aldosterone system blockers	ACE inhibitors: All patients, especially those with left ventricular ejection fraction <40% and in those with hypertension, diabetes, or chronic kidney disease unless contraindicated Angiotensin receptor blockers: Patients who are intolerant of ACE inhibitors and have heart failure or have had a myocardial infarction with left ventricular ejection fraction <40%; consider in other patients who are ACE inhibitor–intolerant. Aldosterone blockade: Post–myocardial infarction patients without significant renal dysfunction or hyperkalemia who are already receiving therapeutic doses of an ACE inhibitor and beta blocker, have a left ventricular ejection fraction <40%, and have either diabetes or heart failure.
Beta blockers	All patients who have had myocardial infarction, acute coronary syndrome, or left ventricular dysfunction with or without heart failure symptoms unless contraindicated. Consider chronic therapy for all other patients with coronary or other vascular disease or diabetes unless contraindicated.
Influenza vaccine	All patients with cardiovascular disease.

Source: From Smith SC Jr, Allen J, Blair SN, et al., and the AHA/ACC/NHLBI. AHA/ACC guidelines for secondary prevention for patients with coronary and other atherosclerotic vascular disease: 2006 update: endorsed by the National Heart, Lung, and Blood Institute. *Circulation* 2006;113(19): 2363–2372, with permission.

TABLE 10-9	ATP III LDL-C GOALS AND CUTPOINTS FOR TLC AND DRUG THERAPY IN DIFFERENT RISK CATEGORIES AND PROPOSED MODIFICATIONS BASED ON RECENT CLINICAL TRIAL EVIDENCE		
Risk Category	LDL-C Goal	Initiate TLC	Consider Drug Therapy
High risk: CHD or CHD risk equivalents (10-year risk >20%)	<100 mg/dL (optional goal: <70 mg/dL)‖	≥100 mg/dL	≥100 mg/dL (<100 mg/dL: consider drug options)
Moderately high risk: 2 + risk factors (10-year risk 10% to 20%)§§	<130 mg/dL	≥130 mg/dL	≥130 mg/dL (100–129 mg/dL: consider drug options)
Moderate risk: 2 + risk factor (10-year risk <10%)	<130 mg/dL	≥130 mg/dL	≥160 mg/dL
Lower risk: 0–1risk factor	<160 mg/dL	≥160 mg/dL	≥190 mg/dL (160–189 mg/dL: LDL-lowering drug optional)

Source: From Grundy SM, Cleeman JI, Merz CN, et al. Coordinating Committee of the National Cholesterol Education Program. Implications of recent clinical trials for the National Cholesterol Education Program Adult Treatment Panel III Guidelines. *J Am Coll Cardiol* 2004;44(3):720–732, with permission.

low HDL-C), or acute coronary syndromes. These recommendations and others are shown in Table 10-9. Additional recommendations include the following:

- When the target of LDL-C <70 mg/dL is chosen, it may be prudent to increase statin therapy in a graded fashion to determine a patient's response and tolerance.
- If it is not possible to attain LDL-C <70 mg/dL because of a high baseline LDL-C, it is generally possible to achieve LDL-C reductions of >50% with either statins or LDL-C–lowering drug combinations.
- The recommendation of a level of <70 mg/dL LDL-C does not apply to other types of lower-risk individuals who do not have coronary heart disease (CHD) or other forms of atherosclerotic disease; in such cases, recommendations contained in the 2004 ATP III update still pertain.

Cardiac Rehabilitation. Comprehensive cardiac rehabilitation services include long-term programs involving medical evaluation, prescribed exercise, cardiac risk-factor modification, education, and counseling. These programs are designed to limit the physiologic and psychological effects of cardiac illness, reduce the risk of sudden death or reinfarction, control cardiac symptoms, and enhance the psychosocial and vocational status of selected patients. Enrollment in a cardiac rehabilitation program after discharge can enhance patient education and compliance with the medical regimen and assist with the implementation of a regular exercise program. Exercise training can generally begin within 1 to 2 weeks after unstable angina/non–ST-segment-elevation myocardial infarction

TABLE 10-10 EXERCISE PRESCRIPTIONS FOR CAD PATIENTS

Patients	Intensity	Frequency	Duration
Aerobic Exercise			
General CAD	70%–85% peak HR	≥3 times weekly	≥20 minutes per session
With asymptomatic ischemia	70%–85% ischemic HR	≥3 times weekly	≥20 minutes per session
With angina	70%–85% ischemic HR or angina onset	≥3 times weekly	≥20 minutes per session
With angioplasty ± stent	As for general CAD patient		
With claudication	Walking to pain tolerance	≥3 times weekly	≥30 minutes per session
With NYHA class I-III HF	As for general CAD patient		
Resistance Exercise			
For most CAD patients	30%–50% RM	2–3 times weekly	12–15 repetitions

RM indicates 1-repetition maximal weight.

Source: From Thompson PD. Exercise prescription and proscription for patients with coronary artery disease. *Circulation* 2005 Oct 11;112(15):2354–2363, with permission.

(UA/NSTEMI) treated with percutaneous coronary intervention (PCI) or coronary artery bypass grafting (CABG) to relieve ischemia. Unsupervised exercise may target a heart rate range of 60% to 75% of maximal heart rate; supervised training may target a somewhat higher heart rate (70%–85% of maximal heart rate). Additional restrictions apply when residual ischemia is present (see Table 10-10).

Patients with CAD should undergo symptom-limited exercise testing before referral to an exercise program to establish a baseline exercise ability, determine maximal heart rate, and exclude important ischemia, symptoms, or arrhythmias that would alter the therapeutic approach. This testing should be performed with the patient on his or her usual medications to match the conditions likely to be encountered during the exercise sessions.

The simplest approach for clinicians prescribing exercise for patients with CAD is to refer them to an established cardiac rehabilitation program. Patients in such programs exercise three times a week for $\geq$30 minutes, including 5 minutes of warmup and cool-down calisthenics and $\geq$20 minutes of exercise at an intensity requiring 70% to 85% of the predetermined peak heart rate ($\sim$60%–75% of VO_2max). Most rehabilitation programs recommend other activities such as light yard work or brisk walking on other days.

Patients in medically supervised and unsupervised programs should include some resistance exercises in their training regimens. These exercises should be performed at least twice weekly with dumbbells light enough to permit 12 to 15 repetitions of each exercise.

Hormone Replacement Therapy. For several years it was thought that hormone replacement therapy was protective against cardiovascular events in postmenopausal women. However, both the HERS (secondary prevention) study and the Women's Health Initiative (primary prevention) showed higher rates of cardiovascular events. Therefore, the AHA guidelines in 2007 recommend that hormone replacement therapy *not* be used for primary or secondary prevention of CAD in women.

Antibiosis. Epidemiologic and animal studies suggest a relationship between *Chlamydia pneumoniae* and atherogenesis. In a secondary prevention study in patients with stable CAD, there was no difference in cardiac events between groups that were given either azithromycin weekly or placebo for 1 year. Antibiotics, therefore, have no specific role in the secondary prevention of CAD.

Additional Risk Factors

There are numerous additional risk factors for CVD that are currently under investigation, including:

- **C-reactive protein (hs-CRP)**, a marker of systemic inflammation that has been shown to be an independent risk factor for cardiovascular events. Guidelines for cutoffs for risk assessment include <1 mg/L (low risk), 1 to 3 mg/L (average risk), and >3 mg/L (high risk). Levels >10 mg/L are not helpful and suggest an alternate cause of inflammation. **In primary prevention**, CRP is useful in patients with an intermediate cardiac risk (i.e., those with a Framingham estimated 10-year cardiovascular risk between 10%–20%). These patients may benefit from more intensive risk-factor modification. **In secondary prevention**, elevated CRP indicates higher risk, but no specific recommendations as to therapeutic implications can yet be made.
- **Lipoprotein(a)** is a genetic variation of LDL, and elevated levels (>30 mg/dL) pose a risk for developing premature atherosclerosis. The exact mechanism of this is unclear. Checking these levels is not part of routine screening.
- **Homocysteine** is a product of folate metabolism. Elevated levels (>15 µmol/L) are associated with an increased risk of vascular disease. Data suggest that reducing levels of homocysteine through folate treatment may reduce the rate of coronary restenosis after angioplasty.

- High levels of **fibrinogen** (>350 mg/dL) are associated with increased risk of MI and stroke. There is no drug therapy, but smoking cessation, moderate alcohol intake, and exercise can decrease levels.
- The presence of **coronary calcium** (see Chapter 26) correlates with the presence of atherosclerotic disease. A calcium score of zero has a strong negative predictive value. A high calcium score is associated with an increased risk of cardiovascular events. Currently, calcium screening by electron-beam computed tomography is best used in the intermediate-risk population.

KEY POINTS TO REMEMBER

- Primary prevention is prevention of the atherosclerotic process that leads to heart disease; secondary prevention is the prevention of death and/or progression of heart disease in patients who already have coronary atherosclerosis.
- Assess for cardiac risk factors to tailor your therapeutic recommendations.
- One useful method of assessing risk is to use the Framingham risk assessment, which helps stratify patients into low-, intermediate-, and high-risk categories.
- In intermediate-risk patients, there are additional noninvasive tests (hs-CRP, coronary calcium screening, etc.) that can be useful to further assess risk and help therapeutic recommendations.
- Identify the patient at risk for CAD and aggressively treat all modifiable and clinical risk factors.
- Cardiac rehabilitation is appropriate for patients after an MI, percutaneous revascularization, or bypass as well as for those with stable angina.

REFERENCES AND SUGGESTED READINGS

American Heart Association. Heart Disease and Stroke Statistics—2005 Update. Dallas: American Heart Association, 2005.

Brook RD, Greenland P. Secondary prevention. In Wong ND, Black HR, Gardin JM, eds. *Preventive Cardiology: A Practical Approach.* New York: McGraw-Hill; 2005:515–542.

Chobanian, AV et al. The Seventh Report of the Joint National Committee on Prevention, Detection, Evaluation, and Treatment of High Blood Pressure: the JNC 7 Report. *JAMA* 2003;289:2560–2571.

Expert Panel on Detection, Evaluation, and Treatment of High Blood Cholesterol in Adults. Executive Summary of the Third Report of the National Cholesterol Education Program (NCEP) Expert Panel on Detection, Evaluation, and Treatment of High Blood Cholesterol in Adults (Adult Treatment Panel III). *JAMA* 2001;285:2486–2497.

Grayston JT, Kronmal RA, Jackson LA, et al. Azithromycin for the secondary prevention of coronary events. *N Engl J Med* 2005;352:1637–1645.

Grundy SM et al. Implications of recent clinical trials for the National Cholesterol Education Program Adult Treatment Panel III Guidelines, *J Am Coll Cardiol* 2004;44:720–732.

Haskell WL, Lee I-M, Pate RP, et al. Physical activity and public health: updated recommendation for adults from the American College of Sports Medicine and the American Heart Association. *Circulation* 2007;116:1081–1093.

Hobbs, FD. Cardiovascular disease: different strategies for primary and secondary prevention? *Heart* 2004;90:1217–1223.

Lichtenstein, AH et al. Diet and Lifestyle Recommendations Revision 2006: A Scientific Statement from the American Heart Association Nutrition Committee. *Circulation* 2006;114:82–96.

Mosca L et al. Evidence-based guidelines for cardiovascular disease prevention in women: 2007 update. *Circulation* 2007;115:1–21.

Pearson TA et al. AHA/ACC Guidelines for Secondary Prevention for Patients With Coronary and Other Atherosclerotic Vascular Disease: 2006 Update. Consensus Panel Guide to Comprehensive Risk Reduction for Adult Patients Without Coronary or Other Atherosclerotic Vascular Diseases. *Circulation* 2002;106:388–391.

Smith SC, Allen J, Blair SN, et al. AHA/ACC guidelines for secondary prevention for patients with coronary and other atherosclerotic vascular disease: 2006 update. *Circulation* 2006;113:2363–2372.

Taubert D, Roesen R, Lehmann C, et al. Effects of low habitual cocoa intake on blood pressure and bioactive nitric oxide. *JAMA* 2007;298(1):49–60.

Thompson PD. Exercise prescription and proscription for patients with coronary artery disease. *Circulation* 2005;112;2354–2363.

Wilson MA, Pearsion TA. Primary prevention. In Wong ND, Black HR, Gardin JM, eds. *Preventive Cardiology: A Practical Approach.* New York: McGraw-Hill; 2005: 493–514.

Wilson PWF et al. Prediction of coronary heart disease using risk factor categories. *Circulation* 1998;97:1837–1847.

Management of Acute and Chronic Heart Failure

11

Joel D. Schilling

BACKGROUND

Heart failure (HF) is reaching an epidemic level in the United States. The societal and medical impact of this disorder is likely to continue to grow over the next several decades, given the increasing prevalence of diabetes and hypertension and the aging population. Early recognition and treatment of HF risk factors can curb the expected rise in HF incidence. In addition, the appropriate utilization of evidence-based therapies for acute and chronic HF will be a critical component to improve patient survival and to reduce hospitalizations.

Epidemiology

More than 5 million people in the United States currently have HF, with an estimated 550,000 new diagnoses each year. Despite significant advances in the management of HF, 1- and 5-year mortality is ~30% and 50%, respectively. Of interest, almost half of all patients admitted to the hospital for HF have preserved systolic function (PSF), indicating the clinical importance of this disease entity. Fewer than 5% of patients with HF present with hypotension or cardiogenic shock.

Pathophysiology

Regardless of the initial insult leading to myocardial injury (ischemia, hypertension, viral infection, etc.) a stereotypical pathologic remodeling response occurs. Over time, this negative remodeling leads to progressive cardiac enlargement and deterioration in cardiac function. The current and most accepted explanation for the progression of HF is referred to as the **neurohormonal model of HF.** This theory states that the reduction in cardiac output seen with myocardial dysfunction leads to the activation of compensatory neurohormonal pathways such as the renin-angiotensin-aldosterone system (RAAS) and the sympathetic nervous system. The initial function of these responses is to maintain cardiac output by increasing ventricular filling pressures (preload) and myocardial contractility. However, over time, high levels of angiotensin II, aldosterone, and catecholamines lead to progressive myocardial fibrosis and apoptosis. This secondary injury promotes a further decline in cardiac function and contributes to the increased risk of arrhythmias. The neurohormonal model of HF is the basis for the most effective treatments used for HF management today.

PREVENTION

Many patients with clinically evident HF had preexisting and treatable conditions that increased their probability of developing this disorder. Early treatment and prevention of left ventricular (LV) dysfunction is possible by identifying and treating high-risk individuals. Factors that increase the chance of developing HF are age, hypertension, diabetes, coronary artery disease (CAD), a strong family history of cardiomyopathy, and exposure to cardiotoxins. **The critical modifiable risk factors are diabetes, hypertension, and CAD; aggressive treatment of these entities is paramount.**

- Hypertension (HTN) is present in ~66% of patients with HF and treatment significantly reduces the incidence of HF.
- Diabetes is associated with a two- to fivefold increased risk of developing HF independent of CAD. The term **"diabetic cardiomyopathy"** is used to describe the abnormal diastolic function (with or without systolic abnormalities) seen in diabetics. Up to 33% of patients hospitalized for HF have diabetes.
- CAD accounts for ~60% of patients with systolic dysfunction.

DIAGNOSTIC TESTING

Chapter 4 discusses the clinical presentations of HF. The diagnosis of an acute HF syndrome is based on history, physical exam, laboratory data, and imaging findings. The first stage of the evaluation is focused on confirming the diagnosis of HF and stabilizing the patient. The second stage is directed towards determining the etiology of the patient's HF.

The first stage typically begins in the emergency department when the patient presents with significant dyspnea and/or evidence of volume overload. **A reasonable diagnostic plan is found in Figure 11-1.** An electrocardiogram (**ECG**) should be obtained rapidly to look for evidence of ischemia, infarct, or arrhythmias. Early chest x-ray (**CXR**) is important to assess for evidence of pulmonary edema or cardiomegaly and rule other causes of dyspnea (pneumonia, pneumothorax). It is important to remember that up to 40% of chronic HF patients with significant elevations in pulmonary capillary wedge pressure will have no radiographic evidence of congestion. In some instances, an **urgent echocardiogram** should be performed to assess LV function and rule out acute valvular disease (new murmur) or tamponade (hypotension, low voltage and/or electrical alternans on ECG, bottle-shaped heart on CXR, history of malignancy or viral illness).

Laboratory data also plays an important role in the early assessment of acute HF. The primary questions to address with the initial blood work include: Is there evidence of **cardiac ischemia**? What is the patient's **renal function**? Does the patient have **anemia or leukocytosis**? The presence of an elevated troponin may signify an acute coronary syndrome; however, mild troponin elevations can occur even in the absence of epicardial coronary disease. In either case, the presence of an elevated troponin signifies myocardial injury and identifies a high-risk subset of HF patients.

In addition to the standard labs, a **brain natriuretic peptide (BNP)** level may be helpful, particularly if the **dyspnea is of unclear etiology**. BNP is a small polypeptide released by myocytes in response to increased wall stress. Systemic levels of BNP correlate with invasive intracardiac pressure measurements and are a reliable marker of volume status. However, BNP specificity is reduced in patients with renal dysfunction, and the sensitivity is reduced in obese patients. A BNP level >400 is consistent with HF. Levels ranging from 100–400 may represent underlying left ventricular (LV) dysfunction; however, other diseases such as acute pulmonary embolism must be considered.

In some cases, placement of a pulmonary artery (PA) catheter can help guide therapy. A PA catheter should be considered for patients who present with hypotension and evidence of shock. Invasive hemodynamic data can direct the use of inotropes and pressors

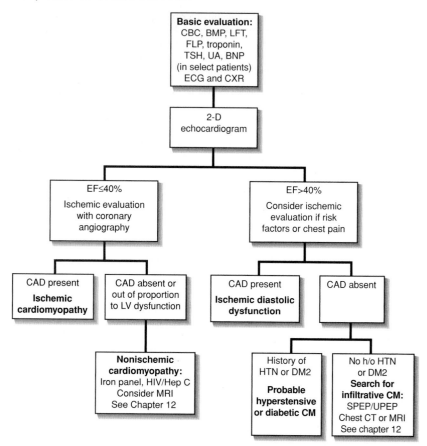

FIGURE 11-1. Diagnostic evaluation of new-onset heart failure.

and can help with volume assessment (Table 11-1). However, the ESCAPE trial demonstrated that routine PA catheter placement does not alter mortality or length of hospital stay in acute decompensated HF. Therefore, placement of a **PA catheter should be reserved for hemodynamically unstable patients or for those not responding to empiric inotrope or diuretic therapy.**

Once the patient is hemodynamically stable, the focus of the evaluation shifts to the diagnostic workup (Fig. 11-1). For patients presenting with new-onset HF, the goal is to determine the etiology of their cardiac dysfunction. A **2D echocardiogram** provides information regarding systolic and diastolic function, valvular disease, left ventricular hypertrophy (LVH), asymmetric septal hypertrophy, and pericardial disease and provides an estimation of pulmonary artery systolic pressure. Further evaluation is directed by the presence or absence of systolic dysfunction. **Patients with new systolic dysfunction should undergo an ischemic evaluation.** For patients with multiple cardiac risk factors, chest pain, and/or segmental wall motion abnormalities on echocardiography, cardiac catheterization is preferred. Coronary angiography or stress testing can be utilized in patients without CAD risk factors or a history of chest pain. Revascularization via

TABLE 11-1	INTERPRETING HEMODYNAMIC DATA IN THE HEART FAILURE PATIENT WITH A PA CATHETER					
Cardiac Index (2.5–4.5 L/min/m^2)	CVP (5–8 mm Hg)	Mean PAP (15–25 mm Hg)	PCWP (5–10 mm Hg)	SBP (100–120 mm Hg)	SVR (800–1200 dynes/sec × cm^{-5})	Diagnosis and Management
↓	↓	↓ or normal	↓	↓	↑	D: Hypovolemia M: IV fluids
↓	↑	↑	↑	↑ or normal	↑↑	D: HF with high vascular tone M: Vasodilators/afterload reduction
↓	↑	↑	↑	↓	↑↑	D: HF with poor systemic perfusion M: Inotropes, diuretics
↓	↑	↑	↑	↓↓	↑	D: HF with shock M: Inotrope, vasopressors, mechanical support
↑↓ or normal	↓ or normal	↓ or normal	↓ or normal	↓	↓	D: Distributive shock (sepsis) M: IV fluids, vasopressors, antibiotics
↓	↑	↑	↓	↓	↑	D: Pulmonary HTN, Right heart failure M: Inotropes, pulmonary vasodilators

CVP, central venous pressure; HF, heart failure; HTN, hypertension; PAP, pulmonary artery pressure; PCWP, pulmonary capillary wedge pressure; SBP, systolic blood pressure; SVR, systemic vascular resistance. Normal values in parentheses.

percutaneous intervention or coronary artery bypass grafting is indicated in patients with reduced ejection fraction (EF) and viable myocardium.

In the absence of significant CAD, **additional blood work** should include an iron panel, a test for human immunodeficiency virus (HIV), and hepatitis C testing (in at-risk individuals). Routine testing for viral infections is not recommended as the results do not alter therapy. However, if performed, the most common viruses associated with myocarditis include coxsackie B, adenovirus, cytomegalovirus (CMV), echovirus, HIV, hepatitis C, and parvovirus B19. In patients with physical findings consistent with a rheumatologic disease, additional testing such as an antinuclear antibody (ANA) and/or antineutrophil cytoplasmic antibody (ANCA) titer can be checked. If the patient has episodic hypertension, tachycardia, and/or headaches, pheochromocytoma should be ruled out. Consideration can be given to genetic testing and counseling if a strong family history of cardiomyopathy is present. Ultimately, up to 40%–50% of patients will have no identifiable etiology of their HF and are classified as idiopathic (see Chapter 12).

For patients who have HF with PSF, the diagnostic workup is slightly different. An ischemic evaluation should be considered, particularly if the patient has ECG changes, elevated troponin, or significant chest pain. Blood glucose testing and assessment of hypertension history is mandatory as diabetes and hypertension are significant risk factors for diastolic cardiac dysfunction. In patients without diabetes or hypertension, a restrictive cardiomyopathy or constrictive pericarditis should be considered. Findings concerning for an infiltrative process include left ventricular hypertrophy (LVH) on echocardiography with low voltage on the ECG, an elevated protein gap, and proteinuria. Laboratory testing should include an serum protein electrophoresis (SPEP)/urine protein electrophoresis (UPEP) and an iron panel. Endomyocardial biopsy and/or magnetic resonance imaging (MRI) can play a role. In patients with a history of previous pericarditis, cardiac surgery, or exposure to chest radiation, a computed tomography (CT) scan or MRI should be performed to look for pericardial thickening. Pericardial constriction can be further assessed hemodynamically via a simultaneous right and left heart catheterization (see Chapter 13). In patients with recurrent episodes of significant HTN and pulmonary edema, it is reasonable to assess for renal artery stenosis with ultrasound or MRA.

TREATMENT

Acute Decompensated HF

The treatment goals during a hospitalization for acute decompensated HF (ADHF) are: (1) **to improve patient symptoms,** (2) **correct hemodynamic and volume status,** (3) **minimize renal and cardiac injury,** and (4) **initiate lifesaving medical therapies.** The treatment strategies for ADHF continue to evolve, as very few randomized controlled trials have been performed to guide therapy. Therefore many of the current recommendations are based more on professional opinion and experience rather than on evidence-based medicine. As discussed in Chapter 4, patients presenting with acute heart failure syndromes can be divided into subgroups based on their clinical presentation (Fig. 11-2).

Acute Pulmonary Edema and Hypertension
Up to 50% of patients with ADHF present with an elevated blood pressure and acute pulmonary edema. **The immediate goal is to stabilize respiratory status by lowering blood pressure and removing fluid from the lungs.** These patients should receive oxygen, IV vasodilators, and IV diuretics. As high vascular tone rather than marked volume overload characterizes this presentation, vasodilators are more important than diuretics to rapidly lower cardiac filling pressures and improve patient symptoms. The VMAC study is one of the few randomized controlled trials evaluating vasodilator therapy in patients with ADHF. In this study, both nitroglycerin and nesiritide infusions were effective at reducing patient symptoms and cardiac filling pressures compared to diuretics alone; however, nesiritide infusion led to a more rapid and sustained improvement in these parameters. Thirty-day mortality was not significantly different between the treatment arms. These short-term data and clinician experience have led to the recommendation that one of these two vasodilator medications be used in the treatment of patients with acute pulmonary edema. Importantly, the dose of nitroglycerin required to induce a significant hemodynamic effect on pulmonary capillary wedge pressure (PCWP) was >100 μg/minute. Nitroprusside can also be considered. Renal dysfunction with nesiritide has been a concern; however, recent studies in the operative and outpatient settings showed no evidence of increased renal failure with this medication. Additional studies of nesiritide for ADHF are ongoing.

In addition to vasodilators, diuretics are useful for reducing preload and improving patient volume status and symptoms. An initial dose of IV furosemide (Lasix) should be administered. However, overaggressive diuresis can lead to renal dysfunction. IV morphine

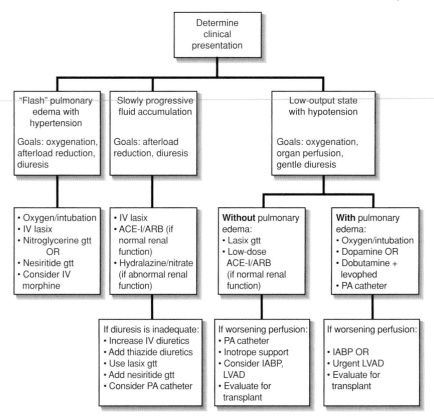

FIGURE 11-2. General approach to the management of acute decompensated heart failure (ADHF).

can also be considered in these patients, as it has venodilating properties and can reduce anxiety. If the respiratory status remains tenuous, noninvasive positive-pressure ventilation (BiPAP) or intubation may be necessary to improve oxygenation until the hemodynamic and volume status can be improved. Rapid assessment to rule out acute valvular disease or ischemia is indicated, as these patients may benefit from early surgery or revascularization, respectively.

Slowly Progressive Volume Overload
In patients with volume overload without respiratory distress, the primary goal is to **maximize afterload reduction and remove excess fluid without promoting kidney dysfunction**. Angiotensin converting enzyme (ACE)-inhibitor therapy should be initiated or continued if renal function is not significantly impaired (Cr <2.0–2.5 mg/dL) and the potassium level is not ≥5.0 mEq/L. If the patient is ACE inhibitor–naïve, it is reasonable to start with a short-acting agent such as captopril. Prior to discharge, patients should be transitioned to a long-acting ACE inhibitor. In the setting of impaired renal function (Cr >2.0–2.5 mg/dL) or hyperkalemia (K ≥5.0 mEq/L), a combination of hydralazine and nitrates can be used for afterload reduction. If renal function improves or stabilizes prior to discharge, patients should be initiated on an ACE inhibitor or angiotensin receptor blocker (ARB).

With diuretic therapy, the goal is to remove between 1.5 and 3.0 L/day, depending on the degree of volume overload. As an initial strategy, bolus IV furosemide is reasonable. For patients on home oral furosemide, administer the same dose IV and assess response (for example, 40 mg PO twice daily can become 40 mg IV twice daily). If the diuresis is inadequate, then the IV dose can be increased or a thiazide diuretic can be added. The addition of a thiazide diuretic can cause profound potassium and magnesium depletion, so aggressive monitoring and repletion are mandatory. If the patient is still resistant to diuretic therapy, then a furosemide or nesiritide infusion can be considered. The presence of continued difficulties with fluid mobilization and/or progressive renal dysfunction should lead to the PA catheter placement and/or the use of inotropes or ultrafiltration. The routine use of inotropes in ADHF was challenged by the OPTIME trial where milrinone infusion did not improve diuresis, but did lead to an increase in adverse events. In addition, the ADHERE database shows an association between inotrope use and worse clinical outcomes. Therefore inotropes should be reserved for patients with reduced cardiac output, refractory edema, and evidence of end-organ hypoperfusion.

In addition to diuretic therapy, maintenance of a 2-g sodium diet and fluid restriction to 1.5 to 2 L is important to attain euvolemia. This is particularly true if the patient is hyponatremic.

Low-Output State ± Volume Overload

Patients who present with ADHF and evidence of hypoperfusion represent <5% of hospital admissions for HF. However, these patients are generally the sickest and are often in overt cardiogenic shock. Acute renal failure, elevated liver enzymes, metabolic acidosis, and peripheral vasoconstriction are common. This situation is most frequently encountered in the setting of an acute MI, acute myocarditis, or at the end stage of a chronic cardiomyopathy. **Patients in early or overt cardiogenic shock require rapid triage and admission to an ICU for stabilization**. Urgent revascularization may be required if the underlying cause of the shock state is an acute MI.

If the systolic blood pressure is between 80 and 100 mm Hg, empiric treatment with dobutamine or milrinone can often help improve end-organ perfusion and facilitate diuresis. A continuous furosemide infusion is often the most effective means to remove fluid from such patients without promoting further hypotension. If the patients fail to respond to empiric therapy quickly, right heart catheterization is warranted.

In the situation where the systolic blood pressure is <80 mm Hg, patients are unlikely to tolerate the hypotension that dobutamine or milrinone can cause. Options include dopamine or the combination of low-dose norepinephrine (Levophed) with dobutamine or milrinone. These patients should receive a PA catheter to direct therapy, as their hemodynamic status is very precarious (Table 11-1). A significant percentage of patients in shock will require additional mechanical support, which includes an intra-aortic balloon pump (IABP) or a LV assist device (LVAD). For critically ill patients who are poor surgical candidates, the TandemHeart percutaneous LVAD (Cardiac Assist, Inc.; Pittsburgh, PA) has been shown to have superior hemodynamic effects compared to the IABP.

In-Hospital Monitoring

It is critical to continually reassess the patient's volume status throughout the hospitalization, which is done by monitoring daily weights, fluid intake and urine output, and physical exam findings (jugular venous pulse, edema). A basic metabolic panel should also be checked daily to monitor electrolytes and renal function. Additionally, close attention should be paid to the BUN and HCO_3 levels as they often climb with intravascular volume contraction. This is a sign to decrease the intensity of diuretic therapy before overt renal dysfunction develops. Prior to discharge, patients should be transitioned to a stable oral diuretic regimen. In general, the lowest dose of diuretic needed to maintain euvolemia should be used.

Transition to Outpatient Management

The key components to long-term success in HF management are patient education, optimal medical and device therapy, and adequate patient follow-up. The inpatient hospitalization provides an opportunity to ensure these issues are addressed. The **ABCs checklist for hospital discharge** is a useful device:

- **A:** ACE inhibitor or ARB
- **B:** Beta blocker
- **C:** Counseling (smoking cessation, exercise)
- **D:** Dietary education (low-sodium diet, fluid restriction), device therapy (if appropriate)
- **E:** Euvolemia achieved
- **F:** Follow-up appointment established

Since patients' symptoms often improve rapidly with diuresis and afterload reduction, it can be tempting to discharge patients prior to achieving optimal volume status and transitioning to a stable oral regimen. This results in increased rates of readmission for recurrent volume overload or overdiuresis. Before patients are discharged, they should be euvolemic and off all IV medications.

Chronic HF

The treatment goals for chronic HF are different than those for ADHF and include (1) **reduction of mortality,** (2) **improvement of symptoms,** and (3) **reduction of hospitalizations.** Also, unlike the case for ADHF, there are several large randomized, controlled trials that guide management decisions for patients with chronic HF. As an understanding of these trials is critical to the implementation of proper medical treatment, they are included herein. Patients with chronic HF can be classified both by disease stage and NYHA functional class (Fig. 4-1).

For patients with stage A HF, the primary goal is risk-factor reduction in an effort to prevent the development of HF. Stage B patients have preclinical HF, and the use of an ACE inhibitor or ARB and beta blocker should be started to delay the progression of adverse myocardial remodeling. Once patients progress to stage C HF, controlling symptoms and reducing hospitalizations becomes a larger focus. Optimal doses of ACE inhibitor or ARB and beta blocker are mandatory; however, certain patients will also benefit from aldosterone antagonists (spironolactone, eplerenone), digoxin, and oral diuretics. Implantable device therapy [implantable cardiac defibrillator (ICD), cardiac resynchronization therapy (CRT)] should be considered in appropriate patients with stage C HF. Stage D HF represents the end-stage of the cardiomyopathic process. These patients generally have severe physical limitations and markedly reduced survival secondary to their cardiac disease. Hypotension and renal dysfunction often limit attempts at afterload reduction and beta blockade. In some instances, cardiac transplantation or LVAD implantation is appropriate. In other patients, relieving symptoms and avoiding hospitalization may be the primary goals; therefore continuous inotrope infusion and/or hospice care may be reasonable. In patients who are not candidates for more aggressive HF therapy, discussions regarding end-of-life issues, including turning off ICD therapy, should be undertaken.

ACE Inhibitors and ARBs

ACE inhibitors have become the cornerstone of medical treatment for patients with systolic dysfunction. Although known for their blood pressure–lowering effects, much of the benefit of ACE inhibitors in HF comes from their action in blocking the effects of angiotensin II by inhibiting its formation. Angiotensin II is a potent vasoconstrictor that also stimulates profibrotic and proinflammatory pathways and promotes adverse myocardial remodeling. V-HEFT 2 was the first clinical trial of ACE inhibitors in HF. In this study, enalapril therapy led to a 28% decrease in mortality as compared with hydralazine/nitrate therapy despite similar levels of blood pressure control. Several subsequent randomized trials have established the benefit of ACE inhibitors in patients with chronic LV dysfunction (SOLVD, CONSENSUS) and with post-MI LV dysfunction (SAVE, TRACE, AIRE). ACE inhibitors were **consistently associated with a mortality reduction of** ~20%–25% at 1 to 5 years. When initiating an ACE inhibitor, low doses should be used at first and then gradually titrated upward. Plasma creatinine and potassium should be checked at 1 to 2 weeks after initiation or uptitration of an ACE inhibitor. Small increases in creatinine (up to 30%) are common and should not prompt discontinuation of therapy. Side effects include cough (~10%), hyperkalemia, hypotension, renal insufficiency, angioedema, and teratogenicity.

ARBs act downstream of ACE inhibitors by inhibiting the type-1 angiotensin receptor, thereby attenuating the biologic effects of angiotensin II. The largest clinical trials of ARBs in patients with chronic HF are Val-HEFT and CHARM. Both of these studies showed that ARBs were equivalent to ACE inhibitors with regard to HF mortality reduction. Similar findings were seen in VALIANT for patients with LV dysfunction post-MI. **Therefore ARBs are an acceptable alternative for patients who are ACE inhibitor–intolerant (usually secondary to cough).** ARBs should be initiated in a similar manner to ACE inhibitors. The expected side effects are the same as with ACE inhibitors with the exception of cough, which is not seen with ARB therapy.

Given their distinct mechanisms of action, it was hypothesized that combination therapy with an ACE inhibitor and an ARB could further improve outcomes in HF patients. This theory was investigated in CHARM-added, a subgroup from Val-HEFT, and VALIANT. In CHARM-added, combination ACE inhibitor/ARB reduced HF hospitalizations and cardiac mortality by 15% compared with ACE inhibitor monotherapy. In contrast, the addition of ARB to ACE inhibitor in VALIANT and Val-HEFT failed to improve clinical outcomes. Moreover, hypotension and hyperkalemia were increased with combination therapy. At present, combination therapy can be considered in stable HF patients already on goal doses of an ACE inhibitor and beta blocker who have stable renal function. Frequent monitoring for hyperkalemia is mandatory. Triple therapy with an ACE inhibitor, ARB, and spironolactone (Aldactone) is not recommended.

Beta Blockers

In addition to inhibitors of the RAAS, beta-blocker therapy is mandatory for all patients with LV dysfunction. Once considered contraindicated in HF, beta blockers have become the most effective drugs for managing this condition. Carvedilol (Coreg) has been studied in patients with mild to moderate HF (U.S. carvedilol studies) or severe HF (COPERNICUS) and in the post-MI setting (CAPRICORN). **All-cause and cardiovascular mortality was consistently reduced by 25% to 48%.** Similar benefit was seen with metoprolol succinate (Toprol XL) in the MERIT-HF trial, where all-cause mortality was reduced by 34% at 1 year in class II–III HF patients. The use of bisoprolol is also supported by clinical data from CIBIS I and II; however, this drug is not commonly used in the United States.

Beta blockers should be started at low doses and titrated every 1 to 2 weeks until goal doses are achieved. Patients should be stable, largely euvolemic, and already on an ACE inhibitor or ARB prior to the initiation of a beta blocker. Caution should be used in patients with underlying bradycardia or conduction system disease. Fatigue is also common with beta-blocker treatment, but it generally improves after 1 to 2 weeks of treatment. If bronchospasm or low blood pressure is an issue, then beta-1–selective agents (metoprolol succinate) are often better tolerated.

Aldosterone Antagonists

Aldosterone is an adrenal hormone whose production is stimulated through angiotensin II–dependent and –independent pathways. In the myocardium, aldosterone leads to fibrosis and progressive pathologic remodeling. The effects of inhibiting aldosterone in HF were first investigated in the RALES trial, where treatment with spironolactone (Aldactone) led to a **30% mortality reduction** and 36% decrease in hospitalizations in patients with NYHA class III–IV HF. Subsequently the EPHESUS trial demonstrated mortality benefit with the more selective aldosterone antagonist eplerenone (Inspra) in patients with post-MI LV dysfunction already taking an ACE inhibitor and beta blocker. Based on these data, aldosterone antagonists are recommended in patients with severe HF and those with LV dysfunction post-MI. The major side effect is hyperkalemia, especially in the setting of reduced renal function or concomitant ACE inhibitor/ARB therapy; thus frequent monitoring is required. Aldosterone antagonists should be avoided in patients with a baseline potassium ≥5.0 mEq/L or with a baseline Cr >2.0 to 2.5 mg/dL. Gynecomastia can also be seen with spironolactone.

Hydralazine/Nitrates
The V-HEFT I study was the first trial to investigate hydralazine combined with nitrates in chronic HF. This vasodilator combination improved patient symptoms and reduced mortality when compared to placebo and doxazosin. V-HEFT I was also the first study showing that medical treatment could modify the disease process in HF, making it a landmark trial in HF management. Further subgroup analysis of V-HEFT I and its counterpart V-HEFT II suggested that African Americans treated with this combination derived particular benefit. These observations lead to the A-HEFT trial which demonstrated a **43% decrease in mortality and a 33% decrease in HF hospitalizations in African American patients** with class III–IV HF already treated with ACE inhibitor and beta blocker. Thus, the combination of hydralazine and nitrates is recommended in African American patients with severe HF symptoms already on aggressive medical therapy. This vasodilator combination can also be used as an alternative to ACE inhibitor/ARB therapy in patients intolerant of these medications. The most common side effects are headache and hypotension. Patient compliance can also be an issue, given the number of pills required per day.

Digoxin
Digoxin was one of the first medical treatments used for HF. It is a cardiac glycoside that inhibits the Na-K- exchange ion channel, leading to increased intracellular calcium and enhanced contractility. The DIG trial demonstrated that digoxin therapy, in addition to ACE inhibitors and diuretics, **decreased HF hospitalizations but did not alter mortality.** Of note, the best outcomes were seen in patients with digoxin levels <1 ng/mL. Based on these results and other studies demonstrating that digoxin can improve HF symptoms, this agent is used for patients on optimal medical therapy who still have frequent hospitalizations for HF. In patients with atrial fibrillation and HF, the addition of digoxin to beta-blocker therapy can be useful for rate control. Caution must be used in patients with renal dysfunction as digoxin has a narrow therapeutic index and toxicity can occur. Adverse reactions with digoxin include cardiac arrhythmias (atrial tachycardia with AV block, bidirectional VT, AF with regular ventricular response), gastrointestinal symptoms, and neurologic complaints (confusion, visual disturbances). Digoxin toxicity usually manifests when serum levels exceed 2 ng/mL; however, hypokalemia and hypomagnesemia can lower this threshold.

Diuretics
Despite the lack of randomized studies to guide the optimal approach to diuretic therapy, diuretics are a mainstay of medical therapy for volume management in chronic HF. The general consensus is to prescribe the lowest dose of diuretic that is necessary to maintain euvolemia. The loop diuretics furosemide (Lasix), torsemide (Demadex), and bumetanide (Bumex) are the primary options for volume control. If they are used in combination with ACE inhibitors and aldosterone antagonists, scheduled potassium repletion may not be necessary. Torsemide or bumetanide should be considered in patients with significant right-sided HF and abdominal venous congestion, where the absorption of furosemide is frequently unpredictable. **The conversion from furosemide to torsemide to bumetanide**

is ~40:20:1. At times, loop diuretics may not be sufficient to maintain euvolemia. In these cases a thiazide diuretic can be added to overcome distal tubular hypertrophy and induce diuresis. Given the potency of combining a thiazide with a loop diuretic, it is recommended to use only short-term dosing or a 3 day/week dosing schedule. Electrolytes and renal function must be followed carefully as significant volume depletion can occur with any diuretic use.

Inotropes

Continuous inotrope infusion should only be considered for **AHA stage D/NYHA HF class III–IV patients with refractory HF symptoms and evidence of end-organ hypoperfusion**. Frequently, these patients are listed for cardiac transplantation. To qualify for continuous inotrope infusion, a patient's cardiac index must be <2 L/minute per square meter and must improve with inotropes. Thus, initiation of inotropes for possible home infusion requires the placement of a PA catheter. The two inotropes available in the United States are the nonselective beta-agonist dobutamine and the phosphodiesterase inhibitor milrinone. Both of these medications increase cardiac output by increasing contractility and reducing afterload. The hemodynamic effects of these agents are similar; however, dobutamine is favored when renal function is impaired and/or the systolic blood pressure is low (85–90 mm Hg). In addition, the half-life of dobutamine is very short, which can be useful in determining how well a patient will tolerate inotrope infusion. Milrinone can be more effective for patients with elevated pulmonary artery pressures, given its potent vasodilating action. The adverse events associated with inotrope infusion include hypotension (particularly when the patient is hypovolemic), atrial and ventricular arrhythmias, and acceleration in the decline of ventricular function. The risks and benefits must be considered very carefully before initiating inotrope therapy.

Implantable Cardiac Defibrillators (ICD)

Sudden cardiac death (SCD) is a major cause of mortality in patients with HF. The ICD represents a significant advance in the primary prevention of death from ventricular arrhythmias in HF. The MADIT-I and MADIT-2 trials established the survival benefit of ICDs in patients with ischemic cardiomyopathy and an ejection fraction (EF) ≤30%. Subsequently, the SCD-HEFT trial demonstrated a similar benefit for ICDs in patients with ischemic cardiomyopathy (ICM) and nonischemic cardiomyopathy (NICM) with EF ≤35%. The absolute survival benefit of ICD therapy based on these trials is ~1% to 1.5% per year. Therefore **ICD implantation should be considered for all HF patients with EF ≤35%.**

In addition to understanding the indications for ICD implantation, it is equally important to understand when primary prevention ICD therapy should be delayed or deferred. Many patients with NICM will experience a significant improvement in EF when treated with an ACE inhibitor and a beta blocker. Thus at least 3 months of optimal medical therapy and echocardiographic evidence of persistently decreased EF is required prior to implanting an ICD in these patients. Based on the DINAMIT trial, which showed no improvement in mortality for ICDs implanted early after acute MI, recent revascularization and/or acute MI also mandates a waiting period of 40 days prior to implanting an ICD. If patients are of advanced age or have significant, life-shortening comorbidities (severe chronic obstructive pulmonary disease, cancer, end-stage renal disease) the benefit of an ICD is reduced. The primary risks of ICD implantation include device infection, generator-site hematoma, cardiac rupture, pneumothorax, and inappropriate shocks. For further discussion of ICD and ventricular arrhythmias, see Chapter 20.

Cardiac Resynchronization Therapy (CRT)

Ventricular dyssynchrony is present in up to one-third of patients with cardiomyopathy and is associated with decreased cardiac efficiency. Dyssynchrony is currently defined electrically as a QRS duration >120 ms. However, echocardiographic parameters are currently being studied for assessing mechanical dyssynchrony. Biventricular pacemakers (BiV) are designed to resynchronize LV contraction and improve cardiac function. They consist of a right atrial, right ventricular ± ICD and epicardial left ventricular lead (placed via the coronary sinus). The two largest randomized trials in CRT are COMPANION and CARE-HF. BiV pacing was associated with an improvement in symptoms and a reduction in hospitalizations compared to patients receiving optimal medical therapy (OMT) alone. The CARE-HF trial also demonstrated a marked decrease in mortality associated with BiV pacing. The patients in these trials had an EF ≤35%, NYHA class III–IV HF symptoms, were on OMT, and were largely in normal sinus rhythm. **CRT should be considered in patients with dyssynchrony (QRS >120) who have severe HF symptoms and frequent hospitalizations despite OMT.**

LV Assist Devices (LVADs)
LVADs can be considered in select patients with acute or chronic end-organ hypoperfusion from cardiac dysfunction. These devices extract oxygenated blood from either the LA or LV, shuttle it though a pulsatile or continuous-flow pump, and then return it to the aorta. LVADs are designed for short- or long-term ventricular support. The short-term devices include the percutaneously inserted TandemHeart and the surgically implanted Abiomed Biventricular System (Abiomed Cardiovascular; Danvers, MA) and Biomedicus Biopump (Medtronic-Biomedicus; Eden Prarie, MN). These devices can provide cardiac support for 1 to 2 weeks or 1 to 2 months, respectively. The long-term LVADs currently approved in the United States are all pulsatile devices [Thoratec VAD and Heart Mate IP, VE, and XVE (Thoratec Laboratories; Pleasanton, CA) and Novocor (World Heart; Ottawa, Canada)].

In most situations, LVADs are used as a "bridge" to transplant. However, LVAD implantation can also be considered in select patients who are not transplant candidates. This is referred to as "destination" therapy. Two randomized trials of destination therapy in end-stage HF patients are the REMATCH and INTrEPID studies, which compared LVAD to standard medical therapy. Although mortality was significantly reduced in the LVAD arm of both trials, over half of the treated patients died within 1 year. Device failure, sepsis, and embolic events are the primary causes of death in patients with LVADs. Continuous axial flow pumps, totally implantable pulsatile devices, and total artificial heart technologies continue to improve and are exclusively available in clinical trial settings.

Heart Transplantation
Heart transplantation is the definitive therapy for end-stage HF. Successful transplantation became possible in the 1980s, when the immunosuppressant cyclosporine was used to control rejection. Currently there are ~2000 heart transplants in the United States each year. **Survival following heart transplantation is very good with 85%, 70%, and 50% of patients alive at 1, 5, and 10 years, respectively.**

The selection of candidates for cardiac transplantation is a critical determinant of transplant outcomes. Patients considered for transplantation have severe HF symptoms despite maximal medical therapy and also have a limited life expectancy. A VO_2max ≤14 mL/kg per minute on cardiopulmonary exercise testing portends a significantly reduced 1-year survival, and this criterion has been used to identify patients with the greatest need for transplant. Contraindications to transplant, some of which are relative, include severe, irreversible pulmonary hypertension, active infection, severe chronic obstructive pulmonary disease(COPD), significant renal impairment (not related to poor cardiac output), severe peripheral vascular disease or carotid disease, severe psychiatric disease, primary liver disease with coagulopathy, advanced age (>70–75), diabetes with end-organ dysfunction, and active malignancy.

Vigilant posttransplant follow-up is mandatory to ensure good outcomes. During the first year after transplant, acute rejection and infection (from both common and opportunistic pathogens—CMV, *Nocardia*, *Pneumocystis*) are the primary complications. Patients receive three-drug immunosuppression, infection prophylaxis, and routine endomyocardial biopsies during this time period to reduce adverse events. After the first year, coronary artery vasculopathy, renal insufficiency, and malignancy are the primary factors that limit survival. Aggressive treatment of hypertension, statin therapy, routine coronary angiography or intravascular ultrasound, lower doses of immunosuppression, and cancer screening are all important to maximize long-term survival.

Prognosis

HF is associated with significant morbidity and mortality. Up to 30% of patients admitted with HF will be dead within 1 year. However, there are many factors that alter prognosis in an individual patient. These factors can be grouped into broad categories including HF symptoms (NYHA class), laboratory tests (troponin, BNP, sodium, hemoglobin, creatinine), cardiac physiology (LVEF, diastolic function, pulmonary pressures, wedge pressure), HF etiology (ICM versus NICM), associated conditions (atrial fibrillation, renal insufficiency), medication and device therapy, and age. **The Seattle HF model** is a comprehensive risk-prediction tool for assessing survival probability in a given individual. A user-friendly calculator for the Seattle HF model is available on the web at http://depts.washington.edu/shfm/index.php. The ability to risk-stratify patients with HF is useful to direct the aggressiveness of therapy and to guide discussions with patients and their families.

Special Topics in HF

HF with Preserved Systolic Function

Nearly 50% of patients hospitalized for acute HF have preserved systolic function (PSF). Most of these patients have abnormal diastolic function. Patients with this condition are more likely to be elderly, female, hypertensive, and diabetic. In addition, atrial fibrillation and renal insufficiency are commonly associated comorbidities. LV hypertrophy and/or abnormal relaxation patterns are common findings on echocardiography. HF with PSF has a similar prognosis to systolic HF and mortality at 3 years, approaching 60% in some series. Unlike in HF with decreased systolic function, there are very few clinical trials to direct optimal medical therapy in these patients. One subset of the CHARM trial, referred to as CHARM-preserved, demonstrated that candesartan therapy resulted in a 15% relative risk reduction in hospitalizations, but did not affect mortality. At present, the guidelines are largely based on professional opinion and include:

- Control blood pressure (favoring the use of ACE inhibitor/ARB and beta blocker).
- Control heart rate and consider attempts to maintain sinus rhythm for patients in atrial fibrillation.
- Use diuretics to control signs and symptoms of volume overload.
- Consider revascularization when ischemia is felt to be factor in impaired cardiac function.

Beta-Blocker Therapy in ADHF

The issue of what to do with beta-blocker therapy during a HF exacerbation is a controversial and frequently discussed topic. As the benefits of beta blocker are realized over the long term, it has been general practice to discontinue these medications during ADHF, given their negative inotropic effects. However, HF exacerbations are associated with high levels of systemic catecholamines, and there are data to suggest that the withdrawal of beta blocker during ADHF can worsen outcomes. Therefore the guidelines have been continually evolving. In a beta blocker–naïve patient, it is reasonable to defer treatment until euvolemia has been achieved and the patient is on an afterload reduction regimen. However, it is critical that all patients be started on a beta blocker prior to discharge from the hospital, as this has been associated with improved long-term outcomes. In patients already receiving beta-blocker therapy, every attempt should be made to continue the medication at its current dose. If the patient is in a low-output state, the dose can be decreased. In the event that the patient requires inotropic therapy it is appropriate to discontinue the beta blocker.

Ultrafiltration and Volume Control in ADHF

Although diuretics are the mainstay of therapy for volume overload in HF, their use has numerous adverse effects such as RAAS activation, electrolyte depletion, and renal dysfunction. Ultrafiltration (UF) allows for fluid removal at a consistent rate without these negative consequences. The UNLOAD trial was a small study that compared UF to standard therapy in patients admitted with ADHF. Fluid removal was more effective and efficient using UF, and the risk of future hospitalizations for HF was reduced. The downside of UF is that it requires specialized peripheral venous access and the machines/equipment can be costly.

Remote Monitoring and Volume Assessment

The physical exam assessment of volume status in HF patients can be challenging, even for HF specialists. In an effort to identify subclinical volume overload, when intervention can prevent hospitalization, several monitoring strategies have been developed. Blood pressure, weight, and symptoms can be monitored wirelessly and remotely via the Internet (Latitude; Boston Scientific, Natick, MA), helping clinicians direct medical therapy. Thoracic impedance levels recorded from an implantable defibrillator/CRT device can assess trends in fluid balance (OptiVol; Medtronic, Minneapolis, MN). Although these monitoring approaches have the potential to improve volume assessment in patients with HF, there are limited data at this point to suggest that HF hospitalization or mortality is altered.

KEY POINTS TO REMEMBER

- Early treatment and prevention of LV dysfunction is possible by identifying and treating high-risk individuals, especially those with diabetes, hypertension, or CAD.
- Most patients admitted to the hospital with HF can be categorized into one of three phenotypes: (1) acute pulmonary edema and hypertension; (2) slowly progressive volume overload; (3) low-output state ± volume overload.
- The treatment goals during a hospitalization for acute decompensated HF (ADHF) are (1) to improve patient symptoms, (2) correct hemodynamic and volume status, (3) minimize renal and cardiac injury, and (4) initiate lifesaving medical therapies.
- The key components to long-term success in HF management are patient education, optimal medical and device therapy, and adequate patient follow-up, as described by the following alphabet mnemonic: **A**—ACE inhibitor or ARB; **B**—Beta blocker; **C**—Counseling (smoking cessation, exercise); **D**—Dietary education (low-sodium diet, fluid restriction), Device therapy (if appropriate); **E**—Euvolemia achieved; **F**—Follow-up appointment established.

REFERENCES AND SUGGESTED READINGS

Bardy GH et al. Amiodarone or an implantable cardioverter-defibrillator for congestive heart failure. *N Engl J Med* 2005;352(3):225–237.

Binanay C et al. Evaluation study of congestive heart failure and pulmonary artery catheterization effectiveness: the ESCAPE trial. *JAMA* 2005;294(13):1625–1633.

Bristow MR et al. Cardiac-resynchronization therapy with or without an implantable defibrillator in advanced chronic heart failure. *N Engl J Med* 2004;350(21):2140–2150.

Chakko S et al. Clinical, radiographic, and hemodynamic correlations in chronic congestive heart failure: conflicting results may lead to inappropriate care. *Am J Med* 1991;90(3):353–359.

Chen HH et al. Diastolic heart failure in the community: clinical profile, natural history, therapy, and impact of proposed diagnostic criteria. *J Card Fail* 2002;8(5):279–287.

Cleland JG et al. The effect of cardiac resynchronization on morbidity and mortality in heart failure. *N Engl J Med* 2005;352(15):1539–1549.

Cohn JN, Tognoni G. A randomized trial of the angiotensin-receptor blocker valsartan in chronic heart failure. *N Engl J Med* 2001;345(23):1667–1675.

Cohn JN et al. A comparison of enalapril with hydralazine–isosorbide dinitrate in the treatment of chronic congestive heart failure. *N Engl J Med* 1991;325(5):303–310.

Cohn JN et al. Effect of vasodilator therapy on mortality in chronic congestive heart failure. Results of a Veterans Administration Cooperative Study. *N Engl J Med* 1986;314(24):1547–1552.

Costanzo MR et al. Ultrafiltration versus intravenous diuretics for patients hospitalized for acute decompensated heart failure. *J Am Coll Cardiol* 2007;49(6):675–683.

Dargie HJ. Effect of carvedilol on outcome after myocardial infarction in patients with left-ventricular dysfunction: the CAPRICORN randomized trial. *Lancet* 2001;357 (9266):1385–1390.

Drakos SG et al. Ventricular-assist devices for the treatment of chronic heart failure. *Expert Rev Cardiovasc Ther* 2007;5:571–584.

Effect of metoprolol CR/XL in chronic heart failure: Metoprolol CR/XL Randomised Intervention Trial in Congestive Heart Failure (MERIT-HF). *Lancet* 1999;353(9169): 2001–2007.

Fonarow G. When to initiate beta-blocker in heart failure: is it ever too early? *Curr Heart Fail Rep* 2005;96:47E–53E.

Garg R, Yusuf S. Overview of randomized trials of angiotensin-converting enzyme inhibitors on mortality and morbidity in patients with heart failure. Collaborative Group on ACE Inhibitor Trials. *JAMA* 1995;273(18):1450–1456.

Gheorghiade M et al., Congestion is an important diagnostic and therapeutic target in heart failure. *Rev Cardiovasc Med* 2006;7(Suppl 1):S12–S24.

Hasan A, Abraham WT. Cardiac resynchronization treatment of heart failure. *Annu Rev Med* 2007;58:63–74.

Hohnloser SH et al. Prophylactic use of an implantable cardioverter-defibrillator after acute myocardial infarction. *N Engl J Med* 2004;351(24):2481–2488.

Horwich TB et al. Cardiac troponin I is associated with impaired hemodynamics, progressive left ventricular dysfunction, and increased mortality rates in advanced heart failure. *Circulation* 2003;108(7):833–838.

Hunt S, Abraham WT, Chin MH, et al. ACC/AHA 2005 Guideline Update for the diagnosis and management of chronic heart failure in the adult: a Report of the American College of Cardiology/American Heart Association Task Force on Practice Guidelines. *Circulation* 2005;112:e154–e235. Available at http://www.acc.org/qualityandscience/clinical/guidelines/failure/update/index.pdf.

Intravenous nesiritide versus nitroglycerin for treatment of decompensated congestive heart failure: a randomized controlled trial. *JAMA* 2002;287(12):1531–1540.

Levy D et al. The progression from hypertension to congestive heart failure. *JAMA* 1996;275(20):1557–1562.

McMurray JJ et al. Effects of candesartan in patients with chronic heart failure and reduced left-ventricular systolic function taking angiotensin-converting-enzyme inhibitors: the CHARM-Added trial. *Lancet* 2003;362(9386):767–771.

Mehra MR. Optimizing outcomes in the patient with acute decompensated heart failure. *Am Heart J* 2006;151:571–579.

Moe GW. B-type natriuretic peptide in heart failure. *Curr Opin Cardiol* 2007;21:208–214.

Moss AJ. MADIT-I and MADIT-II. *J Cardiovasc Electrophysiol* 2003:14(9 Suppl): S96–S98.

Nohria A, Mielniczuk LD, Stevenson LW. Evaluation and monitoring of patients with acute heart failure syndromes. *Am J Cardiol* 2005;96:32G–40G.

Packer M et al. Effect of carvedilol on the morbidity of patients with severe chronic heart failure: results of the carvedilol prospective randomized cumulative survival (COPERNICUS) study. *Circulation* 2002;106(17):2194–2199.

Packer M et al. The effect of carvedilol on morbidity and mortality in patients with chronic heart failure. U.S. Carvedilol Heart Failure Study Group. *N Engl J Med* 1996;334(21):1349–1355.

Pfeffer MA et al. Effects of candesartan on mortality and morbidity in patients with chronic heart failure: the CHARM-Overall programme. *Lancet* 2003:362(9386): 759–766.

Pfeffer MA et al. Valsartan, captopril, or both in myocardial infarction complicated by heart failure, left ventricular dysfunction, or both. *N Engl J Med* 2003;349(20): 1893–1906.

Pitt B et al. Eplerenone, a selective aldosterone blocker, in patients with left ventricular dysfunction after myocardial infarction. *N Engl J Med* 2003;348(14):1309–1321.

Pitt B et al. The effect of spironolactone on morbidity and mortality in patients with severe heart failure. Randomized Aldactone Evaluation Study Investigators. *N Engl J Med* 1999;341(10):709–717.

Reis SE et al. Treatment of patients admitted to the hospital with congestive heart failure: specialty-related disparities in practice patterns and outcomes. *J Am Coll Cardiol* 1997;30(3):733–738.

Rogers JG, Butler J, Lansman SL, et al. Chronic mechanical circulatory support for inotrope-dependent heart failure patients who are not transplant candidates: results of the INTrEPID Trial. *J Am Coll Cardiol* 2007;50:741–747.

Rose EA et al. Long-term mechanical left ventricular assistance for end-stage heart failure. *N Engl J Med* 2001;345(20):1435–1443.

Taegtmeyer H, McNulty P, Young ME. Adaptation and maladaptation of the heart in diabetes: part I. general concepts. *Circulation* 2002;105(14):1727–1733.

Taylor AL et al. Combination of isosorbide dinitrate and hydralazine in blacks with heart failure. *N Engl J Med* 2004;351(20):2049–2057.

The Digitalis Investigation Group. The effect of digoxin on mortality and morbidity in patients with heart failure. *N Engl J Med* 1997;336(8):525–533.

Yusuf S et al. Effects of candesartan in patients with chronic heart failure and preserved left-ventricular ejection fraction: the CHARM-Preserved Trial. *Lancet* 2003:362 (9386):777–781.

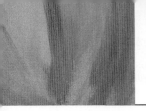

Assessment and Management of the Dilated, Restrictive, and Hypertrophic Cardiomyopathies

12

Jennifer L. Peura

INTRODUCTION

Although ischemic cardiomyopathy is the most common etiology for heart failure (HF), almost half of HF cases do not fit into this category. This chapter discusses other causes of systolic dysfunction (dilated cardiomyopathy) and diastolic dysfunction (restrictive and hypertrophic cardiomyopathy). Management of these disorders is focused on the primary dysfunction (systolic or diastolic), and is discussed in detail in Chapter 11. Treatment of hypertrophic cardiomyopathy is specific and is discussed in detail below.

DILATED CARDIOMYOPATHY

Dilated cardiomyopathy (DCM), or nonischemic cardiomyopathy (NICM) is responsible for 10,000 deaths and 46,000 hospitalizations each year. **For the majority of patients with DCM, the etiology will be deemed idiopathic** (Table 12-1). When possible, however, primary diseases associated with DCM should be diagnosed, as reversible causes provide opportunity for tailored treatment. Etiologies to consider include those discussed below.

Infectious

- Viral infection is most common [human immunodeficiency virus (HIV), cytomegalovirus (CMV), coxsackievirus, influenza, adenovirus, echovirus].
- Chagas' disease (*Trypanosoma cruzi*) can cause severe ventricular enlargement (often apical aneurysm) complicated by thromboembolic stroke, arrhythmias and sudden death. Megaesophagus and megacolon are frequently seen as well.

Toxic

- Alcoholic cardiomyopathy is common, accounting for one-third cases of DCM. Patients with alcoholic CM who do not abstain from alcohol suffer a 5-year mortality of 50%.
- Cocaine is associated with DCM; however, ischemic cardiomyopathy (ICM) (due to vasospasm) is more common.
- Chemotherapeutic agents, particularly anthracyclines (doxorubicin), are well known to cause DCM. Total cumulative dose is important; patients who receive >700 mg/m^2 risk developing DCM. Therapy with trastuzumab (monoclonal antibody against Her2/neu) also carries risk for developing CM. Before treatment with these chemotherapeutic agents, patients should have a baseline echocardiogram. They also need periodic cardiac evaluation during treatment.

TABLE 12-1	RELATIVE FREQUENCY OF DILATED CARDIOMYOPATHY IN REVIEW OF 1230 PATIENTS

Idiopathic 50%
Myocarditis 9%
Ischemic heart disease 7%
Infiltrative disease 5%
Peripartum cardiomyopathy 4%
Hypertension 4%
HIV infection 4%
Connective tissue disease 3%
Substance abuse 3%
Doxorubicin 1%
Other 10%

High-Output

- Intracardiac left-to-right communications include ventricular septal defects (VSDs), atrial septal defects, patent ductus arteriosus, or ruptured sinus of Valsalva.
- Extracardiac communications may be iatrogenic (dialysis fistula), genetic (hereditary hemorrhagic telangiectasias, Osler–Weber–Rendu disease) or secondary to trauma (penetrating injury). Compression of the fistula should result in a decrease in heart rate in a substantial shunt.
- Patients with anemia or asymptomatic tachycardias such as atrial fibrillation can present with a tachycardia-induced cardiomyopathy.
- Unique physical findings in high-output HF include increased pulse pressure, hyperdynamic apical impulse, warm extremities, and a systolic flow murmur due to increased flow across the aortic valve.

Endocrine/Metabolic

- Hyperthyroidism may cause a tachycardia-mediated cardiomyopathy as well. A bruit over the thyroid or the presence of a goiter can aid in the diagnosis.
- Excess sympathomimetic amines in pheochromocytoma can lead to direct myocyte injury.
- A similar phenomenon is seen in stress-induced cardiomyopathy (takotsubo cardiomyopathy), where, following an acute stress, patients present with HF symptoms and an echocardiogram with reversible apical ballooning.
- Excess cortisol (Cushing's syndrome) or growth hormone can cause a DCM.
- Carnitine is necessary for normal fatty acid oxidation, and carnitine deficiency leads to fatty acid accumulation and myocyte dysfunction.
- Selenium deficiency can lead to DCM, particularly among patients who have undergone bariatric surgery or among those receiving total parenteral nutrition.

Autoimmune

- Patients with systemic lupus erythematosus often develop myocarditis, but they can also have valvular, conduction, and pericardial disease.
- Celiac disease (commonly with GI symptoms, weight loss, and iron-deficiency anemia) may account for 5% of patients with idiopathic DCM. A gluten-free diet can bring improvement of GI symptoms and cardiac function in these patients.

Congenital

- Familial DCM is associated with mutations to genes encoding sarcomeric proteins.
- Left ventricular noncompaction is characterized by arrest of normal ventricular development leading to HF, thromboembolism, and ventricular arrhythmias.
- Muscular dystrophies (Duchenne's, Becker's, myotonic dystrophy) that arise from mutations in dystrophin-glycoprotein complex and lamin A/C gene mutations are associated with DCM.
- Inborn errors of fatty acid metabolism are known to affect estimated 1:15,000 live births annually. The disorder leads to DCM and sudden cardiac death (SCD).

Clinical Presentation

Idiopathic DCM is the most common cause of HF in young patients; 90% of these have severe symptoms at presentation (New York Heart Association class III or IV). The natural history of the disease is difficult to determine given the unknown length of asymptomatic disease. Symptomatic patients have a poor prognosis, with 5-year mortality rates averaging 20%. Further details regarding the presentation and management of dilated cardiomyopathies are discussed in Chapters 4 and 11.

RESTRICTIVE CARDIOMYOPATHY

Background

The restrictive heart is rigid and is characterized by poor ventricular filling. Myocardial restrictive disease is classified as infiltrative (amyloidosis or sarcoidosis) or noninfiltrative (diabetic or idiopathic restrictive cardiomyopathy). Diseases of the pericardium (constrictive pericarditis) can present similarly but have a considerably different prognosis and treatment. Therefore it is important to exclude pericardial disease (see Chapter 13).

Etiology

Myocardial Infiltrative Disease

Amyloidosis can affect the heart when normal myocardial contractile elements are replaced by interstitial deposits, causing restrictive cardiomyopathy. There are many types of amyloidosis; cardiac involvement is seen most commonly in primary amyloidosis. Amyloid deposits are seen histologically as insoluble amyloid fibrils in all chambers of the heart (Congo red stain). Amyloid deposits found in the conduction system result in cardiac arrhythmias. The electrocardiogram (**ECG**) **classically shows low voltage with poor R-wave progression**. Echocardiographic findings characteristic of cardiac amyloidosis include a granular, sparkling appearance of thickened ventricular walls and significant biatrial enlargement. The degree of wall thickness predicts survival; patients with normal wall thickness have an average survival of 2.4 years, and those with markedly increased wall thickness have an average survival of <6 months.

Cardiac involvement occurs in 5% of **sarcoidosis**. Myocardial restriction may result from patchy scar formation around infiltrating, noncaseating granulomas; however, the most common manifestation of cardiac sarcoid is **conduction system disease**. The disease course is variable, with the most dramatic presentations being SCD due to ventricular tachyarrhythmias or high-degree heart block.

Hemochromatosis results in restrictive cardiomyopathy secondary to abnormal iron metabolism and myocardial iron deposition. Hemochromatosis may be primary, due to an autosomal recessive genetic abnormality, or secondary, due to iron overload. Patients present with diabetes, skin discoloration, and diastolic dysfunction. Workup includes iron studies, with an elevated transferrin saturation being most suggestive, followed by biopsy of an accessible organ (often the liver). Treatment of underlying disease is of utmost importance to prevent progression of disease; this may include phlebotomy and chelation therapy.

Gaucher's and Hurler's cardiomyopathies are rare genetic disorders that may be associated with an infiltrative cardiomyopathy. Gaucher's cardiomyopathy is an autosomal recessive disease produced by mutations of the glucocerebrosidase gene that result in the accumulation of the lipid glucocerebroside in the heart. Hurler's cardiomyopathy is a genetic disorder caused by a mutation in the chromosome pair responsible for producing alpha-l-iduronidase. This results in a mucopolysaccharide accumulation in the heart.

Myocardial Noninfiltrative Disease

Idiopathic restrictive cardiomyopathy is characterized by a mild to moderate increase in cardiac weight. Biatrial enlargement occurs commonly, with a 10% incidence of atrial appendage thrombi. Patchy endocardial fibrosis is present and may extend into the conduction system, resulting in complete heart block.

Patients with **diabetes** have an increased incidence of HF. The metabolic derangements seen in diabetes are thought to lead to myocyte apoptosis and interstitial fibrosis (see Chapter 29).

Endomyocardial Disease

Hypereosinophilic syndrome (Löffler's endocarditis, parietalis fibroblastica) is an obliterative, restrictive cardiomyopathy thought to result from toxic damage from the intracytoplasmic granular content of activated eosinophils. It occurs in temperate climates and is associated with a hypereosinophilic syndrome. Patients have endocardial thickening and obliteration of the cardiac apex. It is usually an aggressive disease, more common in men than in women. Use of corticosteroids and cytotoxic drugs in the early phase of disease may improve symptoms and survival.

Carcinoid heart disease results from untreated carcinoid syndrome, where lesion formation correlates with the concentration of serotonin and 5-hydroxyindoleacetic acid. Lesions are predominantly in the right ventricular (RV) endocardium, where tricuspid insufficiency is prominent. Tricuspid and pulmonic stenosis can also be seen. Occasionally left-sided valvular lesions can be seen in patients with either pulmonary metastases or a patent foramen ovale (or other intracardiac shunt).

HYPERTROPHIC CARDIOMYOPATHY

Introduction

Hypertrophic cardiomyopathy (HCM) is characterized by myocardial hypertrophy in the absence of an identifiable cause or underlying etiology. This disease was previously called (and often still referred to as) hypertrophic obstructive cardiomyopathy (HOCM) or idiopathic hypertrophic subaortic stenosis (IHSS). Unlike the concentric hypertrophy of pressure overload or the eccentric hypertrophy of volume overload, patients with HCM often develop asymmetric hypertrophy of the ventricular septum. Obstruction of blood exiting the heart can occur, as the aortic outflow tract is geometrically narrowed due to the thick septum abutting against the mitral valve apparatus (**systolic anterior motion**). This dynamic process of LV outflow tract (LVOT) obstruction is present in approximately 30% of patients and produces a characteristic murmur (described below). Identification of this disorder during sports physicals is critical, as HCM is a **common cause of SCD among young athletes in the United States.**

HCM is the most common inheritable cardiac disease and is transmitted in an autosomal dominant fashion with variable penetrance and severity. The prevalence of HCM is approximately 1 in 500. HCM is caused by mutations in genes encoding proteins of the cardiac sarcomere. Mutations of β-myosin heavy-chain, cardiac troponin T, and myosin-binding protein C are the most common; however, several others have also been reported. Histologic analysis of affected myocardium reveals **disorganized myocytes** with unusual shapes in chaotic alignment. The coronary arteries may also be affected, with arteriolar wall thickening leading to small-vessel coronary disease. Myocyte disorganization and small-vessel disease both contribute to ventricular dysfunction and arrhythmogenic substrate.

Clinical Presentation

The majority of patients with HCM are asymptomatic. The diagnosis of HCM is often made upon screening of affected relatives or by recognition of a murmur on routine physical. The onset of symptoms is variable and can occur at any stage of life. The classic presentations of HCM include **angina** (from myocardial oxygen mismatch due to increased myocardial mass, small-vessel disease or wall stress), **HF** (usually due to LVOT obstruction with activity), and **arrhythmia** (manifesting as palpitations, syncope, or sudden death). It is important to elicit a family history of sudden death for risk stratification (see below).

On physical exam, the characteristic systolic ejection murmur of HCM is heard at the left-lower sternal border. This murmur is preload-dependent and intensifies with maneuvers that decrease preload, such as standing and the Valsalva maneuver. Conversely, the murmur of HCM decreases with squatting (which increases preload and afterload) and handgrip (which increases afterload). Amyl nitrite decreases systemic vascular resistance and decreases LV volume, which increases the murmur of HCM. Other physical findings may include a bisferiens (bifid) carotid pulse, split S2, and a prominent S4 (Table 12-2). Because only one-third of HCM patients manifest obstruction, most will have a normal exam.

Differential Diagnosis

Prior to diagnosis of HCM, concentric LV hypertrophy due to systemic hypertension or aortic stenosis must be excluded. Other less common causes of fixed outflow tract obstruction—such as subvalvular obstruction (subaortic membrane or muscular subaortic stenosis) or supravalvular stenosis—should be considered. Hypertrophy can be a physiologic adaptation to training in the athlete, differentiated from pathologic HCM by the absence of wall stress or physiologic obstruction. At times, the systolic anterior motion of the mitral valve can be detected in normal small hearts and under severe conditions that cause significant underfilling of the left ventricle.

TABLE 12-2	PHYSICAL FINDINGS OF LEFT VENTRICULAR OUTFLOW TRACT OBSTRUCTION IN HYPERTROPHIC CARDIOMYOPATHY
Systolic ejection murmur, left lower sternal border	
Squatting	↓
Handgrip	↓
Valsalva	↑
Stand from squat	↑
Amyl nitrate	↑
Split S2	
Prominent S4	
Bisferiens carotid pulse	

Diagnostic Testing

Close to 95% of all HCM patients have an abnormal ECG, including a pattern of LV hypertrophy (LVH), ST–T-wave abnormalities, deep Q waves involving inferior and precordial leads (**pseudoinfarct pattern**), and left atrial enlargement. Prominent T-wave inversions in the precordial leads are characteristic of apical HCM.

Echocardiography usually confirms the diagnosis. **LV wall thickness greater than 15 mm in any segment** of the LV satisfies criteria for the diagnosis of HCM. When the septum is affected, the term "asymmetric septal hypertrophy" is applied. Other morphologic characteristics of HCM can be assessed by echocardiography, including mitral regurgitation (MR), diastolic dysfunction, and quantification of a LVOT gradient. Turbulent flow through the LVOT leads to MR via the Venturi effect, causing **systolic anterior motion** (SAM) of the mitral valve and a posteriorly directed MR jet. Inhaled amyl nitrite can be helpful in provoking a latent LVOT gradient, corresponding to a gradient that may be unveiled with activity.

There is diverse heterogeneity among the phenotypic expression of HCM. The majority of patients have involvement of the interventricular septum and anterolateral wall. Other areas of hypertrophy include the posterior septum, posterobasal free wall, and even concentric patterns of wall thickness. One variant of HCM is Yamaguchi's apical HCM, which accounts for 25% of HCM in Japan but only 1% of cases outside of Japan. It is distinguished by a localized apical hypertrophy in the distal LV, resulting in a spade-like configuration.

With an initial diagnosis of HCM, patients should undergo **ambulatory cardiac monitoring** for ventricular arrhythmias. Additionally, a monitored **exercise stress test** can evaluate for high-risk features such as ventricular arrhythmia, hypotension, or chest pain with exertion.

Left- and right heart catheterizations are primarily reserved for those patients referred for invasive intervention or if the question of epicardial coronary disease warrants evaluation. On coronary angiography, systolic compression of the septal perforator branches of the left anterior descending artery (septal milking) is classically seen. Hemodynamic assessment is very important; in the setting of a resting gradient, the intraventricular systolic pressure is greater than that in the aorta (normally these are equal). The **Brockenbrough–Braunwald sign** is considered the most specific sign of dynamic LVOT obstruction. By stimulating a premature ventricular contraction (PVC), a compensatory pause will occur, with the following beat having greater contractility. In normal hearts, the aortic pulse pressure increases with this post-PVC beat; however, in HCM, the post-PVC aortic pulse pressure will decrease or remain the same, and the pressure gradient between the LV and aorta will increase (Fig. 12-1).

Treatment

Pharmacologic therapy can provide relief of the congestive symptoms associated with LVOT obstruction. Negative inotropic agents such as β-**blockers and calcium-channel blockers** can be used to control the heart rate and increase diastolic filling time. Up to one-third of patients have a clinical response to β-blockers. Angiotensin converting enzyme (ACE) inhibitors are not recommended unless there is significant hypertension, as these drugs can worsen the gradient by peripheral vasodilatation. Nitrates are contraindicated because they decrease preload and thereby increase the gradient across the LVOT. Diuretics must be used with caution. Inotropes such as dobutamine are ineffective and sometimes harmful, as the positive inotropy increases the gradient across the LVOT and can yield significant hypotension. This is an important consideration and must be remembered in evaluating these patients in the peri- and postoperative settings.

Because right ventricular (RV) apical pacing causes a left bundle-branch block (LBBB) ventricular activation pattern, there is a theoretical physiologic reduction in LVOT gradient with dual-chamber pacing. However, because of mixed results from clinical trials, the

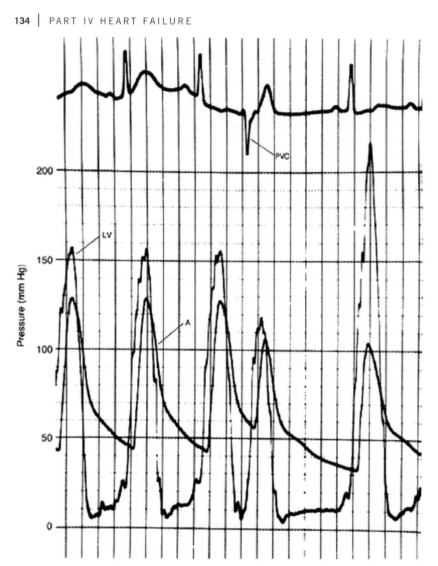

FIGURE 12-1. Brockenbrough–Braunwald sign. Simultaneous arterial (A) and left ventricular (LV) pressures recorded in a patient with HCM. The first three beats show a peak systolic gradient of 25 mm Hg. On the first sinus beat after the premature ventricular contraction (PVC), the peak-systolic gradient increases to over 100 mm Hg, but the pulse pressure (arterial systolic pressure minus diastolic pressure) decreases. This characteristic pattern is known as the Brockenbrough–Braunwald sign. The decrease in pulse pressure after PVC is due to reduced stroke volume caused by increased dynamic obstruction. (From Pollock SG. Pressure tracings in obstructive cardiomyopathy. *N Engl J Med* 1994;331:238, with permission.)

role of pacing for the treatment of obstructive symptoms is limited. Nevertheless, pacemaker implantation eliminates the concern for drug-associated bradycardia and consequently allows maximization of pharmacologic rate control.

Patients with a LVOT gradient greater than 50 mm Hg and severe symptoms refractory to medical therapy are candidates for surgery. **Septal myotomy-myectomy (Morrow procedure)** is the "gold standard" for relief of obstructive symptoms. For this procedure, a transaortic approach is used to resect a small amount of septal muscle, relieving the subaortic obstruction. In experienced centers, operative mortality is 1% to 2%, and long-term data shows a reduction in congestive symptoms and increase in exercise capacity for most patients. Concomitant mitral valve replacement may be necessary if there is no relief of SAM with myectomy alone.

Alcohol septal ablation is an emerging alternative to surgery. It is performed by injecting 2 to 5 mL of 95% to 100% alcohol into the first major septal perforator of the left anterior descending artery. By inducing an infarct in this area of the ventricular septum, volume of muscle is reduced. As a result, localized wall thinning occurs, thereby enlarging the outflow tract and reducing the intraventricular gradient. Risks to alcohol septal ablation include atrioventricular (AV) block, requiring a permanent pacemaker (occurs approximately 30%) and potential increased risk of SCD due to myocardial scar.

Prognosis

The annual mortality for HCM is reported to be from 1% to 6%, with death more likely in symptomatic patient populations. **The most common cause of death is SCD.** Owing to the heterogeneous nature of HCM, the disease can follow several clinical courses. These include (1) high risk for SCD, (2) development of congestive symptoms requiring drug treatment/surgery/ablation, (3) development of AF and risk of stroke, or (4) an asymptomatic course. The role of routine genetic testing for individual patients to establish a diagnosis is extremely limited, but genetic testing can be useful in familial cohorts to assess prognosis as well as in genetic counseling for future generations.

Complications

Atrial Fibrillation

- Occurs in 22% of HCM patients; more frequently in patients with congestive symptoms, increased left atrial size, and advanced age.
- Rate control can be achieved through the use of β-blockers or verapamil. Although the effectiveness of amiodarone therapy in maintaining sinus rhythm after electrical or pharmacologic cardioversion is unproven, it is currently the agent of choice for this indication.
- Anticoagulation with warfarin should be used in patients with paroxysmal or chronic atrial fibrillation (AF) to prevent thromboembolic complications.

Heart Failure

- Progression to HF occurs in 5% of patients with nonobstructive HCM.
- With severe decreased left ventricular ejection fraction (LVEF), conversion from HCM-directed therapy to standard HF therapy is warranted.
- Heart transplantation can be considered in a subset of patients.

Sudden Cardiac Death

Risk stratification for SCD is important in the management of HCM. Major risk factors for SCD are listed in Table 12-3.

TABLE 12-3   RISK FACTORS FOR SUDDEN CARDIAC DEATH IN HCM

Previous SCD/ventricular arrhythmias
Family history of SCD
Unexplained syncope
LV thickness >30 mm
Abnormal exercise blood pressure
Nonsustained ventricular tachycardia

- Patients who have received an implantable cardiac defibrillator (ICD) after a resuscitated cardiac arrest or sustained ventricular tachycardia have had appropriate ICD therapy at a rate of 10.6% per year. Thus it is the standard of care to provide survivors of SCD with HCM with an ICD.
- Use of ICDs for primary prevention in high-risk patients is controversial although widely accepted. The yearly rate of appropriate ICD therapy in patients with one or more risk factors has been reported as 3.6%.
- Intense physical exertion can be a trigger for sudden death; therefore the current recommendation is to disqualify patients with HCM from participation in organized competitive athletics.

KEY POINTS TO REMEMBER

- Dilated, restrictive, and hypertrophic cardiomyopathies should be considered when HF symptoms are present in the absence of ischemia.
- The majority of cases of DCM are idiopathic. While determining the cause of DCM can be important, it rarely affects course of treatment.
- Restrictive cardiomyopathy must be distinguished from constrictive cardiomyopathy, as treatment and prognosis for these differ considerably.
- Hypertrophic cardiomyopathies can cause angina, HF, syncope, and fatal arrhythmias.
- Treatment of obstructive symptoms with beta blockers or calcium channel blockers and risk-stratifying for SCD are the most important features in caring for patients with hypertrophic cardiomyopathies.

REFERENCES AND SUGGESTED READINGS

Caforio AL, Bonifacio E, Stewart JT, et al. Novel organ-specific circulating cardiac autoantibodies in dilated cardiomyopathy. *J Am Coll Cardiol* 1990;15(7):1527–1534.

Felker GM, Thompson RE, Hare JM, et al. Underlying causes and long-term survival in patients with initially unexplained cardiomyopathy. *N Engl J Med* 2000;342(15): 1077–1084.

Ferrans VJ, Morrow AG, Roberts WC. Myocardial ultrastructure in idiopathic hypertrophic subaortic stenosis. A study of operatively excised left ventricular outflow tract muscle in 14 patients. *Circulation* 1972;45(4):769–792.

Frustaci A, Cuoco L, Chimenti C, et al. Celiac disease associated with autoimmune myocarditis. *Circulation* 2002;105(22):2611–2618.

Frustaci A, Kajstura J, Chimenti C, et al. Myocardial cell death in human diabetes. *Circ Res* 2000;87:1123.

Kabbani SS, LeWinter MM. Diastolic heart failure. Constrictive, restrictive, and pericardial. *Cardiol Clin* 2000;18(3):501–509.

Kamisago M, Sharma SD, DePalma SR, et al. Mutations in sarcomere protein genes as a cause of dilated cardiomyopathy. *N Engl J Med* 2000;343(23):1688–1696.

Kelly DP, Strauss AW. Inherited cardiomyopathies. *N Engl J Med* 1994;330(13):913–919.

Kim CH, Vlietstra RE, Edwards WD, et al. Steroid-responsive eosinophilic myocarditis: diagnosis by endomyocardial biopsy. *Am J Cardiol* 1984;53(10):1472–1473.

Kushwaha SS, Fallon JT, Fuster V. Restrictive cardiomyopathy. *N Engl J Med* 1997;336(4):267–276.

Manolio TA, Baughman KL, Rodeheffer R, et al. Prevalence and etiology of idiopathic dilated cardiomyopathy (summary of a National Heart, Lung, and Blood Institute workshop). *Am J Cardiol* 1992;69(17):1458–1466.

Maron BJ, Estes NA III, Maron MS, et al. Primary prevention of sudden death as a novel treatment strategy in hypertrophic cardiomyopathy. *Circulation* 2003;107(23):2872–2875.

Maron BJ, McKenna WJ, Danielson GK, et al. American College of Cardiology/European Society of Cardiology clinical expert consensus document on hypertrophic cardiomyopathy. A report of the American College of Cardiology Foundation Task Force on Clinical Expert Consensus Documents and the European Society of Cardiology Committee for Practice Guidelines. *J Am Coll Cardiol* 2003;42(9):1687–1713.

Maron BJ, Nishimura RA, McKenna WJ, et al. Assessment of permanent dual-chamber pacing as a treatment for drug-refractory symptomatic patients with obstructive hypertrophic cardiomyopathy. A randomized, double-blind, crossover study (M-PATHY). *Circulation* 1999;99(22):2927–2933.

Maron BJ. Hypertrophic cardiomyopathy: a systematic review. *JAMA* 2002;287(10):1308–1320.

Maron BJ. Sudden death in young athletes. *N Engl J Med* 2003;349(11):1064–1075.

Maron BJ, Spirito P, Shen W-K, et al. Implantable cardioverter-defibrillators and the prevention of sudden cardiac death in hypertrophic cardiomyopathy. *JAMA* 2007;298:405–412.

McNally EM, MacLeod H. Therapy insight: cardiovascular complications associated with muscular dystrophies. *Nat Clin Pract Cardiovasc Med* 2005;2(6):301–308.

Nishimura RA, Holmes DR Jr. Clinical practice. Hypertrophic obstructive cardiomyopathy. *N Engl J Med* 2004;350(13):1320–1327.

Obrador D, Ballester M, Carrio I, et al. Presence, evolving changes, and prognostic implications of myocardial damage detected in idiopathic and alcoholic dilated cardiomyopathy by ^{111}In monoclonal antimyosin antibodies. *Circulation* 1994;89(5):2054–2061.

Olivotto I, Cecchi F, Casey SA, et al. Impact of atrial fibrillation on the clinical course of hypertrophic cardiomyopathy. *Circulation* 2001;104(21):2517–2524.

Robiolio PA, Rigolin VH, Wilson JS, et al. Carcinoid heart disease. Correlation of high serotonin levels with valvular abnormalities detected by cardiac catheterization and echocardiography. *Circulation* 1995;92(4):790–795.

Sardesai SH, Mourant AJ, Sivathandon Y, et al. Phaeochromocytoma and catecholamine induced cardiomyopathy presenting as heart failure. *Br Heart J* 1990;63(4):234–237.

Spirito P, Seidman CE, McKenna WJ, et al. The management of hypertrophic cardiomyopathy. *N Engl J Med* 1997;336(11):775–785.

Sugrue DD, Rodeheffer RJ, Codd MB, et al. The clinical course of idiopathic dilated cardiomyopathy. A population-based study. *Ann Intern Med* 1992;117(2):117–123.

Tai PC, Ackerman SJ, Spry CJ, et al. Deposits of eosinophil granule proteins in cardiac tissues of patients with eosinophilic endomyocardial disease. *Lancet* 1987;1(8534): 643–647.

Thompson PD, Klocke FJ, Levine BD, et al. 26th Bethesda Conference: recommendations for determining eligibility for competition in athletes with cardiovascular abnormalities. Task Force 5: coronary artery disease. *Med Sci Sports Exerc* 1994;26(10 Suppl):S271–S275.

Von Hoff DD, Layard MW, Basa P, et al. Risk factors for doxorubicin-induced congestive heart failure. *Ann Intern Med* 1979;91(5):710–717.

Wittstein IS, Thiemann DR, Lima JA, et al. Neurohumoral features of myocardial stunning due to sudden emotional stress. *N Engl J Med* 2005;352(6):539–548.

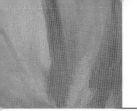

Diseases of the Pericardium

Steven M. Ewer

INTRODUCTION

The pericardium is a fibrous sac surrounding the heart. It consists of two layers: the thin visceral pericardium attached to the epicardium and the thicker parietal pericardium. The two are separated by the **pericardial space**, normally containing 15 to 50 mL of fluid. Pericardial fluid consists of an ultrafiltrate continuously produced from the mesothelial cells of the visceral pericardium and resorbed via lymphatics and venules. Although it is not absolutely essential for cardiac performance, several functions have been attributed to the pericardium:

- Tethering of the heart within the mediastinum
- Lubrication of the movements of the heart
- Augmentation of diastolic function
- Serving as a barrier to infection and inflammation
- Participation in autonomic reflexes and paracrine signaling

This chapter discusses the major pericardial syndromes—including acute pericarditis, pericardial effusion, tamponade, pericardial constriction—and pericardial tumors.

ACUTE PERICARDITIS

Background

Acute pericarditis is the most common pericardial syndrome, diagnosed in 1 in 1000 hospital admissions. Inflammation of the pericardium results in characteristic clinical features. Because inflammation of adjacent myocardium is nearly always present (explaining ECG changes and elevation of serum cardiac markers), some prefer the term "myopericarditis." Large pericardial effusions are uncommon among patients with acute pericarditis, especially those with idiopathic or viral etiology.

Causes

Table 13-1 lists the most common categories and specific causes of acute pericarditis. Idiopathic causes account for the greatest number of cases, with viral infections the as next most frequent. Autoimmune phenomena collectively represent a major cause of acute pericarditis, including collagen vascular diseases, drug-induced, postpericardiotomy, and **Dressler's syndrome**, which is pericarditis that occurs in 1% of patients in the weeks to months after a myocardial infarction (MI). Uremic pericarditis occurs in one-third of patients with chronic uremia, most of whom are on hemodialysis. It is often associated with a pericardial effusion. Tuberculous pericarditis should be suspected in high-risk patients (history of exposure, immunocompromised state).

TABLE 13-1	ETIOLOGIES OF ACUTE PERICARDITIS

1. Infectious
   a. Viral (coxsackie, echovirus, Epstein–Barr virus, HIV)
   b. Tuberculosis
   c. Lyme disease
   d. Miscellaneous (other viral, bacterial, fungal, parasitic)
2. Uremia
3. Collagen vascular disease
4. Myocardial infarction, acute or subacute (Dressler's syndrome)
5. Post–cardiac surgery
6. Trauma
7. Cancer, chemotherapy, radiation
8. Drugs (hydralazine, procainamide, isoniazid, phenytoin, penicillin)
9. Hypothyroidism
10. Idiopathic

Clinical Presentation

Patients with acute pericarditis almost universally complain of recent-onset chest pain. The pain is usually sharp, retrosternal or left-sided, and radiates to the back, neck, and shoulders. It may be pleuritic in nature. **Classically, the pain is worse when the patient is supine and improves when the patient leans forward.** Some patients may remember a recent viral illness or complain of fever, dyspnea and cough. Initially, distinction from myocardial ischemia can be quite challenging.

Physical exam of patients with acute pericarditis is unimpressive unless a pathognomonic **pericardial friction rub** is present. This is a specific but not very sensitive finding caused by friction between the inflamed, juxtaposed visceral and parietal pericardia. The rub is high-pitched, grating, and scratching. Classically, it has three components per cardiac cycle (ventricular systole, early diastole, and atrial systole), but only one or two components may be present. Pericardial rubs can be fleeting and dynamic, often changing by the hour in the early stages of the disease.

Diagnostic Testing

Serial electrocardiograms (ECGs) during the initial hours to days of acute pericarditis reveal a characteristic evolution; these signs are present in most cases (Fig. 13-1):

- Stage 1: Diffuse ST-segment elevation and PR depression
- Stage 2: Normalized ST segment, decreased T-wave amplitude
- Stage 3: T-wave inversion
- Stage 4: Normalization

Of these changes, only stage 1 is diagnostic for acute pericarditis, with the others being too nonspecific to be useful. Progression through the stages can help confirm the diagnosis, however. The crucial distinction between stage 1 ECG changes and acute ST-segment-elevation MI, which requires immediate diagnosis and treatment, lies in the **noncoronary distribution of the ST changes** (leads I, II, and III) and the presence of PR depression with pericarditis. Because there can be considerable overlap in the ECG findings in these two

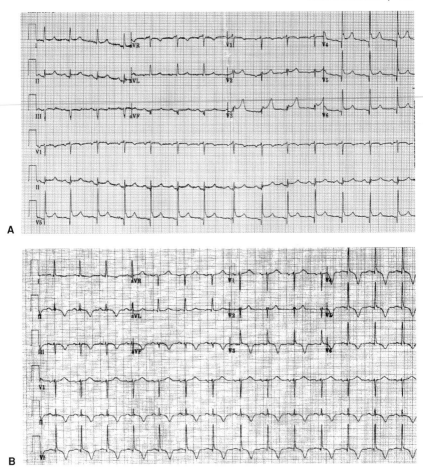

FIGURE 13-1. ECG in pericarditis. **A:** Stage 1 pericarditis, exhibiting diffuse concave ST-segment elevations and PR depression except in aVR, where the abnormalities are reversed. **B:** Stage 3 pericarditis, 1 day later in the same patient, showing diffuse T-wave inversion after ST segments had normalized.

entities, urgent echocardiography can be useful to rule out segmental wall motion abnormalities, which would be expected with ischemia.

Transthoracic echocardiography (TTE) is obtained at diagnosis and usually 1 to 2 weeks after initiation of treatment to rule out significant pericardial effusion. Large effusions are not typical in uncomplicated viral or idiopathic pericarditis; the presence of such alerts the physician to a broader differential diagnosis and a higher likelihood of complications, such as chronic inflammation, constriction, or tamponade.

Laboratory tests may reveal nonspecific markers of inflammation, such as an elevated erythrocyte sedimentation rate (ESR), C-reactive protein (CRP), and leukocytosis. Serum cardiac markers are often mildly elevated, indicating some level of myocarditis as well. More specific tests, such as antinuclear antibody (ANA), rheumatoid factor, thyroid function, purified protein derivative (PPD), and blood cultures, should be ordered based on the clinical scenario.

Treatment

Treatment consists of a **short course of a nonsteroidal anti-inflammatory drug** (NSAID) such as aspirin, ibuprofen, naproxen, or indomethacin. A reasonable dose of ibuprofen is 400 to 800 mg every 8 hours. We favor at least a 2-week course even if symptoms resolve, as this may reduce the risk of scarring. Recent evidence suggests that colchicine may also be beneficial, especially in recurrent disease. However, in patients with renal insufficiency, care must be taken to avoid toxicity. Corticosteroids may be needed for refractory cases but are generally avoided, given their substantial side-effect profile and the possible increased likelihood of recurrence. Further therapy is tailored to the underlying disease when appropriate. **Anticoagulants are generally avoided to decrease the risk of hemopericardium**, a rare complication. Other complications include recurrent or chronic pericarditis; pericardial constriction (usually resulting from chronic pericarditis); and pericardial effusion and tamponade (including hemopericardium).

PERICARDIAL EFFUSION

Background
Pericardial effusion is an increased amount of fluid in the pericardial space. Effusions become clinically detectable around 50 mL and can reach up to 2L. The significance of pericardial effusions is determined by their size, rate of accumulation, and cause. Etiology can be categorized mechanistically:

- Increased fluid production (chronic inflammation)
- Decreased resorption (disruption of lymphatics and veins)
- Altered oncotic balance [congestive heart failure (CHF), renal failure, hypoalbuminemia]
- Foreign substance (blood, pus, lymph, tumor infiltration)

Causes

Differential diagnosis of a pericardial effusion overlaps substantially with that of acute pericarditis (Table 13-1), but the relative frequencies differ. Acute idiopathic and viral pericarditis are less common, whereas chronic inflammation, renal disease, and cancer move higher on the list. An underlying diagnosis is often established prior to development of the pericardial effusion.

Clinical Presentation

Fluid in the pericardial sac can present variably. It can be asymptomatic—noticed incidentally on diagnostic testing—or it can present as life-threatening cardiac tamponade, in which the intrapericardial pressure compresses the heart (discussed separately below). Symptoms of pericardial effusion, when present, are often vague and nonspecific. Fatigue, decreased exercise capacity, and dyspnea are common. Occasionally patients may complain of a dull ache or chest pressure. Large effusions may compress extrinsic structures and lead to complaints of dysphagia, hiccups, hoarseness (due to recurrent laryngeal nerve impingement), or cough.

Physical exam often yields no unique findings unless tamponade is present, but large effusions may cause decreased heart sounds and dullness at the left lung base due to compression of the left lung (**Ewart's sign**). Despite a substantial effusion, a pericardial rub may still be present.

TABLE 13-2	ESTIMATION OF PERICARDIAL EFFUSION BY ECHOCARDIOGRAPHY	
Effusion Size	**Volume (mL)**	**Posterior Effusion Thickness**
Physiologic	<50	<10 mm, systole only
Small	50–100	<10 mm, seen in systole and diastole
Moderate	100–500	10–20 mm, seen anteriorly as well
Large	>500	>20 mm, seen anteriorly, posteriorly, and apically

Diagnostic Testing

ECG may reveal **low voltage of the QRS complex** with flattening of the T waves. Chest x-ray may reveal enlargement of the cardiac silhouette if >250 mL of fluid has accumulated. The classic **globular or water bottle–shaped heart** may occasionally be seen. CT and MRI are capable of determining size of effusion, estimating pericardial thickness, and have the added advantage of imaging surrounding structures.

Transthoracic echocardiography is the study of choice for diagnosis and follow-up of pericardial effusions. The size of an effusion can be estimated by evaluating the posterior echo-free space on the parasternal long-axis view during diastole (Table 13-2). In addition to size and location of the effusion, echo can detect other features, such as pericardial thickness, fibrinous stranding, and fluid loculations or masses. When large effusions are present, findings of tamponade should be specifically excluded.

Diagnostic pericardiocentesis can be considered if an effusion is large and readily accessible and if further diagnostic information would affect management decisions. This is particularly important if there is a high suspicion for neoplastic or purulent pericarditis. After noting the gross features of the effusion, fluid should be sent for cell count, differential, Gram's stain, culture, and cytology. Further specific testing (acid-fast staining) is based on the clinical scenario. Malignant pericardial effusion is defined by an effusion associated with pathologic evidence for tumor invasion of the pericardium and portends a very poor prognosis. However, of patients with known cancer and a pericardial effusion, only one-third to one-half will have a malignant effusion. Because many patients will have a nonmalignant and potentially treatable etiology, the correct diagnosis is of utmost importance. Cytology is positive in 80% to 90% of malignant effusions, with sensitivity increased further when pericardial biopsy is performed.

Treatment

Therapy for pericardial effusion is directed at the underlying cause, with drainage indicated for symptomatic or refractory cases and where infection is present. Specific drainage procedures are discussed below and in Chapter 6. Anticoagulation is generally avoided until the effusion resolves.

CARDIAC TAMPONADE

Background
Cardiac tamponade is a condition that exists when the pericardial space contains fluid under sufficient pressure to interfere with cardiac filling, resulting in decreased cardiac output and the inability to sustain vital functions. **Tamponade is a medical emergency**, as cardiogenic

shock and death can rapidly ensue. The intrapericardial pressure depends on the **amount of fluid** present, its **rate of accumulation,** and the **compliance** of the pericardium. A large effusion is generally a prerequisite for tamponade, exceptions being tamponade associated with trauma or cardiac surgery, which can cause small, localized hemorrhages.

Causes

Any condition that can lead to pericardial effusion can cause tamponade. The most common causes are idiopathic, malignancy, uremia, cardiac rupture, iatrogenic disease, bacterial infection, tuberculosis, radiation, myxedema, dissecting aortic aneurysm, postcardiotomy, and lupus.

Clinical Presentation

Symptoms of tamponade include dyspnea, cough, extreme fatigue, presyncope, and anxiety. With progression, evidence of shock is found with decreased urine output, mental status changes, obtundation and pulseless electrical activity. Physical exam findings of tamponade include the following:

- Jugular venous distention (JVD)
- Tachycardia and hypotension
- Pulsus paradoxus >10 mm Hg
- Decreased heart sounds
- Signs of cardiogenic shock

The most sensitive sign of tamponade is **JVD.** The neck veins may also show a **prominent *x* descent and lack of *y* descent** (Fig. 13-2), characteristic of tamponade. **Pulsus paradoxus,** an exaggerated drop in systolic pressure on inspiration, should be assessed. While inspiration normally increases right ventricular (RV) filling, the pressure constraints of tamponade require a compensatory decrease in LV filling and hence lower systemic blood pressure. Pulsus paradoxus can be checked by inflating the blood pressure cuff above the systolic pressure and deflating until Korotkoff sounds are heard only during expiration. Then the cuff is further deflated until Korotkoff sounds are heard with both inspiration and expiration. The pulsus paradoxus is the difference between these pressures. A drop in

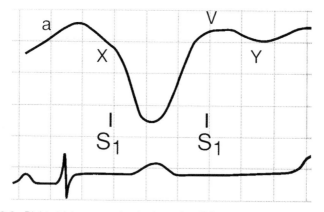

FIGURE 13-2. Right atrial pressure tracing in pericardial tamponade. Note the prominent *x* descent and absent *y* descent. (From Murphy JG. *Mayo Clinic Cardiology Review,* 2nd ed. Philadelphia: Lippincott Williams & Wilkins; 2000:854, with permission.)

pressure of >10 mm Hg is considered significant. Other disorders that may be associated with an abnormal pulsus paradoxus include obstructive pulmonary disease, constrictive pericarditis, and RV failure from infarction and pulmonary embolism.

Diagnostic Testing

The ECG may show low precordial voltages. **Electrical alternans** is a more specific finding of tamponade and is caused by the heart swinging within the pericardium. Because the heart usually moves back and forth over two cardiac cycles, a beat-to-beat alternation in the voltage appears on the ECG.

As soon as tamponade is suspected, **transthoracic echocardiography (TTE) should be performed urgently** to confirm the diagnosis, clinical status permitting. TTE reveals a large effusion and may show swinging of the heart, as mentioned above. There are four echo findings that suggest the hemodynamic alterations of tamponade:

- Right atrial notching in systole
- RV collapse in diastole
- Dilated, noncompressible inferior vena cava (IVC)
- Variation of tricuspid valve inflow velocities of >50% or mitral valve inflow velocities of >25% with respiration

Right atrial compression and a dilated IVC are more sensitive findings; RV compression and abnormal Doppler inflow velocities tend to occur later and are more specific. Note that echocardiography reveals only a snapshot in time and therefore cannot assess the rate of progression or predict onset of fatal hemodynamic collapse. Tamponade is a clinical diagnosis, and echocardiography has a confirmatory role. The decision of how and when to best perform drainage is best determined by the patient's clinical status and not the specific echo findings.

If tamponade is suspected in cases of postcardiotomy or cardiac trauma, transthoracic echo provides inadequate assessment because of the possibility of localized effusions and usually poor echocardiographic windows. Indeed, the most common location of hemorrhage postcardiotomy is posterior to the left atrium, which is virtually invisible by TTE. Transesophageal echocardiography (TEE) should be used instead to confirm the diagnosis.

Treatment

Patients with clinical tamponade need to be drained expediently. Options for treatment include percutaneous needle pericardiocentesis and surgical drainage. Different drainage procedures should be selected on an individual basis determined by the clinical situation (degree of exigency, location of effusion, likelihood for recurrence). Before drainage, patients must be **resuscitated with volume-expanding agents** to delay RV diastolic collapse. Norepinephrine (Levophed) may be added for blood pressure support if absolutely necessary. Additionally, endotracheal intubation must be undertaken with caution owing to the decrease in preload both with sedative agents and with positive-pressure ventilation.

Percutaneous needle pericardiocentesis is a rapid method for draining pericardial fluid and is appropriate for all emergent and most urgent cases involving some hemodynamic compromise. It can be performed at the bedside or in a cardiac catheterization lab. Most operators use echocardiographic guidance and agitated saline injected through the pericardiocentesis needle to visually confirm entry in to the pericardial space. There is a low but significant risk of complications, including cardiac puncture. A pericardial drain is usually left in place for several days postprocedure until drain output tapers off to prevent short-term reaccumulation.

If the patient is not experiencing imminent hemodynamic collapse, **subxiphoid pericardiotomy** is a minimally invasive surgical procedure that can provide a more definitive treatment and reduced risk of recurrence. Additionally, a pericardiotomy allows for visualization, thorascopic inspection, and tissue biopsy. A pleuropericardial window may also be created. Complication rates are low.

More definitive surgical management of malignant pericardial disease requires partial or complete **pericardiectomy**. This requires general anesthesia for anterior thoracotomy or sternotomy and is associated with significant morbidity and mortality. Less invasive treatments are usually preferred, but pericardiectomy can be considered in those with a relatively good prognosis in whom more definitive therapy is desired.

CONSTRICTIVE PERICARDITIS

Background
Constrictive pericarditis occurs when chronic inflammation renders the pericardium thickened and scarred. The pericardial space is usually obliterated, and the hallmark feature of constriction is **loss of normal pericardial compliance**. This exerts an external volume constraint on the heart, thus interfering with cardiac filling. At the onset of diastole, ventricular filling begins unimpeded, but pressures rapidly increase and filling ceases owing to the noncompliance. Because of the external volume limit, there is **equalization of pressures across all four cardiac chambers** during late diastole. Knowing this pathophysiology is important to understanding the classic findings of constriction.

Causes
Any chronic insult to the pericardium (including host immune response) can result in constriction. The most common causes include:

- Idiopathic or viral pericarditis (smoldering, chronic, recurrent)
- Postcardiotomy
- Chest irradiation (e.g., mantle radiation for lymphoma)
- Collagen vascular disease
- End-stage renal disease/hemodialysis
- Malignancy (e.g., lung, breast, lymphoma)
- Tuberculosis (most common cause in developing countries)

Idiopathic/viral causes account for about 45% of cases; postcardiotomy, 25%; and radiation, 20%; with other causes being fairly uncommon.

Clinial Presentation
The signs and symptoms of constrictive pericarditis are due to elevated filling pressures and left- and right-sided failure. In early stages, patients may complain of **fatigue, weakness, and decreased exercise tolerance**. As filling pressures continue to rise, patients complain of right-sided symptoms, such as **lower extremity edema, increased abdominal girth and ascites**, and eventually left-sided symptoms, such as dyspnea on exertion, orthopnea, paroxysmal nocturnal dyspnea, and cough. Because there are many other more common causes of these symptoms, the diagnosis of constrictive pericarditis requires a high degree of clinical suspicion.

Physical exam in constriction typically reveals impressive findings of right-sided heart failure, including **hepatomegaly, ascites, and markedly elevated JVP**. Findings of left-sided heart failure, such as frank pulmonary edema, are less common. Physical exam findings more specific for constriction include:

- Increased JVP with **prominent *y* descent** (rapid early diastolic filling) (Fig. 13-3)
- **Kussmaul's sign** (lack of expected decrease or obvious increase of JVP on inspiration)

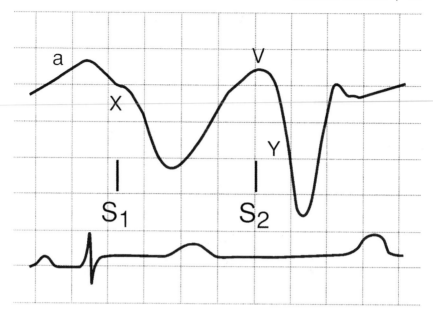

FIGURE 13-3. Right atrial pressure tracing in constrictive pericarditis. Note the prominent *y* descent. (From Murphy JG. *Mayo Clinic Cardiology Review,* 2nd ed. Philadelphia: Lippincott Williams & Wilkins; 2000, with permission.)

- **Pericardial knock** (early, loud, high-pitched S3 derived from rapid pressure equalization after initial ventricular filling)

Diagnostic Testing

No single study provides definitive evidence of constrictive pericarditis; it is often necessary to obtain several different studies to support clinical suspicion. **Chest x-ray may reveal a calcified pericardium** or pleural effusions. ECG findings commonly include low QRS voltage, generalized T-wave inversion or flattening, and left atrial enlargement. Atrial fibrillation is fairly common.

TTE can reveal several indirect features suggestive of constriction:

- Thickened, echogenic pericardium
- Tram-tracking (adherence to and movement with the myocardium during contraction)
- Dilated, noncompressible IVC
- Septal bounce (rapid early diastolic filling)
- Posterior LV wall flattening in diastole (equalization of pressures, equivalent to the "square root" sign)
- Ventricular interdependence on Doppler exam

No findings are particularly pathognomonic, although ventricular interdependence is the closest physiologic correlate. Because of the external volume constraint, right and left ventricles fill at the expense of each other. Mitral inflow velocities decrease with inspiration

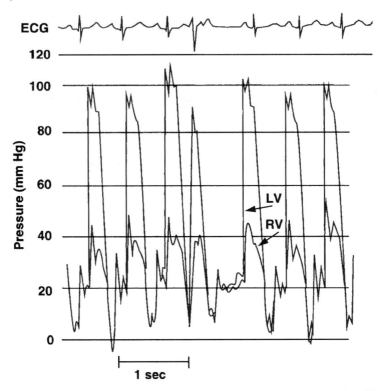

FIGURE 13-4. Simultaneous RV and LV pressure tracings in constrictive pericarditis. Note the prominent dip and plateau (square root sign), particularly post-PVC. (Adapted from Marso SP, Griffin BP, Topol EJ, eds. *Manual of Cardiovascular Medicine*. Philadelphia: Lippincott Williams & Wilkins; 2000, with permission.)

and increase with expiration, and tricuspid velocities conversely increase with inspiration and decrease with expiration.

Right- and left-heart catheterizations are done simultaneously to assess right- and left-sided pressures, determine cardiac output, and help differentiate constrictive from restrictive physiology. Hemodynamic measurements reveal elevated and **equal pressure in all four chambers** in diastole before the a wave. Right atrial measurements reveal a **preserved *x* descent and a steep *y* descent** from the increased flow during early diastole (Fig. 13-3) and **Kussmaul's sign.** Ventricular hemodynamic measurements reveal **the dip-and-plateau (square root sign) during diastole** due to rapid early diastolic filling, which is abruptly halted once the constricted volume is reached (Fig. 13-4).

CT and MRI are useful for detecting pericardial thickening, dilated hepatic veins, dilated right atrium, and other findings that support constrictive pericarditis. These studies are not diagnostic and should be used only to support a diagnosis of pericardial constriction.

A common diagnostic dilemma is the **distinction between pericardial constriction and restrictive cardiomyopathy.** Decreased compliance of either the pericardium and myocardium lead to similar defects in ventricular filling, and substantial overlap exists in signs, symptoms, and hemodynamic measurements. The distinction is critical however, as patients with restrictive cardiomyopathy carry an exceptionally high mortality risk with cardiac surgery. Restrictive

TABLE 13-3	DISTINGUISHING PERICARDIAL CONSTRICTION AND RESTRICTIVE CARDIOMYOPATHY	
Constriction	**Restriction**	
Ventricular interdependence present	Absent	
Abnormal pericardial features (thick, echogenic, adherent, calcified)	Abnormal myocardial features (infiltration, abnormal biopsy, conduction system disease)	
Preserved tissue Doppler velocities	Restrictive diastolic filling pattern	
Pulmonary hypertension mild or absent	Significant pulmonary hypertension	
Septal bounce	Normal septal motion	
LVEDP–RVEDP <5 mm Hg (equalization)	LVEDP-RVEDP >5 mm Hg	
RVEDP/RVSP >1/3	RVEDP/RVSP <1/3	
BNP low or mildly elevated (<200)	BNP elevated (>200)	

BNP, B-type natriuretic peptide; LVEDP, left ventricular end-diastolic pressure; RVEDP, right ventricular end-diastolic pressure; RSVP, right ventricular systolic pressure.

cardiomyopathy and constriction can be present in the same patient (i.e., after chest irradiation). Occasionally endomyocardial biopsy is required to rule out a myocardial process prior to surgery. Table 13-3 highlights some the major differences between these entities.

Treatment

Constrictive pericarditis is a difficult disease to manage medically. If possible, it is desirable to treat underlying cause. Diuretics and a low-salt diet form the cornerstone of therapy but often meet with limited success. **Surgical pericardiectomy** (stripping) is the definitive therapy of choice in surgical candidates; however, the operative mortality rate can be as high as 15%. Some 90% of patients report symptomatic improvement. Surgery should be performed early, as constrictive pericarditis is a progressive disease, and patients with poor functional class are at higher risk of perioperative death.

PERICARDIAL TUMORS

It is not infrequent for a patient to present with a mass (or multiple masses) within the pericardium. Although there is occasionally some overlap in presentation with the pericardial processes discussed above, the spectrum of pericardial tumors could be considered a pericardial syndrome in its own right. Tumors can be categorized as **primary** (derived initially from pericardial tissue) or **metastatic**. Common presentations include incidental findings on imaging, symptoms from compression of the cardiac chambers (usually dyspnea or syncope), pericarditis, effusion/tamponade, and arrhythmias.

Primary Pericardial Tumors

Primary pericardial tumors are very rare. Five entities make up the bulk of tumors in this category:

- Pericardial cyst
- Teratoma

- Mesothelioma
- Angiosarcoma
- Lipoma

Pericardial cysts are fluid-filled fibrous sacs lined with mesothelial cells and represent the most common primary pericardial tumor. They are usually <3 cm in size and are often located at the right heart border. Surgery is curative but is often not necessary, as there is no malignant potential. Teratomas occur more often in young women; although benign, they are quite aggressive and are especially likely to cause compressive symptoms. Mesotheliomas are malignant, with features similar to the better-known pleural mesothelioma. Association with asbestos exposure is still controversial. Angiosarcomas are aggressive malignancies that can be derived from pericardial or myocardial tissue. Pericardial lipomas are similar to lipomas in other locations.

Pericardial Metastases

Pericardial metastases are 100- to 1000-fold more common than primary tumors. This usually represents a late-stage process; thus the diagnosis of malignancy is usually well established at the time of presentation. The most common malignancies found to metastasize to the pericardium include **lung cancer** (33%), **breast cancer** (19%), **and hematologic malignancies** (13%), which together account for about two-thirds of cases. Although less common overall, **melanoma** has the highest propensity to spread to the pericardium. There are three routes of metastasis to the pericardium: lymphatic spread (lung and breast cancer), hematogenous spread (leukemia, lymphoma, melanoma), and direct extension (lung and esophageal cancer). Lymphatic spread is associated with significant pericardial effusion, and hematogenous spread tends to result in hemorrhagic effusion.

Diagnosis typically involves imaging with multiple modalities, pericardial fluid analysis, and, when feasible, tissue biopsy. In addition to systemic antitumor therapy, treatment includes local control with drainage procedures, radiation, and occasionally instillation of chemotherapeutic drugs into the pericardial space. Prognosis is very poor, however, and treatment strategies are generally aimed at palliation.

KEY POINTS TO REMEMBER

- Acute pericarditis often presents with chest pain and ST-segment elevations on the ECG. Acute MI must immediately be ruled out.
- Positional or pleuritic chest pain, friction rub, PR depression on ECG, a noncoronary distribution of ST-segment elevation, and lack of segmental wall motion abnormalities on echocardiography all favor pericarditis over MI.
- Treat pericarditis with NSAIDs or colchicine.
- Pericardial effusions are diagnosed and evaluated with imaging, especially echocardiography; tamponade should be excluded when large effusions are present.
- Diagnostic pericardiocentesis is indicated for accessible effusions if infection or malignancy is suspected or if the underlying etiology is unknown.
- Signs of tamponade include increased JVP, tachycardia, hypotension, pulsus paradoxus, and electrical alternans on ECG.
- Treatment of tamponade includes volume expansion and expedient drainage.
- Consider constrictive pericarditis in patients with fatigue, symptoms of right-sided heart failure, or a history of pericardial disease, cardiac surgery, or chest irradiation.
- Diagnosis of constrictive pericarditis requires a high index of suspicion, and several studies are typically needed to confirm. Restrictive cardiomyopathy must be excluded.

REFERENCES AND SUGGESTED READINGS

Appleton PA, Hatle LK, Popp RL. Cardiac tamponade and pericardial effusion: respiratory variation and transvalvular flow velocities studied by Doppler echocardiography. *J Am Coll Cardiol* 1988;11:1020.

Braunwald E, ed. *Heart Disease: A Textbook of Cardiovascular Medicine,* 5th ed. Philadelphia: Saunders; 1997:1481–1533.

Fuster V, Alexander RW, O'Rourke RA, eds. *Hurst's the heart,* 10th ed. New York: McGraw-Hill, 2000:2064.

Guberman BA, Fowler NO, Engel PJ, et al. Cardiac tamponade in medical patients. *Circulation* 1981;64:633.

Hatle LK, Appleton CP, Popp RL, et al. Differentiation of constrictive pericarditis and restrictive cardiomyopathy by Doppler echocardiography. *Circulation* 1989;79:357–370.

Maisch B, Seferovic PM, Ristic AD, et al. Guidelines on the diagnosis and management of pericardial diseases executive summary; The task force on the diagnosis and management of pericardial diseases of the European Society of Cardiology. *Eur Heart J* 2004;25(7):587–610.

Marso SP, Griffin BP, Topol EJ, eds. *Manual of Cardiovascular Medicine.* Philadelphia: Lippincott Williams & Wilkins; 2000:354–383.

Oh J, Hatle LK, Seward JB, et al. Diagnostic role of Doppler echocardiography in constrictive pericarditis. *J Am Coll Cardiol* 1994;23:154–162.

Spodick DH. *The Pericardium: A Comprehensive Textbook.* New York: Marcel Dekker; 1997.

Pulmonary Hypertension and Right Heart Failure

Raksha Jain

INTRODUCTION

The pulmonary vasculature is typically elastic, highly distensible, and forms a low-resistance circuit, one-tenth that of the systemic vasculature. The normally thin-walled right ventricle thus pumps blood into the lungs against little resistance. Pulmonary hypertension (PH) may develop from processes that cause vasoconstriction, occlusion, or stasis of the pulmonary vascular circulation at the level of the arteries, capillaries, or veins. PH can ultimately result in right heart failure (RHF) and is associated with high morbidity and mortality.

Definition

PH is defined as a mean pulmonary artery pressure of ≥ 25 mm Hg at rest or ≥ 30 mm Hg with exercise as measured by right heart catheterization. PH can be a consequence of left heart failure, defined by having left ventricular end-diastolic pressure (LVEDP) and pulmonary capillary wedge pressure (PCWP) ≥ 15 mm Hg. Alternatively, PH can be independent of left heart failure, with normal LVEDP and PCWP. Pulmonary arterial hypertension (PAH) is a subset of PH (Table 14-1). Many of the specific mechanisms and vasoactive therapies have been studied specifically in patients with PAH.

Etiology

PH can develop acutely or chronically. Causes of acute PH include pulmonary edema due to left heart failure, adult respiratory distress syndrome, or pulmonary embolism. With acute PH, pulmonary artery systolic pressure (PASP) can rise modestly but usually not more than 50 mm Hg. With acute PH, right ventricular (RV) size is normal. When it is exposed to persistently high PA pressures, the RV begins to remodel, hypertrophy, and ultimately dilate. At this point, it is capable of generating higher PA pressures (>50 mm Hg). In evaluating a patient for PH, the **chronicity** and **specific etiology** of the disease are important. The classification of etiologies of PH is found in Table 14-1.

The finding of RHF is most commonly caused by PH due to left heart failure. However, RHF can exist without PH in the following conditions:

- RV infarction: Patients are very dependent on RV preload, so medications that venodilate (nitrates) can cause a dramatic drop in systemic blood pressure.
- Arrhythmogenic right ventricular dysplasia: A fibro-fatty replacement of myocardium, generally affecting the right ventricle. Patients usually present with arrhythmias prior to heart failure.
- Uhl's anomaly: Also known as "parchment heart," this is a congenital absence of the myocardial layer of the RV.

TABLE 14-1   CLASSIFICATION OF PULMONARY HYPERTENSION

Pulmonary arterial hypertension (PAH)

Idiopathic (previously referred to as primary pulmonary hypertension)

Familial

Related to:

 Collagen vascular disease (scleroderma, lupus, mixed connective tissue disease)

 Congenital systemic-to-pulmonary shunts

 Portopulmonary hypertension and hepatopulmonary hypertension

 HIV infection

 Drugs or toxins (anorexigens—fenfluramine, rapeseed oil, methamphetamine, cocaine)

 Thyroid disorders

 Hereditary hemorrhagic telangiectasias

Others: Glycogen storage disease, Gaucher's disease, hemoglobinopathies, myeloproliferative disorders, splenectomy

Associated with significant venous or capillary involvement

 Pulmonary venoocclusive disease

 Pulmonary–capillary hemangiomatosis

Pulmonary venous hypertension

Left heart failure (systolic or diastolic)

Left-sided valvular disease

Pulmonary hypertension associated with hypoxemia

Chronic obstructive pulmonary disease (COPD)

Interstitial lung disease (ILD)

Sleep-disordered breathing (obstructive sleep apnea or obesity hypoventilation syndrome)

Chronic high altitude

Alveolar hypoventilation disorders

Pulmonary hypertension due to chronic thromboembolic disease

Thromboembolic obstruction of distal or proximal pulmonary arteries

Pulmonary embolism (tumor, parasites, foreign material)

Miscellaneous

Sarcoidosis, lymphangioleiomyomatosis, extrinsic compression of pulmonary vessels

Source: From the 1998 World Symposium of Primary Pulmonary Hypertension sponsored by the World Health Organization.

- Massive acute pulmonary embolism: In this situation, the RV may dilate in the absence of elevated PASP, because the RV cannot generate higher pressures. However, with chronic thromboembolic disease, the RV hypertrophies over time, becoming capable of generating higher pressures.

Epidemiology

The incidence of PH varies among patient populations. The incidence of idiopathic PH has been estimated to be 1 to 2 per million. The incidence of PH is particularly high in patients with scleroderma, especially the CREST (calcinosis, Raynaud phenomenon, esophageal dysmotility, sclerodactyly, telangiectasia) variant, with an estimated incidence of 20% to 30%. The incidence of PH in the those infected with human immunodeficiency virus (HIV) has been estimated to be 2% to 4% and in cirrhotic patients to be 2% to 5%.

CAUSES

Pathophysiology

The vascular remodeling of PAH specifically is the culmination of multiple deranged homeostatic pathways, particularly involving pulmonary endothelial cell dysfunction, leading to **vasoconstriction, proliferation of smooth muscle cells, and thrombosis in situ**. Individual factors that play a role include:

- **Nitric oxide (NO)**: Released from the endothelium, NO acts as a pulmonary vasodilator. Low levels of NO have been found in samples of exhaled breath samples from patients with PAH.
- **Endothelin-1 (ET-1)**: Also produced by the endothelium, this peptide is a potent vasoconstrictor. Patients with PAH have increased expression of ET-1 in pulmonary vascular endothelial cells.
- **Prostacyclin**: Produced by the endothelium and systemically, prostacyclin is a vasodilator and inhibitor of platelet aggregation. It is produced at low levels in patients with PAH.
- **Endothelial proliferation and differentiation**: Results in the formation of plexiform lesions, increased numbers of smooth muscle cells and increased deposition of extra-cellular matrix, causing narrowing and stiffening of the pulmonary vasculature. One molecular pathway for this is through **BMPR-II (bone morphogenetic protein receptor II)**. Mutations in this gene have been found in ~50% of patients with familial PAH and ~25% of idiopathic PAH.
- **Platelet activation**: Results in increased propensity for vascular thrombosis.

PRESENTATION

Clinical Presentation and History

The most common presenting symptom is **exertional dyspnea**. However, symptoms of PH and RHF can often be nonspecific and include fatigue, early satiety, and anorexia. Patients may also present with palpitations, syncope, chest pain, hemoptysis, and cough. When RHF has developed, patients will also often complain of lower extremity edema, weight gain, and increased abdominal girth from ascites. A modified New York Heart Association (NYHA) classification is one way to characterize symptom severity (Table 14-2).

Risk factors for PH to specifically ask about include:

- Family history of PH
- Smoking history
- Collagen vascular disease (particularly scleroderma)
- HIV infection
- Liver disease or cirrhosis
- History of use of anorexigens or of illicit drugs such as cocaine or methamphetamines
- Hereditary disorders such as hereditary hemorrhagic telangiectasia or sickle cell disease
- Risk factors for thromboembolic disease (hypercoaguable state)
- Congenital heart disease, with a systemic-to-pulmonary cardiac shunt

TABLE 14-2	FUNCTIONAL ASSESSMENT OF PATIENTS WITH PULMONARY HYPERTENSION: MODIFIED NEW YORK HEART ASSOCIATION

Classification for Patients with PH

- Class I—No limitation of physical activity. Ordinary physical activity does not cause undue dyspnea or fatigue, chest pain, or near syncope.
- Class II—Slight limitation of physical activity. Comfortable at rest. Ordinary physical activity causes undue dyspnea or fatigue, chest pain, or near syncope.
- Class III—Marked limitation of physical activity. Comfortable at rest. Less than ordinary activity causes undue dyspnea or fatigue, chest pain, or near syncope.
- Class IV—Unable to carry out any physical activity without symptoms. Dyspnea and/or fatigue may be present at rest. Discomfort is increased by any physical activity. Signs of right heart failure are present.

Source: From the 1998 World Symposium of Primary Pulmonary Hypertension sponsored by the World Health Organization.

Physical Examination

Physical signs of PH include **RV heave** and **accentuated P$_2$**. When RHF is present, jugular venous distention (JVD) is usually apparent, along with a right-sided S3, a pulsatile and congested liver, ascites, and lower extremity edema. Tricuspid regurgitation often develops and causes a large v wave.

MANAGEMENT

Diagnostic Studies

When PH and RHF are suspected, **Doppler echocardiography with agitated saline bubble study** is the initial test of choice. This gives estimates of systolic PA pressures and reveals the appearance of the RV, which can help determine chronicity of the disease. It is important to understand the limitation of echocardiography in estimating PA pressure (see Chapter 25), as not all patients have a reliable tricuspid regurgitation (TR) jet with which to estimate PA systolic pressure. End-systolic flattening of the interventricular septum indicates RV pressure overload. A saline contrast bubble study can suggest intracardiac shunts (atrial septal defect, patent foramen ovale [PFO]), arteriovenous shunts, or intrapulmonary shunting (liver disease or hereditary hemorrhagic telangiectasia). Echocardiography can also reveal whether left-sided heart failure or valvular abnormalities such as mitral regurgitation or stenosis may be the driving force for PH or RHF. Other common diagnostic studies are outlined in Table 14-3.

The electrocardiogram (**ECG**) may provide useful clues to PH and RHF, including:

- Right axis deviation: QRS axis >90 degrees
- RV hypertrophy: dominant R wave in V1 (>7 mm or R/S ratio >1)
- Right atrial abnormality: P waves >2.5 mm in leads II, III, and aVF
- RV infarction: ST-segment elevation in II, III, aVF and ST-segment elevation in V4R (and occasionally in V1)
- S1Q3T3 pattern: indicative of RV strain, classically described with acute pulmonary embolism

TABLE 14-3	DIAGNOSTIC TESTING FOR PATIENTS WITH PULMONARY HYPERTENSION

- Doppler echocardiography with agitated saline bubble study
- Chest x-ray: evaluate for parenchymal abnormalities (emphysema, interstitial lung disease)
- V̇/Q̇ scan: evaluates for chronic thromboembolic disease
- ECG: provides evidence of right ventricular hypertrophy, right atrial enlargement
- Pulmonary function test with 6-minute-walk oximetry: evaluates for obstructive or restrictive lung disease; provides a functional assessment of exercise tolerance and identifies unmet oxygen demands (O_2 saturation <90%)
- Arterial blood gas: detects chronic hypercapnea and hypoxemia that would either be causative of PH or contribute to its progression
- Laboratory evaluation: HIV, ANA, ENA panel, anti-Scl 70, anticentromere Ab, RNP, TSH, hemoglobin electrophoresis
- Right heart catheterization with vasodilator challenge: "gold standard" study

Additional studies based on initial testing:

- Transesophageal echocardiography: evaluates for intracardiac shunt (PFO, ASD)
- Chest CT: evaluates for thromboembolic disease and parenchymal disease
- Pulmonary angiogram: evaluates for thromboembolic disease if prior testing is nondiagnostic
- Polysomnogram: evaluates for sleep-disordered breathing when history of excessive snoring, daytime somnolence, or morning headache and other causes has not been determined
- Hypercoaguable panel: evaluates for unexplained thromboembolic disease (lupus anticoagulant, anticardiolipin antibody, protein S and C, factor V Leiden, prothrombin gene mutation, homocysteine, and antithrombin III)

ANA, antinuclear antibody; ASD, atrial septal defect; CT, computed tomography; ECG, electrocardiogram; ENA, extractable nuclear antigen; HIV, human immunodeficiency virus; PFO, patent foramen ovale; RNP, ribonucleoprotein; TSH, thyroid-stimulating hormone; V̇/Q̇, ventilation/perfusion.

The "gold standard" for diagnosing PH and RHF is **right heart catheterization,** and it remains an essential part of the evaluation and management of PAH. Right heart catheterization can confirm the diagnosis of PH and RHF, reveal pulmonary venous hypertension with elevated wedge pressures, measure cardiac output, and characterize left-to-right shunts. If PAH is confirmed, the patient should undergo vasodilator testing with short-acting intravenous adenosine, intravenous epoprostenol, or inhaled nitric oxide as long as severe RHF is not present [mean right atrial pressure (RAP) <20 mm Hg and cardiac index >1.5 L/minute per square meter]. Calcium channel blockers (CCBs) are no longer recommended for use in the determination of vasoreactivity because they may induce systemic hypotension, syncope, and cardiovascular collapse, particularly in patients with severe right heart failure. Vasodilator responsiveness is defined as a reduction in the mean pulmonary artery pressure of at least 10 mm Hg to <40 mm Hg and without a decline in the cardiac output.

Treatment

The underlying cause of PH often guides therapy. For example, pulmonary venous hypertension secondary to left heart failure requires appropriate heart failure medications, including diuretics and angiotensin converting enzyme (ACE) inhibitors, but it rarely requires vasoactive therapy. PH secondary to thromboembolic disease should be managed with anticoagulation and thromboendarterectomy when appropriate.

Major advances have been made in the treatment of PAH in the past several years, which reduce symptoms, improve functional class, improve quality of life, and prolong survival in some cases. However, none of these therapies are curative.

General Therapy

- **Supplemental oxygen** is required if O_2 saturation is $<89\%$. The goal is to maintain oxygen saturations of $\geq90\%$ 24 hours a day to avoid hypoxic vasoconstriction.
- **Inotropic therapy** (digoxin) may improve right heart function, cardiac output, and symptoms, but data supporting an effect on survival are lacking.
- Anticoagulation with **warfarin** is appropriate for many patients with severe PH to prevent recurrent thromboembolic events as well as thrombosis in situ. It may also prevent strokes in patients with right-to-left shunts. Anticoagulation is contraindicated, however, in certain types of Eisenmenger's syndrome because of the risk of hemoptysis and pulmonary hemorrhage. Anticoagulation risks may also be prohibitive in other subtypes of PAH due to chronic GI blood loss (scleroderma and portpulmonary hypertension).
- **Diuretics** are useful in managing ascites and pedal edema but should be used with caution to avoid excessive reduction in RV preload and cardiac output.
- Pregnancy should be avoided. Maternal mortality may be as high as 30% to 50% in patients with PH. Use of **contraception** should be encouraged.
- **Smoking cessation** and drug counseling may be beneficial for patients with a history of tobacco, cocaine, or anorexigen use.

Vasoactive Therapy for PAH

Vasodilator therapy can be extremely beneficial in controlling and relieving symptoms of PAH. Data supporting the use of vasodilator therapy to treat PAH has primarily come from patients with NYHA functional class III or IV who have idiopathic PAH or scleroderma associated PAH. Caution should be used in extrapolating the data to other patient populations. Treatment can be complex and is individualized based on the patient's age, comorbidities, psychosocial situation, and disease severity as judged by functional class and hemodynamics (Fig. 14-1). Patients need to be followed closely for initiation and titration of medications. Thus referral to a specialist should be made when vasoactive agents are being considered.

Calcium-channel blockers (nifedipine/Procardia, Adalat, diltiazem/Cardizem): If a significant vasodilator response is seen on right heart catheterization, CCBs may be beneficial. They cause smooth muscle relaxation and thus vasodilate the pulmonary and systemic vasculature, but they can also have a negative inotropic effect and cause a reflex increase in alpha-adrenergic tone. Nifedipine is the most commonly used CCB, but diltiazem may be more appropriate for patients with resting tachycardia. Verapamil should be avoided owing to its negative inotropic effect. If a sustained response is not achieved, other vasodilators should be considered.

Prostanoids (epoprostenol/Flolan, treprostinil/Remodulin, iloprost/Ventavis, beraprost): Prostacyclin causes vasodilation by relaxing vascular smooth muscle cells through the production of cAMP. It also inhibits smooth muscle proliferation and platelet aggregation. Epoprostenol, a synthetic prostacyclin, improves exercise tolerance, hemodynamics, and survival in patients who are in NYHA functional class III or IV. Epoprostenol

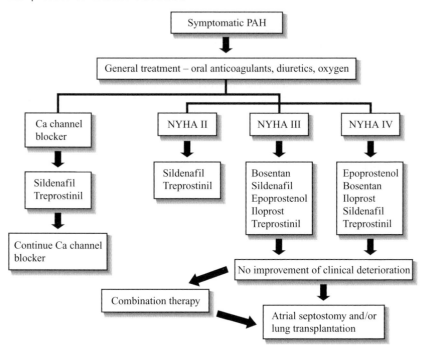

FIGURE 14-1. Approach to treating patients with PH. (Adapted from Badesch DB, Abman SH, Simonneau G, et al. Medical therapy for pulmonary arterial hypertension. *Chest* 2007;131:1925, with permission.)

must be initiated in the hospital and carefully titrated over months. Drug-related side effects include jaw pain, headache, diarrhea, and musculoskeletal pain. Because of its very short half-life ($\sim$2 minutes), sudden discontinuation can be dangerous by causing rebound hypertension and/or RV failure; therefore therapy should never be discontinued abruptly. New and more stable analogs with longer half-lives, such as treprostinil and iloprost, are compatible with subcutaneous and inhaled dosing but appear to have less potency.

Endothelin antagonists (bosentan/Tracleer, sitaxsentan, ambrisentan): Endothelin-1 acts as a direct vasoconstrictor and causes proliferation of smooth muscle cells through the ET_A receptor. Activation of the ET_B receptor promotes ET-1 clearance and induces production of NO and prostacyclin from endothelial cells, which may cause vasodilation. Bosentan is a dual ET_A and ET_B receptor antagonist, which improves exercise capacity and time to clinical worsening as compared with placebo in patients with PAH. Bosentan is metabolized by the liver and should be used with caution in patients with elevated liver function tests. Sitaxsentan and ambrisentan are selective ET_A receptor blockers and show benefits as well.

Phosphodiesterase inhibitors (sildenafil/Viagra, Revatio): The phosphodiesterase inhibitors cause vasodilation by enhancing NO-dependent cGMP activation by inhibiting breakdown of cGMP by phosphodiesterase type 5 inhibition. Sildenafil has shown improved hemodynamics and clinical improvement in patients with PAH.

Nitric oxide (NO): NO is a potent vasodilator that directly relaxes smooth muscle though cGMP. Inhaled NO has shown short-term benefits in patients with PAH, but its role as a long-term treatment agent remains investigational.

Surgical Options

Atrial septostomy: Atrial septostomy is the creation of an atrial septal defect used for select patients with refractory RHF, particularly in the setting of recurrent syncope. By creating a hole between the right and left atria, the high pressures of the right atrium and right ventricle can be "decompressed," improving left ventricular filling and cardiac output. However, this essentially creates an Eisenmenger physiology, with worsening systemic oxygen saturations due to the creation of a right-to-left shunt. Since the mortality associated with this procedure is high, it should be performed only at highly experienced centers.

Lung or heart–lung transplantation is an option for some patients who are refractory to pharmacologic treatment. A criterion for lung transplantation in PH patients is NYHA functional class III or IV despite optimal medical management. Concomitant heart transplant is rarely necessary in PAH because the RV will recover in vast majority of cases; the main indication for a heart–lung transplant is complex congenital heart disease. Single-lung and bilateral lung transplantation has been successful for patients with idiopathic PH. The 5-year survival of patients with idiopathic PH has been 40% to 45%, slightly lower than the survival of patients who undergo lung transplantation for other diseases.

Prognosis

Individual responses to vasodilator therapy for PAH are variable and often difficult to predict, although dramatic clinical improvements are common. Systemic hypotension is the most common complication of therapy. Treatment regimens should be managed by a specialist and be titrated and reevaluated frequently. Overall, the prognosis in patients with PH is highly variable and depends on the underlying disease and degree of RHF. Mean duration of survival after diagnosis of idiopathic untreated PAH is 2.8 years.

KEY POINTS TO REMEMBER

- In evaluating a patient with PH, it is important to determine the chronicity of symptoms and to look for clues to the etiology of the PH.
- The initial test for evaluating PH is a Doppler echocardiogram with agitated saline bubble study. The gold standard for diagnosing PAH is a right heart catheterization with nitric oxide vasoreactivity testing.
- In addition to treating the underlying cause, specific treatment of PAH can include oxygen, digoxin, diuretics, contraception, smoking cessation, warfarin, and pulmonary vasoactive therapy.
- Patients' quality of life has improved significantly with the advancement in medical treatment for PAH. However, these therapies are still not curative, and morbidity and mortality remain high.

ACKNOWLEDGMENTS

Special thanks to Murali Chakinala, MD; Assistant Professor, Division of Pulmonary and Critical Care, Washington University School of Medicine, for reviewing this chapter.

REFERENCES AND SUGGESTED READINGS

Badesch DB, Abman SH, Simonneau G, et al. Medical therapy for pulmonary arterial hypertension. *Chest* 2007;131:1917–1928.

Farber HW, Loscalzo J. Mechanisms of disease – pulmonary arterial hypertension. *N Engl J Med* 2004;351:1655–1665.

Ghamra ZW, Dweik RA. Primary pulmonary hypertension: an overview of epidemiology and pathogenesis. *Cleve Clin J Med* 2003;70:S2–S7.

Humbert M, Sitbon O, Simonneau G. Treatment of pulmonary arterial hypertension. *N Engl J Med* 2004;351:1425–1436.

Krowka MJ. Pulmonary hypertension: diagnostics and therapeutics. *Mayo Clin Proc* 2000;75:625–630.

Nauser TD, Stites SW. Diagnosis and treatment of pulmonary hypertension. *Am Fam Physician* 2001;63:1789–1798.

Rubin LJ, Badesch DB. Evaluation and management of the patient with pulmonary arterial hypertension. *Ann Intern Med* 2005;143:282–292.

Rubin LJ. Primary pulmonary hypertension. *N Engl J Med* 1997;336:111–117.

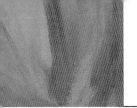

Adult Congenital Heart Disease

Phillip S. Cuculich

INTRODUCTION

Children with congenital heart disease (HD) have benefited from decades of pioneering effort and now more frequently are living into their adult years. Major advances in cardiac imaging, surgical techniques, catheter-based technologies, medical therapy, and our understanding of the natural history of specific cardiac lesions have all contributed to this success story. It is estimated that there are over a million adult survivors of congenital HD. In caring for an adult patient with congenital HD, there are three important pieces of information to know:

- The original cardiac condition
- The specific surgical repair(s) that the patient has undergone
- The anticipated natural history associated with both the condition and the repair

The following sections briefly review some of the most important features of various types of congenital HD anatomies, organized by major anatomic defect (septal, left ventricular outflow, right ventricular outflow, univentricular heart, and major blood vessels). Particular emphasis is placed on the expected natural history and specific screening/prevention efforts for each condition as it relates to caring for an adult with these conditions.

SEPTAL DEFECTS

Atrial Septal Defect

Atrial septal defects (ASDs) can be classified into one of several types based on anatomic location (Fig. 15-1):

- Ostium secundum, the **most common form of ASD** (75%), is a defect in the true fossa ovalis. It occurs more frequently in women and can be associated with mitral valve prolapse.
- Ostium primum, a less common defect (15%), is located in the lower aspect of the atrial septum. It is **associated with Down's syndrome, arteriovenous (AV) canal defects, and cleft mitral valve.**
- Sinus venosus is a rare defect (10%) found where the superior vena cava joins the right atrium near the intra-atrial septum. It is frequently **associated with anomalous pulmonary venous return.**
- Inferior vena cava (IVC) sinus venosus and "unroofed" coronary sinus are the rarest forms of ASD. The former occurs at the junction of the IVC and the right atrium, while the latter uses the coronary sinus as a conduit between the left and right atria.

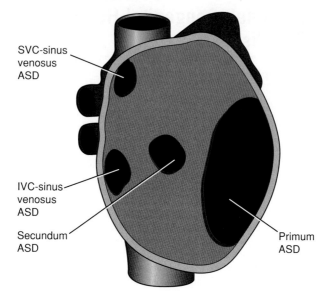

SVC-sinus
venosus
ASD

IVC-sinus
venosus
ASD

Secundum
ASD

Primum
ASD

FIGURE 15-1. Anatomic location of common atrial septal defect.

ASD is distinct from patent foramen ovale (PFO), which is far more common (occurs in nearly one-quarter of the general population) and usually does not allow a left-to-right shunt.

Physiology
In usual circumstances, the hole in the atrial septum can cause mild left-to-right shunting from the higher-pressure left atrium (LA) into the lower pressure right atrium (RA). Over time, this can cause dilatation in the right-sided chambers, which is typically the time when patients develop symptoms. At the extreme end of the disease process, pulmonary hypertension develops as a result of increased right-sided blood volume, ultimately causing a reversal of the shunt flow and cyanosis, a phenomenon described as Eisenmenger syndrome (see below).

Clinical Presentation
In general, many adults with an ASD are asymptomatic. First symptoms often include **dyspnea** with exertion or **fatigue**. **Atrial arrhythmias** usually arise in the third or fourth decade. Heart failure or systemic thromboembolic disease is usually a later manifestation of uncorrected disease.

Physical Exam
Patients are pink (not cyanotic) and often demonstrate a **fixed, split S2 with a loud P2 component** (due to elevated pulmonary pressures). A soft systolic murmur can be heard at the left upper sternal border (due to increased flow in the pulmonary arteries). With more advanced disease, one can palpate a right-ventricle (RV) heave or a pulmonary artery (PA) tap, as the pulmonary pressures rise considerably.

Diagnostic Studies
The ECG can demonstrate atrial tachyarrhythmias, thought to be due to increased atrial stretch. A common finding in all ASDs is an **incomplete right bundle-branch pattern**

(rSR' pattern). A patient with ostium secundum ASD may have right axis deviation with right atrial enlargement, right ventricular hypertrophy, and a first-degree atrioventricular (AV) block. Patients with an ostium primum ASD can develop extreme right- or left-axis deviation, biventricular enlargement, and AV block. On chest x-ray, dilatation of the right heart chambers can be seen, particularly on the lateral film.

Echocardiography is the "gold standard" for defining both the specific type of ASD and the chamber enlargement. Transthoracic views are adequate for screening for most ASDs (ostium secundum and primum), particularly if **agitated saline bubbles are injected** and a right-to-left shunt is seen (bubble study). A transesophageal approach is usually necessary to diagnose a sinus venosus ASD and can specifically measure the size of any ASD. Cardiac magnetic resonance imaging (MRI) has excellent sensitivity and specificity and is often used when the diagnosis is unclear after echocardiographic studies. In addition to anatomic information, cardiac catheterization offers the ability to directly **quantify the flow of blood across the shunt ($\dot{Q}p{:}\dot{Q}s$).**

Management Decisions
The ASD is considered "significant" (and should be treated) if any one of the following is present:

- $\dot{Q}p{:}\dot{Q}s$ shunt ratio $>1.5{:}1.0$.
- Evidence of dilatation of the right heart chambers (RV volume overload)
- Symptoms attributed to the ASD

Contraindications to closure include irreversible pulmonary arterial hypertension or poor left ventricular (LV) function.

Treatment options consist of open surgical repair or placement of a catheter-based closure device. Surgical closure is required for ostium primum ASD, especially in the setting of AV canal defect and/or cleft mitral valve and for sinus venosus ASD, where the anomalous pulmonary veins can be rerouted at the same time. Transvenous catheter-based device closure has been widely used for closure of appropriately-sized ostium secundum ASD.

Additional management considerations that frequently arise in treating adults with ASD are as follows:

- In general, pregnancy is well tolerated with most ASDs. There is a slightly increased risk for paradoxical embolism with an unrepaired ASD, although the overall risk is small. Pregnant patients with a newly discovered ASD can often defer repair until after delivery.
- The estimated risk of congenital HD for a child with an affected parent is 5% to 10%.
- Sudden cardiac death from ventricular arrhythmia is extremely rare in patients with an ASD in the absence of other structural HD.
- Prophylaxis for bacterial endocarditis is not routinely recommended unless the patient is cyanotic, has a residual leak near a site of prior repair with prosthetic material, or has had a recent repair (within 6 months).
- Thromboprophylaxis with aspirin or warfarin is not routinely indicated unless the patient has had suspected transient ischemic attack/cerebrovascular accident (TIA/CVA) symptoms or a recent repair (within 6 months).

Ventricular Septal Defect

Background
Ventricular septal defects (VSDs) are the **most common form of congenital HD in children**, involved in nearly 50% of all congenital HD presentations. By age 10, a vast majority of small VSDs have closed spontaneously. Most of the children with large VSDs surviving into adulthood have undergone surgical repair.

Physiology

VSDs can occur in the membranous or muscular septa. Blood flows preferentially from the higher-pressure LV into the lower pressure RV. If the volume of blood returning to the LV via the pulmonary vasculature is significantly large, it can cause **LV volume overload** and eventual heart failure. In an uncorrected heart with a large enough VSD, pulmonary vascular remodeling leads to increased right heart pressures, reversal of shunt flow, and development of the dreaded Eisenmenger physiology.

Clinical Presentation

Adult patients may be referred for evaluation of a loud murmur without symptoms. The most common symptom, if present, is increasing **dyspnea and fatigue** with exertion. An association with recurrent upper respiratory infections has been described. Rarely, patients develop aortic regurgitation (perimembranous VSD), endocarditis near the areas of turbulent flow (smaller VSD), or left heart failure.

Physical Exam

The hallmark finding on physical exam is a **loud, harsh holosystolic murmur**. Often a thrill can be palpated near the area of the VSD. With LV chamber enlargement, the point of maximum impulse (PMI) becomes laterally displaced. If pulmonary hypertension is present, a loud second heart sound is often found. A clinical pearl: If the intensity of the murmur decreases over time, why is this bad for the patient? A decrease in the murmur's intensity means that the pressures in the ventricles are becoming equal, signaling higher RV pressures and the early development of Eisenmenger physiology.

Diagnostic Studies

The ECG normally reveals LA and LV enlargement related to LV volume overload. Transthoracic echocardiography often confirms the diagnosis and offers additional information such as location and size of the VSD, presence of aortic valve regurgitation, and heart chamber size. Cardiac MRI can offer detailed anatomic imaging and an estimation of flow across the VSD. Cardiac catheterization directly measures the $\dot{Q}p:\dot{Q}s$ and the pulmonary vascular resistance.

Management Decisions

In general, small VSDs do not cause symptoms and do not require intervention. One exception to this is in the setting of recurrent endocarditis, when repair of any size VSD would be warranted. Larger VSDs usually **require closure if there is evidence of LV chamber dilatation, elevated PA vascular resistance, or if the $\dot{Q}p:\dot{Q}s$ exceeds 1.5.** In the absence of these findings, the VSD is termed "restrictive" and observation is warranted.

As in the case of ASDs, both surgical repair and catheter-based devices have been used successfully to treat VSDs, although percutaneous techniques are considered investigational. Decisions on the type of intervention are individualized based on clinical experience, type/location/shape of the VSD, and presence of aortic insufficiency. Surgical repair carries a higher risk of heart block (3%), while catheter-based closure is associated with a higher incidence of valve damage (aortic valve, tricuspid valve) particularly if deployed across a perimembranous VSD.

Other answers to questions that patients frequently ask:

- Pregnancy is well tolerated if the VSD has been repaired or is a "restrictive" VSD. The risk of maternal (up to 50%) and fetal (up to 60%) mortality increases dramatically in the setting of Eisenmenger physiology.
- The estimated risk of congenital HD for a child with an affected parent or sibling is 1% to 5%.

- The risk of sudden cardiac death is low in the absence of other structural HD. Patients with small "restrictive" VSDs or with repaired VSDs generally have normal life expectancies.
- Prophylaxis for bacterial endocarditis is recommended only for patients with a residual leak near a site of prior repair or with a recent repair (within 6 months).
- Thromboprophylaxis with aspirin or warfarin is not routinely indicated unless the patient has had suspected TIA/CVA symptoms or a recent repair (within 6 months).

LEFT VENTRICULAR OUTFLOW TRACT (LVOT)

Subaortic Stenosis

This lesion is usually a **fibrous or fibromuscular ring in the LV outflow tract**. Patients are usually referred for evaluation of a systolic murmur or suspected aortic stenosis/regurgitation. Associated conditions include membranous VSD (37%) and bicuspid aortic valve (23%). The diagnosis is best made with echocardiography, although cardiac MRI can be helpful if echo is nondiagnostic. This lesion generally progresses slowly; over time, however, the accelerated turbulent blood flow can take a toll on the aortic valve apparatus, causing acquired aortic regurgitation. The major dilemma in treating this condition involves the timing of surgery. Surgical resection is usually deferred until:

- Peak LVOT gradient >50 mm Hg
- LV systolic dysfunction
- Moderate/severe aortic regurgitation or presence of VSD
- Symptoms of outflow obstruction (angina, dyspnea, syncope)
- Peak LVOT gradient >30 mm Hg along with plans to start competitive sports or to become pregnant

Recurrence of the fibromuscular band after surgery is seen in at least one-third of patients. Concomitant aortic valve replacement may be warranted for a bicuspid valve or severe aortic regurgitation. In patients with a more diffuse, tunnel-type lesion, a Konno-Rastan LVOT reconstruction procedure may be necessary.

BICUSPID AORTIC VALVE (BAV)

Background

BAV is **the most common congenital malformation**, occurring in ~1% of the general population, with a 4:1 male predominance. First-degree relatives and offspring are at increased risk of LVOT lesions.

Clinical Presentation

Symptoms of BAV physiology develop slowly over time. Over two-thirds of patients develop **symptoms related to aortic stenosis** (angina, dyspnea, syncope), **usually around the fifth decade**. Patients with BAV have abnormal aortic root tissue structure, prone to dilating and causing aortic regurgitation. The ascending aorta gradually dilates at mean rate of ~1 mm/year. Although aortic dissection is rare, it is a serious complication. Patients with BAV are at a five- to ninefold **increased risk of aortic dissection** compared with the general population.

Physical Exam

Early in the disease, a crescendo–decrescendo midsystolic murmur can be heard at the upper sternal borders, radiating to the neck. An ejection sound can be heard as long as the valve is mobile. **As the aortic stenosis progresses, the murmur becomes more late-peaking, the ejection sound disappears, and the peripheral pulses become diminished and delayed.** Aortic regurgitation can be heard at the midsternal border, often with the patient leaning forward.

Diagnostic Studies

Practically speaking, BAV should be strongly considered in any 40- to 60-year-old patient with symptoms of aortic stenosis (AS) and a loud systolic murmur. Transthoracic echocardiography often suggests the presence of a BAV and can measure the severity of AS and presence of aortic insufficiency (AI). Often the anatomy of the valve is best confirmed by the transesophageal approach. Cardiac MRI has proven to be an accurate alternative to echocardiography, with a specific benefit of sizing the entire ascending aorta.

Management Decisions

There are no proven medical therapies to alter the course of aortic valve disease or aortic dilatation in BAV. Beta blockers have been shown to slow the progression of aortic root disease in Marfan's syndrome and are frequently used in BAV, though caution must be exercised with severe AR. Other medications have been used to delay valve sclerosis (statins and aspirin) and adverse LV remodeling (angiotensin converting enzyme [ACE] inhibitors) with varying success.

The ultimate decision in BAV is the timing and type of surgical repair. If the **aortic root diameter exceeds 5 cm or if the yearly growth exceeds 5 mm, it is generally recommended to repair or replace the aortic root.** Surgical repair or replacement of the BAV is considered for patients with severe AS (>4 m/second peak Doppler velocity) and:

- Symptoms of AS (angina, dyspnea, syncope)
- LV systolic dysfunction
- Moderate to severe AR
- Desire to become pregnant or to start vigorous exercise
- Dilated aortic root (>4.5 cm)

If the valve is not calcified, a repair is an option. If a valve replacement is required, a bioprosthetic valve is generally preferred in older patients, young women wishing to become pregnant, and patients at a high risk of serious bleeding complications related to warfarin. Otherwise, a mechanical prosthetic valve provides better longevity than a bioprosthesis. The Ross procedure involves excision of the diseased aortic valve, autograft of the patient's pulmonary valve (PV) and pulmonary trunk into the aortic valve position, coronary artery reimplantation, and placement of an allograft pulmonary valve. This procedure has fallen out of favor at some centers due to the risks of progressive neoaorta dilatation, AR, pulmonary homograft degeneration, and risk of myocardial ischemia. It has been said that the Ross procedure doubles the patient's long-term risk by converting a one-valve disease to a two-valve disease.

Other Considerations

- In general, pregnancy is well tolerated with most BAVs. Maternal and fetal risks increase significantly in the presence of significant AS or aortic root dilatation.
- The estimated risk of congenital HD for a child with an affected parent or sibling is can be as high as 10% to 15%. Because of this strong inheritance pattern, echocardiographic screening of first-degree family members is warranted.
- Sudden cardiac death from ventricular arrhythmia is extremely rare in patients with a BAV in the absence of other structural HD.
- Despite an increased risk for endocarditis, antibiotic prophylaxis is not routinely recommended for patients with BAV.

Supra-aortic Stenosis

This rare lesion is most often **associated with Williams syndrome**, a multisystem autosomal dominant mutation of chromosome 7, in the region near the elastin gene. Patients are developmentally delayed and often have characteristic elf-like facial features. Associated aortic valve abnormalities are found in nearly half the patients and supravalvular lesions can be found in the pulmonary arteries as well.

Echocardiography can be useful, but computed tomography (CT) or MR angiography often more clearly delineate the extent of the lesion. Cardiac catheterization can directly measure the gradient across the obstruction. Surgical repair is the treatment of choice and is recommended when outflow obstruction symptoms develop or the mean pressure gradient exceeds 50 mm Hg.

RIGHT VENTRICULAR OUTFLOW TRACT (RVOT)

Pulmonary Stenosis (PS)

A dome-shaped PV with mobile valves and a narrow central opening is the pathology classically described and most commonly found in congenital PS. This condition makes up 7% to 12% of cases of all congenital HD and a vast majority of right-sided congenital lesions (80%–90%). Associations of valvular PS and supravalvular stenosis exist with Noonan, William, Alagille, and DiGeorge syndromes.

Most patients are asymptomatic; but with advanced disease, symptoms of fatigue, dyspnea, angina, and palpitations can occur. The diagnosis is made with echocardiography, with cardiac MRI reserved for cases in which the diagnosis is in doubt. The **management decisions are largely driven by the peak Doppler gradient across the diseased valve**: gradients <25 mm Hg rarely progress and warrant observation; gradients >50 mm Hg often cause symptoms and warrant intervention. Based on the valve morphology and severity of pulmonary insufficiency (PI), treatment can consist of percutaneous balloon valvuloplasty, surgical commissurotomy, or valve replacement. Percutaneous valve replacement is a new technique with promising results in the RVOT. **The common long-term complication to look for is PI.** Unexplained enlargement of the RV any time after an intervention should warrant an investigation for PI.

TETRALOGY OF FALLOT (ToF)

Background

The four major defects that define this syndrome are pulmonary stenosis, VSD, RV hypertrophy, and an overriding aorta. An atrial septal defect is present in ~5% of patients; it is called the pentalogy of Fallot. ToF represents ~10% of all congenital HD. Unlike previously presented conditions, ToF is a cyanotic condition (deoxygenated blood cannot exit out the stenotic pulmonary outflow tract, so it crosses the VSD and enters the overriding aorta). **In the adult population, ToF is the most common cyanotic congenital HD encountered.**

Clinical Presentation

Adult survivors have almost exclusively undergone a surgical repair early in life. Depending on the era during which the repair was done, patients may have had a previous palliative arterial-to-pulmonary shunt (Table 15-1), followed by a definitive repair consisting of a VSD patch and RV outflow reconstruction (Fig. 15-2). Adult patients are generally asymptomatic, although common symptoms to ask about include **exertional fatigue and dyspnea, palpitations, syncope, and lower extremity edema.** Ventricular arrhythmias,

TABLE 15-1 COMMON SURGICAL PROCEDURES PERFORMED ON ADULTS WITH CONGENITAL HEART DISEASE

Type	Name	Description	Advantage	Disadvantage	Consequences
Arterioplumonary Shunt	Classic Blalock–Taussig	Subclavian artery to PA	Predictable blood flow into pulmonary circulation. Easy to close during corrective surgery	Thrombosis. Risk of damaging the recurrent laryngeal nerve. Mutilates the subclavian artery	Reduced radial pulse on ipsilateral side Rarely used currently
	Potts	Descending aorta to left PA	Low risk of thrombosis	Pulmonary hypertension Unilateral PA flow Distorted PA	Heart failure in up to 20% No longer used
	Waterston	Ascending aorta to right PA	Low risk of thrombosis	Pulmonary hypertension Unilateral PA flow Distorted PA	Heart failure in up to 20% No longer used
	Central	PTFE graft from descending aorta to main PA	Low failure rate	Requires a PDA Pericardial entry	Used only in specific situations, primarily with small branch PAs
	Sano Modification	PTFE graft from RV to main PA	Low failure rate	Pericardial entry	Used with the Norwood procedure (see below)
	Modified Blalock–Taussig	PTFE graft from subclavian artery to PA	Predictable blood flow Easy to close during corrective surgery Long patency	Pseudoaneurysm Fatal hemoptysis	Reduced radial pulse on ipsilateral side **Currently the AP shunt of choice**

Cavopulmonary Shunt	**Glenn**	SVC to RPA	Does not increase volume load on ventricle (venous flow).	Unilateral PA flow. Requires low PA pressures.	No longer used
	Bidirectional Glenn	SVC to bilateral PA	Does not increase volume load on ventricle (venous flow).	Requires low PA pressures.	Currently in use
	Fontan	SVC and IVC to bilateral PA	Bypasses right heart. Versatile procedure for many anatomies.	Arrhythmia. Thromboembolism. Obstruction. Protein-losing enteropathy.	**Commonly used, usually after bidirectional Glenn.**

(continued)

TABLE 15-1	COMMON SURGICAL PROCEDURES PERFORMED ON ADULTS WITH CONGENITAL HEART DISEASE (*Continued*)				
Type	Name	Description	Advantage	Disadvantage	Consequences
Transposition Repairs	**Mustard**	Intra-atrial baffle (pericardium or PTFE)	Low mortality.	Arrhythmia. Sinus node dysfunction. Baffle leak or obstruction. Ventricular failure.	**Most common TGA repair in adult population,** though largely supplanted by Jatene.
	Senning	Intra-atrial baffle (atrial septum)	Low mortality.	Arrhythmia. Sinus node dysfunction. Baffle leak or obstruction. Ventricular failure.	Seen in adult populations, though supplanted by Jatene.
	Jatene	Arterial switch (PA and aortic root)	Establishes LV as systemic ventricle. Fewer arrhythmia than atrial switch.	Coronary artery closure. Neoaortic root dilatation.	**Currently the surgery of choice for TGA,** although long-term results are pending.
	Rastelli	Ventricular switch (RV to PA conduit and LV to aorta baffle)	Establishes LV as systemic ventricle.	High-risk procedure.	Used when a VSD and pulmonary stenosis are present with D-TGA.
	Rashkind	Balloon atrial septostomy	Rapidly creates an ASD, allowing for mixing of arterial and venous blood.	Palliative maneuver.	Used in the first few days of life for D-TGA to allow mixing of blood.

Aortic valve	Ross	1. Aortic valve replaced with pulmonary autograft 2. Pulmonary valve replaced with homograft valve 3. Coronary arteries resewn into the neoaortic root	Avoids the need for anticoagulation (no mechanical valves)	Often requires reintervention Coronary artery closure Neoaortic root dilatation	**Used primarily in patients wishing to avoid anticoagulation** (i.e., young women wishing to become pregnant)
Univentricular heart	Norwood	Stage 1: Modified BT or Sano shunt (to establish pulmonary circuit) and joining main PA with aorta (to create a univentricular systemic circuit). Stage 2: Bidirectional Glenn. Stage 3: Fontan.	Only set of procedures that create both a systemic and pulmonary circuit.	Multiple surgeries	Used primarily for HLHS.
ToF	Tetralogy repair	Closure of VSD and reconstruction of RVOT.	Can be performed as a primary repair in infants with a durable response.	Pulmonary insufficiency Sudden death Arrhythmia Progressive ventricular failure	Used in tetralogy of Fallot.

AP, Arteriopulmonary; ASD, atrial septal defect; BT, Blalock–Taussig; D-TGA, dextrotransposition of the great arteries; HLHS, hypoplastic left heart syndrome; IVC, inferior vena cava; LV, left ventricle; PA, pulmonary artery; PDA, patent ductus arteriosus; PTFE, polytetrafluoroethylene; RPA, right pulmonary artery; RV, right ventricle; RVOT, right ventricular outflow tract; SVC, superior vena cava; VSD, ventricular septal defect.

171

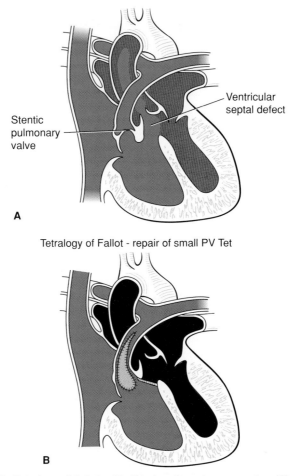

Stentic pulmonary valve

Ventricular septal defect

A

Tetralogy of Fallot - repair of small PV Tet

B

FIGURE 15-2. A: Tetralogy of Fallot, with (1) stenotic pulmonary valve, (2) ventricular septal defect, (3) right ventricular hypertrophy, and (4) overriding aorta with mixing of oxygenated and deoxygenated blood. **B:** Primary repair of the condition, with closure of the ventricular septal defect and patch reconstruction of the right ventricular outflow tract. (Images from the American Heart Association, with permission.)

likely originating from the surgical repair site, can cause syncope and sudden death in 1% to 5% of patients.

Physical Exam

A **prior arterial-to-pulmonary shunt often causes reduced or absent arm pulses on the ipsilateral side**. The location and size of the surgical scars can often tell the story of the surgical history. Tricuspid regurgitation (as demonstrated by the v wave in the jugular veins) and an RV heave are often present. Special attention should be paid to the presence of a diastolic murmur (PI, see below).

Diagnostic Studies

An ECG demonstrates right ventricular hypertrophy (RVH) with varying degrees of right bundle-branch block (RBBB). **Patients with a QRS >180 ms are at increased risk for ventricular arrhythmias and sudden death**. A chest x-ray often demonstrates a classic "boot-shaped" horizontal heart. Transthoracic echocardiography confirms the lesions described above, including the completeness of the surgical repair. It is especially useful for routine follow-up of pulmonary insufficiency, the size of the right heart chamber, and ventricular systolic function.

Management Decisions

The three primary concerns of treating adult patients with repaired ToF are **pulmonary insufficiency, sudden death, and bacterial endocarditis**. PI is common, particularly if the repair involved a transannular patch. Severe PI manifests as RV dilatation and systolic dysfunction; the echocardiographic findings often predate symptoms of heart failure. Timing of reintervention in ToF is a source of considerable debate. Some of the common indications for late PV replacement include:

- Symptoms of right heart failure
- RV chamber enlargement or RV dysfunction
- Clinically significant arrhythmias
- Progressive dilatation of the RVOT

Arrhythmias generally herald a problem with hemodynamics, so PI and residual VSD are usually evaluated prior to any treatment for the arrhythmia. The role for an implantable cardioverter/defibrillator for primary prevention of sudden death in patients with wide QRS on ECG remains controversial. Catheter ablation of ventricular tachycardias related to ToF repair has shown promising results.

Follow-up considerations include:

- Pregnancy is fairly well-tolerated by most women with a repaired ToF, although increased risks of heart failure (up to 20%) and miscarriage (up to 30%) exist, particularly for those with pulmonary hypertension, severe PI, or ventricular dysfunction.
- There is an association between deletions on chromosome 22q11 and ToF. The estimated risk of ToF for a child with an affected parent depends on the presence of this mutation; preconception genetic counseling may be beneficial in this case.
- Sudden cardiac death does occur in patients with a ToF. Syncopal events should be considered aborted sudden death unless proven otherwise.
- Bacterial endocarditis prophylaxis is generally not recommended for patients with successful ToF repairs. Cyanotic patients or patients who have undergone only palliative surgical procedures warrant antibiotic endocarditis prophylaxis.

EBSTEIN ANOMALY

Background

This rare disease of the tricuspid valve (TV) and right ventricle accounts for <1% of congenital HD. It consists of an **apically displaced, malformed TV with an "atrialized" portion of the RV**. The classic pathophysiology involves severe tricuspid regurgitation and inability to fill the RV during atrial systole, leading to underfilling of the pulmonary circulation and subsequently underfilling of the LV.

Over 50% of patients will have an ASD or PFO, which, in conjunction with severe tricuspid regurgitation, may lead to cyanosis in the absence of pulmonary arterial hypertension. Over 25% will have **accessory AV conduction pathways**, usually near the diseased TV annulus. Ebstein anomaly has been linked to maternal lithium use.

Clinical Presentation

The classic symptoms of Ebstein anomaly are **cyanosis, right heart failure, atrial arrhythmia**, and **sudden death**. The severity of the disease varies greatly. A severely diseased TV often leads to death in utero. Roughly one-third of infants with Ebstein anomaly do not live beyond the first year of life. Those that survive into adulthood usually have had successful surgical repairs and/or have favorable physiology.

Physical Exam

This lesion is difficult to discover on exam, as the tricuspid regurgitation jet is often difficult to auscultate. A widely split second heart sound may be the only significant finding suggesting this diagnosis. Cyanosis may be present.

Diagnostic Studies

ECG can show marked RA enlargement (known as "Himalayan" P waves), first-degree AV block, various degrees of RBBB, and an abnormal QRS configuration with notching in the terminal portion of the QRS, likely due to delayed conduction through the atrialized RV. Up to one-third of patients have an accessory AV pathway. Echocardiography makes the diagnosis, with an **apically displaced septal leaflet of the TV, marked enlargement of the RA, and an atrialized RV.**

Management Decisions

Surgical treatment for Ebstein anomaly is pursued for **increasing cyanosis, New York Heart Association (NYHA) functional class III–IV heart failure, or paradoxical embolism.** Recurrent supraventricular arrhythmias refractory to medical and catheter ablation treatment is a relative indication for surgical repair. Valve repair is preferred over replacement if the anatomy is favorable. A concomitant maze procedure and accessory pathway ablation can address the arrhythmias.

- Pregnancy is usually well tolerated in the absence of cyanosis, heart failure, and significant arrhythmia.
- The estimated risk of congenital HD for a child with an affected parent is 1% to 5%.
- Most arrhythmias are supraventricular, although sudden cardiac death has been reported; this is thought to be due to rapid AV conduction over the accessory pathway (Wolff–Parkinson–White physiology).
- Bacterial endocarditis prophylaxis is not routinely recommended unless the patient is cyanotic, has a residual leak near a site of prior repair with prosthetic material, or has had a recent repair (within 6 months).

UNIVENTRICULAR HEART—FONTAN PROCEDURE

Background

Patients presenting with various anatomic abnormalities that ultimately fall under a similar physiologic condition are described as having a univentricular heart. Common forms include hypoplastic left heart syndrome (HLHS), tricuspid atresia, double-inlet ventricle, and other conditions with a large, nonrestrictive VSD acting as a "functional" single ventricle. Surgical correction happens at a young age, usually by using the ventricle as a systemic pump and **diverting venous return directly to the pulmonary arteries,**

known as the Fontan procedure. Caring for these adult patients requires familiarity with Fontan-related sequelae; therefore the remainder of this section is devoted to this topic exclusively.

Physiology

Patients with decreased pulmonary blood flow will have received an aortopulmonary shunt (Blalock–Taussig) or a bidirectional cavopulmonary shunt (Glenn) early in life. Patients with HLHS (decreased systemic blood flow) will have received a series of operations to restore systemic and pulmonary circulations (Norwood stages 1–3). The culmination of either set of procedures is the establishment of adequate blood flow to the pulmonary arteries (Table 15-1).

The Fontan procedure (Fig. 15-3) has evolved over decades from (1) a valved conduit between the right atrium and pulmonary artery to (2) a direct connection between the RA and PA (modified Fontan) to (3) a connection between the IVC and pulmonary artery within the right atrium (intracardiac lateral tunnel Fontan) to (4) an extracardiac conduit from the IVC to the PA (extracardiac Fontan).

Clinical Presentation

As a rule, adult patients with a Fontan procedure experience a progressive decline in functional status over time. Other important late sequelae of the Fontan procedure include:

- **Arrhythmia.** Sinus node dysfunction (15%) and atrial tachyarrhythmias [atrial fibrillation and intra-atrial reentry tachycardia (IART), 20% at 5 years] are common. Atrial tachyarrhythmias are usually poorly tolerated and often require prompt cardioversion.
- **Thromboemboli** (6%–25%). Patients at high risk for RA thrombus include those with atrial arrhythmias, fenestrated Fontan connections, or spontaneous echo contrast ("smoke") seen in the RA, signaling very slow flow. These patients should be anticoagulated.
- **Hepatic dysfunction.** Due to congestion and cirrhosis, often not clinically significant.
- **Protein-losing enteropathy** (4%–13%). Due to chronically elevated venous pressure, causing intestinal lymphangiectasia and loss of albumin and immunoglobin into the GI tract.
- **Fontan obstruction.** Can lead to exercise intolerance, right-sided heart failure, and sudden death.
- **Right pulmonary vein compression.** Due to enlarged RA and/or atrial baffle, compressing the pulmonary vein inflow into the LA.
- **Ventricular dysfunction.** A progressive process, particularly troublesome if the systemic ventricle is a morphologic right ventricle.
- **Systemic aortic valve regurgitation.** Can cause progressive deterioration of exercise ability and, if severe, may warrant a surgical repair or replacement.

Physical Exam

Patients often have an elevated jugular venous pulse (JVP), normal S1, and a single S2 (no functioning pulmonary valve). A diastolic murmur may be present if there is systemic aortic valve regurgitation.

Diagnostic Studies

ECG can vary depending on the underlying physiology that triggered the Fontan conversion. Echocardiography is the routine test to evaluate the function of the Fontan circuit, presence of an atrial thrombus, systemic ventricular function, and aortic valve regurgitation.

Total extracardiac conduit fontan palliation of hypoplastic left heart

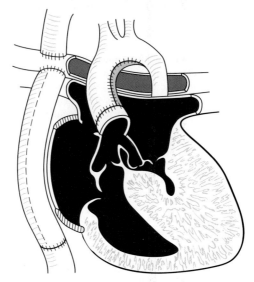

A

Tricuspid atresia palliation with bidirectional Glenn shunt

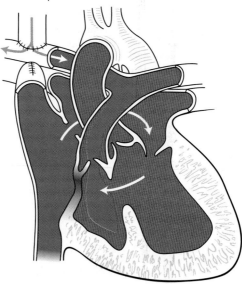

B

FIGURE 15-3. A: Extracardiac Fontan procedure for hypoplastic left heart, resulting in a total cavopulmonary shunt (superior vena cava and inferior vena cava into pulmonary artery). **B:** Bidirectional Glenn shunt (superior vena cava to pulmonary artery) in a patient with tricuspid atresia and an atrial septal defect. (Images from the American Heart Association, with permission.

Cardiac MRI can provide similar information in patients who cannot provide adequate echo images. Cardiac catheterization is usually reserved for patients considering surgical intervention.

Management Decisions

Careful, expert follow-up is recommended, with particular attention to changes in functional status, development of arrhythmias, or development of cyanosis. Any significant change should prompt a search for potential causes, including worsening ventricular function, worsening aortic valve regurgitation, formation of pulmonary arteriovenous malformations, venovenous collaterals decompressing right-sided chambers to the LA with progressive cyanosis, or obstruction of the Fontan circuit.

Other Considerations

- Because of the increased hemodynamic burden on the single ventricle and the slow-flow physiologic properties of the Fontan circuit, pregnancy carries increased risks to both the mother and the fetus. Specific concerns include atrial arrhythmias, thromboemboli, venous congestion, worsening ventricular function, and worsening aortic valve regurgitation.
- The estimated risk of congenital HD for a child with an affected parent varies by underlying condition but is estimated to be 1% to 5% (higher for HLHS).
- Sudden cardiac death from ventricular arrhythmia has been reported, particularly in the setting of prior ventricular repair surgery or a failing ventricle.
- Bacterial endocarditis prophylaxis is warranted for 6 months after surgical repair and lifelong for patients with a fenestrated Fontan repair.

DISORDERS OF THE BLOOD VESSELS

Transposition of the Great Arteries (TGA)

Background

Transpositions can generally be classified into one of two types: D-TGA or L-TGA, based on the direction of the cardiac loop during embryogenesis (dextro- or levorotation). Most patients with D-TGA surviving into adulthood have had a surgical correction.

Physiology

The path of blood flow in uncorrected D-TGA is as follows: venous blood into the right atrium, to the right ventricle, and out the aorta to the body. In the absence of a septal defect or PDA, one can see that this pathway puts deoxygenated venous blood directly back into the systemic circulation, causing immediate cyanosis. Without intervention, one-third of infants die within the first week and nearly 90% die within the first year of life. (Remember that "**D-transpositions Die without correction.**")

In contrast, L-TGA has been called a "double switch" or "congenitally corrected" transposition. Venous blood enters through the RA into the morphologic LV (first switch) but exits out the pulmonary artery (second switch). This yields a normal path for blood flow, albeit through the "wrong" ventricles. (Remember that "**L-transpositions Live.**")

Clinical Presentation

For adults with surgically repaired D-TGA, it is essential to know the natural history and types of late complications of the particular repair (Fig. 15-4). The **atrial switch procedures are the most common in the current adult population.** Blood is redirected across the atrium by the use of baffles made of either Dacron or pericardium (Mustard procedure)

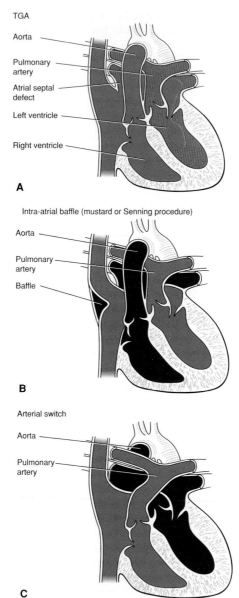

TGA
Aorta
Pulmonary artery
Atrial septal defect
Left ventricle
Right ventricle

A

Intra-atrial baffle (mustard or Senning procedure)
Aorta
Pulmonary artery
Baffle

B

Arterial switch
Aorta
Pulmonary artery

C

FIGURE 15-4. A: Dextrotransposition of the great arteries (D-TGA). Note the systemic and venous systems in parallel, with mixing only through an atrial septal defect. **B:** Atrial switch procedure, bringing venous blood to the morphologic left ventricle and out to the lungs. The right ventricle is the systemic ventricle, which is the cause of many of the long-term sequelae in this repair. **C:** Arterial switch procedure, maintaining the left ventricle as the systemic ventricle. (Images from the American Heart Association, with permission.)

or atrial septum (Senning procedure). Most adults with an atrial switch procedure will have mildly decreased functional capacity and are at risk for:

- **Systemic ventricular dysfunction.** An element of late RV dysfunction and tricuspid regurgitation is almost universal over time, as these structures often struggle to handle systemic pressures. Roughly 10% of patients will have clinical heart failure by age 20.
- **Arrhythmia.** Sinus node dysfunction (50% by age 20) and a type of atrial flutter involving the atrial scar site [intra-atrial reentry tachycardia (IART), 20% by age 20] are common.
- **Atrial baffle obstruction or leak.** Atrial baffle obstructions can occur near the SVC or IVC junctions or near the pulmonary veins (causing pulmonary hypertension and congestion). Small baffle leaks often do not cause symptoms, but large leaks can lead to progressive heart failure or cyanosis if associated with an obstructive lesion.
- **Pulmonary hypertension.** For reasons incompletely understood, 5% to 10% of adult patients with an atrial switch procedure have pulmonary hypertension.

More recently, **the Jatene arterial switch has become the procedure of choice**, where the arterial trunks are transected and sewn to the contralateral root with a transposition of coronary arteries to the neoaorta (Fig. 15-4). The clear advantage of this procedure is the use of the morphologic LV as the systemic ventricle. These patients are beginning to survive into adulthood and have the following late complications:

- Dilatation of the neoaortic root, causing aortic regurgitation.
- Stenosis near the anastomosis sites, causing PS or AS physiology.
- Stenosis at the ostia of transposed coronary arteries, leading to myocardial infarction or sudden death in a minority of patients.

Patients with L-TGA may not be diagnosed until adulthood. Associated cardiac abnormalities are very common (~95%) and are normally discovered first:

- **VSD.** Up to 70% of those with L-TGA have a VSD, usually perimembranous in location.
- Pulmonary stenosis (40%), often subvalvular.
- Regurgitation of the systemic aortic valve (90%).
- AV block (2% yearly), due to abnormalities in AV node location and accelerated conduction system fibrosis.
- Progressive systemic ventricular dysfunction (nearly universal), usually occurring after the third decade. This is usually the most common presentation in an adult patient.

Physical Exam
Many patients who have had an atrial switch procedure will have a midline surgical scar, RV heave, and a single S2 (because of the posterior position, P2 is often not heard). A systemic (tricuspid) regurgitation murmur is heard at the left lower sternal border. In a failing right ventricle, a right-sided S3 can be heard. Physical exam of a patient with the arterial switch should be rather unremarkable except for the surgical scar.

Patients with L-TGA may have a more medial PMI (due to the rotation of the heart) with a single S2. If present, a VSD murmur (harsh, holosystolic), aortic valve regurgitation murmur (softer, systolic, at the left sternal border), or PS murmur (systolic, radiating to the right sternal border) may be heard.

Diagnostic Studies
In D-TGA, ECG findings after an atrial switch procedure include sinus bradycardia or junctional escape rhythm with marked RVH. The classic chest x-ray finding is **an oblong cardiac shadow, described as an "egg on its side."** Echocardiography will demonstrate **parallel great arteries, characteristic of D-TGA.** The systemic ventricular function, degree of

systemic aortic valve regurgitation, and evidence for baffle leak or stenosis can also be evaluated by echocardiography, making this test essential for long-term follow-up. Cardiac MRI provides excellent evaluation of systemic ventricular function. For patients with a high clinical suspicion of baffle malfunction and whose echo images are poor, cardiac catheterization is usually required.

In L-TGA, the classic ECG findings are first-degree AV block (50%) and reversal of the precordial Q-wave pattern due to the reversed septal activation. Echocardiographic identification can be subtle, as the morphologic ventricles can be identified by specific characteristics:

- The RV has a trabeculated apex, moderator band, and a trileaflet apically displaced AV valve (tricuspid) associated with it. In describing valves, a way to remember is: <u>V</u>alves go with <u>V</u>entricles.
- The LV has a smooth endocardial surface and a bileaflet AV valve (mitral).

Management Decisions

For patients with an atrial switch, the **major decisions address the late complications of the repair procedure**:

- Symptomatic bradycardia is treated with a pacemaker
- IART is treated medically and/or with catheter ablation procedure
- A baffle leak resulting in a left-to-right shunt ($\dot{Q}p{:}\dot{Q}s$) of >1.5 or any symptoms warrants a surgical or catheter-based closure procedure.
- Baffle stenosis causing symptoms is usually treated with balloon dilatation and stent placement.
- Although not proven in this population, treatment of RV dysfunction starts with ACE-inhibitor afterload reduction. For severely symptomatic patients, a heart transplant may be necessary.

For patients with L-TGA, the **main decision hinges on the development of systemic ventricular dysfunction**. Again, ACE-inhibitor therapy may provide benefit. Surgical correction with a "double switch" procedure (both an atrial *and* arterial switch, allowing the LV to become the systemic ventricle) has been performed in children successfully but is unproven in adults. Heart transplantation is an option for severely symptomatic patients.

General considerations for patients with TGA:

- Pregnancy after a repair procedure carries a mildly increased risk to the mother and fetus, but it has been tolerated well in many cases. Severe ventricular dysfunction and significant arrhythmia portend a much worse prognosis; pregnancy should be avoided in these settings.
- The estimated risk of congenital HD for a child with an affected parent is 1% to 5%.
- Sudden cardiac death occurs in up to 5% of patients with an atrial switch procedure.
- Bacterial endocarditis prophylaxis is not routinely recommended unless the patient is cyanotic, has a residual leak near a site of prior repair with prosthetic material, or has had a recent repair (within 6 months).

PATENT DUCTUS ARTERIOSUS (PDA)

Background

The ductus arteriosus connects the proximal descending aorta to the roof of the PA. Its patency is essential for fetal circulation, but the ductus should close naturally during a baby's first few weeks. PDAs comprise roughly 10% of congenital HD conditions

($\sim$1:2000 births). There are associations with prematurity, maternal rubella infection, and fetal valproate syndrome.

Physiology

Severity of disease is driven largely by the magnitude of left-to-right blood flow across the PDA. This shunt ultimately results in a *left* chamber volume overload, with left atrial and ventricular enlargement. The increased pulmonary blood flow also can cause remodeling in the pulmonary vasculature, resulting in pulmonary hypertension and Eisenmenger physiology.

Clinical Presentation

In fortunate patients, ther PDA is discovered during childhood. In general, most PDA lesions are well tolerated throughout adolescence. Adult patients can present without symptoms for an evaluation of a murmur or with heart failure symptoms with or without cyanosis. Another common presentation is new atrial fibrillation due to the increased LA size. Patients with a PDA have a higher risk of endarteritis, particularly at the pulmonary end of the PDA. Embolic events are usually found in the lung rather than systemically.

Physical Exam

The classic finding is a **"machinery" continuous murmur at the left upper sternal border which can often radiate to the back.** The PMI may be laterally displaced and the peripheral pulses may be bounding. Patients presenting later in the disease course, with Eisenmenger physiology, may have **differential cyanosis**, with clubbing and cyanosis of the feet but not the hands. This is due to the right-to-left shunt, allowing for deoxygenated blood to be preferentially sent through the PDA and to the lower extremities.

Diagnostic Studies

Consistent with the physical exam, the ECG may show sinus tachycardia or atrial fibrillation, left atrial abnormality, or LVH. In older adults with long-standing disease, calcification of the ductus can be seen on the chest x-ray. Echocardiography confirms the diagnosis and allows for characterization of the shunt, evaluation of chamber size, and estimation of pulmonary artery pressure. Cardiac CT or MR can often delineate the PDA, in addition to other associated abnormalities that may influence the intervention decision. Cardiac catheterization can be both diagnostic and therapeutic.

Management Decisions

Closure of the ductus is indicated for any patient with symptoms or in asymptomatic patients with evidence of left heart enlargement. The management of an asymptomatic patient with a small, incidentally discovered PDA is controversial. In general, closing right-to-left shunts in patients with Eisenmenger physiology is relatively contraindicated, although successful outcomes of PDA closure in these patients has been reported.

Both surgical ligation and transcatheter closure devices have a high success rate for closure of a PDA. Decisions regarding the type of closure should be tailored to the individual and the experience of the center performing the procedure. An open PDA requires endocarditis prophylaxis regardless of the size. A closed PDA requires endocarditis prophylaxis only during the 6 months after the procedure.

- In general, pregnancy is well tolerated with small or asymptomatic PDA. With a larger, hemodynamically significant PDA, the pregnant woman is at risk for heart failure. Women with Eisenmenger physiology have very high maternal and fetal mortality rates.
- The estimated risk of congenital HD for a child with an affected parent is 1% to 5%.

- Bacterial endocarditis prophylaxis is not routinely recommended unless the patient is cyanotic, has a residual leak near a site of prior repair with prosthetic material, or has had a recent repair (within 6 months).

COARCTATION OF THE AORTA (COA)

This discrete narrowing near the ligamentum arteriosum can be seen in 7% of congenital HD, with a slight male predominance. Common **associated conditions include BAV (20%–40%) and intracranial aneurysms in the circle of Willis (10%)**. One-third of patients with Turner syndrome (XO) have CoA.

Clinical Presentation

Adult patients may present with mild symptoms such as headache, epistaxis, or claudication. Patients with unrepaired CoA live an average of 35 years. Common causes of death in the absence of a repair are congestive heart failure (CHF) (25%), aortic rupture (21%), endocarditis (18%), and intracranial hemorrhage (11%).

Physical Exam

Most patients will have systemic hypertension in the upper extremities. Additionally, lower extremity blood pressures will be reduced (normally lower extremity blood pressure is ~10 mm Hg greater than upper extremity) and the pulse will be delayed (palpating brachial and femoral pulses simultaneously). A systolic murmur may be heard between scapulae (from the coarctation) or throughout the chest wall (from intercostal collateral arteries). Attention should also be given to the possibility of a BAV (loud crescendo–decrescendo systolic murmur at the upper sternal borders).

Diagnostic Studies

Chest x-ray has two characteristic findings: **rib notching** (on the inferior surface of the ribs owing to large intercostal collateral arteries) and the "**3 sign**" (shadows of the dilated left subclavian artery and dilated postcoarctation aorta creating the outline of the number). Echocardiographic evaluation should include a suprasternal Doppler study looking for a continuous forward flow across the coarctation throughout diastole. Patients with repaired CoA will inevitably have turbulent flow across the repair site. It is our practice to screen patients with a CoA for BAV and berry aneurysms with a cardiac and cerebral MRI at least once.

Management Decisions

Surgical repair is the mainstay of treatment. Notable complications include spinal cord ischemia with paraplegia (0.4%), recoarctation (7%–60%), and aneurysm formation (2%–27%). Percutaneous balloon angioplasty with or without stent placement has demonstrated promising results.

- Pregnancy is well tolerated in repaired CoA, although there is an increased risk of miscarriage. Significant residual obstruction can lead to worse maternal and fetal outcomes and should be repaired prior to pregnancy if possible. Residual hypertension (18%) and preeclampsia (6%) can complicate the pregnancy.
- The estimated risk of congenital HD in the offspring of an affected parent is ~5%.
- Current guidelines for endocarditis prophylaxis hold that it is warranted in the 6 months after repair and in the setting of residual turbulent flow, particularly with prosthetic graft material.

EISENMENGER PHYSIOLOGY

This dreaded condition is the **end-stage complication for many untreated congenital HDs**. Over time, a left-to-right shunt can lead to vascular remodeling in the pulmonary system and increased right-sided pressures. The ultimate consequence is a reversal of blood flow across the defect such that deoxygenated venous blood moves into the systemic circulation (right-to-left shunt) and systemic cyanosis becomes evident.

Clinical Presentation

Most patients develop exercise intolerance in the second or third decade of life. Heart failure is seen after age 40. Frequent associated conditions include atrial or ventricular arrhythmias (50% of patients), hemoptysis (20%), pulmonary embolism (10%), syncope (10%), endocarditis (10%), hyperviscosity syndromes (fatigue, headache, dizziness, visual changes), and neurologic disease (cerebral hemorrhage, embolism, cerebral abscess). Because of high cell turnover and decreased resorption of uric acid, patients often have gout and cholelithiasis.

Unfortunately, the **survival of patients with Eisenmenger physiology is poor**, with only 42% of patients alive at 25 years of age. **Pregnancy and surgical procedures are generally poorly tolerated.**

Physical Exam

Patients are usually hypoxic, which becomes worse with exertion. Marked cyanosis and clubbing of the nail beds can be quite obvious in some patients. Signs of pulmonary hypertension (RV heave, PA tap, loud P2, right-sided S4) can be heard on cardiac auscultation.

Diagnostic Testing

ECG reflects the increased right-sided pressure (right atrial enlargement, RVH, right axis deviation). Chest x-ray often shows dilated proximal pulmonary arteries with distal "pruning" along with an enlarged right atrium or right ventricle. Echocardiography usually shows an obvious defect with bidirectional shunting of blood and elevated PA pressures. **Agitated saline bubble study during the echo is contraindicated, as this can cause air embolism.** A cardiac catheterization with vasodilator challenge can be particularly useful to assess for pulmonary vasoreactivity. Irreversible pulmonary hypertension portends a grave prognosis.

Management Decisions

Eisenmenger physiology should be considered a fragile hemodynamic system. Swings in intravascular volume can have serious consequences. Conservative, preventive measures include:

- Immunizations
- Avoidance of volume depletion, high altitude, smoking
- Antibiotics for endocarditis prophylaxis
- Avoidance of pregnancy and general anesthesia
- Use of IV filters to minimize possibility of a systemic air embolism
- Phlebotomy (with crystalloid replacement) for hyperviscosity syndromes due to erythrocytosis (rare)
- Cautious iron supplementation for microcytosis

Oxygen therapy can improve symptoms but has not been shown to have an impact on mortality. ACE inhibitors have both theoretical benefits and risks and are not routinely used. Pulmonary vasoreactive medications (calcium-channel blockers, prostacyclin, endothelin receptor blockers) are considered investigational and should be initiated and monitored by pulmonary specialists. Ultimately, the definitive treatment for Eisenmenger physiology is a combined heart–lung transplant (70% one-year survival) or lung transplant with cardiac repair (55% one-year survival).

OUTPATIENT APPROACH TO ADULTS WITH CONGENITAL HD

Caring for patients with congenital HD requires regular follow-up, intensive screening for early symptoms, and clear education for preventing severe complications. Follow-up visits should focus on:

- **Symptoms and signs.**
  - Changes in functional ability.
  - Development of cyanosis, heart failure, palpitations, syncope.
  - New murmurs.

- **Imaging.**
  - When management decisions are based on cardiac chamber size or patency of a surgically created circuit, serial imaging studies should be performed (echocardiography or cardiac MRI are first-line modalities).
  - Serial ECGs for certain lesions if high risk for atrial arrhythmias or sudden death

- **Education.**
  - Bacterial **endocarditis prophylaxis** is recommended for:
    - Unrepaired cyanotic congenital HD, including palliative shunts and conduits.
    - Completely repaired congenital HD with prosthetic material (surgery or device) for first 6 months following procedure.
    - Repaired congenital HD with residual defect at or near the site of prosthetic material (surgery or device).
    - Except for these conditions, antibiotic prophylaxis is no longer recommended for other forms of congenital HD.
  - **Pregnancy planning** (maternal and fetal risks of pregnancy, types of birth control) and fetal cardiac ultrasound (around 20–22 weeks' gestation).
    - High-risk congenital HD includes Eisenmenger physiology, cyanosis or symptomatic heart failure, pulmonary hypertension, significant systemic ventricular dysfunction, or left heart obstructive anatomies (aortic or mitral stenosis).
    - Many of the commonly prescribed heart failure medications are contraindicated in pregnancy (see Chapter 28 for a more detailed discussion).
    - High-risk obstetric care and frequent follow-up with a congenital HD specialist are essential. Usually, a cesarean section is not necessary unless indicated for obstetric reasons.
    - The choice of birth control can be tricky. Patients with complex congenital HD, pulmonary hypertension, or cyanosis should avoid oral contraceptive agents owing to the increased risk of blood clots. Depo-Provera or low-dose estrogens are often the birth control measures of choice.
  - Up-to-date **immunizations** (influenza, Pneumovax).
  - Explain to the patient which specific **symptoms to watch for** and **when to call the physician's office.**
  - Social considerations.
    - Adults with congenital HD often receive medical insurance through their employers, so extra attention to the details of changing jobs can prevent a patient from being deemed "noninsurable" due to a preexisting congenital HD condition.

• Often, adolescents with congenital HD who were "rejected" for life insurance are deemed insurable when they become adults.

KEY POINTS TO REMEMBER

• In caring for an adult patient with congenital HD, the three important pieces of information to know are:
  • The original cardiac condition
  • The specific surgical repair(s) that the patient has undergone
  • The anticipated natural history associated with both the condition and the repair
• Follow-up visits should focus on:
  • New symptoms or signs, especially functional ability, palpitations, or syncope
  • The need for serial imaging, especially when treatment decisions are based on the results
  • Patient education, specifically endocarditis prophylaxis, pregnancy planning, immunizations, and anticipated symptoms for which to call the physician's office.

ACKNOWLEDGMENT

The author is indebted to Dr. Joseph Billadello, Associate Professor of Medicine, Washington University School of Medicine, for his enthusiastic mentorship, superb care for adult patients with congenital HD, and considerate review of this chapter.

REFERENCES AND SUGGESTED READINGS

Aboulhosn J, Child JS. Left ventricular outflow obstruction: subaortic stenosis, bicuspid aortic valve, supravalvular aortic stenosis, and coarctation of the aorta. *Circulation* 2006;114:2412–2422.

Attenhofer Jost CH, Connolly HM, Dearani JA, et al. Ebstein's anomaly. *Circulation* 2007;115:277–285.

Bashore TM. Adult congenital heart disease: right ventricular outflow tract lesions. *Circulation* 2007;115:1933–1947.

Dillar GP, Gatzoulis MA. Pulmonary vascular disease in adults with congenital heart disease. *Circulation* 2007;115:1039–1050.

Khairy P, Poirier N, Mercier LA. Univentricular heart. *Circulation* 2007;115:800–812.

Minette MS, Sahn DA. Ventricular septal defects. *Circulation* 2006;114:2190–2197.

Schneider DJ, Moore JW. Patent ductus arteriosus. *Circulation* 2006;114:1873–1882.

Warnes C. Transposition of the great arteries. *Circulation* 2006;114:2699–2709.

Webb G, Gatzoulis MA. Atrial septal defects in the adult: recent progress and overview. *Circulation* 2006;114:1645–1653.

Webb GD, Smallhorn JF, Therrien J, et al. Congenital heart disease. In Zipes DP, Libby P, Bonow R, et al, eds, *Braunwald's Heart Disease: A Textbook of Cardiovascular Medicine*, 7th ed. Philadelphia: Elsevier Saunders; 2005:1489–1552.

Wilson W, Taubert KA, Gewitz M, et al. Prevention of bacterial endocarditis: Guidelines from the American Heart Association: A Guideline from the American Heart Association Rheumatic Fever, Endocarditis, and Kawasaki Disease Committee, Council on Cardiovascular Disease in the Young, and the Council on Clinical Cardiology, Council on Cardiovascular Surgery and Anesthesia, and the Quality Care and Outcomes Research Interdisciplinary Working Group. *Circulation* 2007;116:1736–1754.

Valvular Heart Disease

Brian R. Lindman

INTRODUCTION

Valvular heart disease encompasses those diseases characterized by abnormal mobility or closure of the heart valves, causing obstruction or regurgitation of (forward) flow through the valve. Valvular diseases can be acquired or congenital and may affect any of the four valves. Because the proper functioning of heart valves reflects a dynamic interplay of the valve, annulus, ventricular shape/size/function, and subvalvular apparatus, an abnormality in any of these can lead to valvular heart disease. Although disease prevalence is not known precisely, valve disease is common. It is estimated that >5 million people in the United States have moderate to severe regurgitant valvular lesions. Aortic stenosis (AS) is present in 2% of people >65 years of age and in 4% of those >85 years of age. Although rheumatic valve disease is quite common worldwide, in the developed world antibiotic usage and the aging of the population has led to degenerative valve lesions as the most common etiology. Although sometimes underappreciated, valvular disease is not benign; numerous studies have shown that various valve lesions are associated with excess morbidity and mortality, even when patients are asymptomatic. Forthcoming studies may show a role for medical therapies in slowing the progression of particular valve lesions; but because valve disease is largely a mechanical problem, the role for mechanical therapies will remain prominent. There is a growing understanding of the adverse consequences of valve disease. This, combined with significant improvements in surgical technique and expanding percutaneous therapies, will hopefully lead to expanded options and more appropriate timing in our efforts to treat valvular heart disease.

AORTIC VALVE

The aortic valve is a trileaflet valve that permits unidirectional flow from the left ventricle (LV) into the aorta. AS is characterized by incomplete opening of the valve during systole, which limits antegrade flow, yielding a systolic pressure gradient between the LV and ascending aorta. Aortic regurgitation (AR) is caused by incompetence of the valve, allowing backward flow of blood from the aorta into the LV during diastole.

Aortic Stenosis

Background
Lesions of the aortic valve are the most common cause for obstruction of flow from the LV into the aorta. Other causes of obstruction and the consequent pressure gradient between the LV and aorta include obstruction above the valve (supravalvular) and below the valve (subvalvular), both fixed (i.e., subaortic membrane) and dynamic (i.e., hypertrophic

cardiomyopathy with obstruction). The focus here is on obstruction at the level of the valve. Aortic sclerosis is thickening of the AV leaflets, which causes turbulent flow through the valve and a murmur but no gradient and therefore no stenosis. Aortic sclerosis is considered a risk factor for progression to stenosis.

Etiology

- **Calcific/degenerative**
  - Most common cause in the United States.
  - Trileaflet calcific AS usually presents in the seventh through ninth decades of life (mean age mid-70s).
  - Risk factors similar to coronary artery disease (CAD), exacerbated by abnormal calcium metabolism.
  - Active biological process with bone formation in the valve.
  - Calcification leading to stenosis affects both trileaflet and bicuspid valves.
- **Bicuspid**
  - Occurs in 1% to 2% of population (congenital lesion).
  - Usually presents in the sixth through seventh decades (mean age mid–late 60s).
  - ~50% of patients needing aortic valve replacement (AVR) for AS have a bicuspid valve.
  - More prone to endocarditis than trileaflet valves.
  - Associated with aortopathies (i.e., dissection, aneurysm) in a significant proportion of patients.
- **Rheumatic**
  - More common cause worldwide, much less common in the United States.
  - Usually presents in the third through fifth decades.
  - Almost always accompanied by mitral valve disease.

Pathophysiology

The pathophysiology for calcific AS involves both the valve and the ventricular adaptation to the stenosis. There is growing evidence for an active biological process within the valve that begins much like the formation of an atherosclerotic plaque and eventually leads to the formation of calcified bone (Fig. 16-1).

Natural History

AS is a progressive disease typically characterized by an asymptomatic phase until the valve area reaches a minimum threshold, generally <1 cm^2. In the absence of symptoms, patients with AS have a good prognosis with a risk of sudden death estimated to be $<1\%$ per year. Predictors of decreased event-free survival (free of AVR or death) include higher peak aortic jet velocity, extent of valve calcification, and coexistent CAD. Once patients experience symptoms, their average survival is 2 to 3 years, with an increased risk of sudden death.

History

Classic symptoms include:

- Angina
- Syncope
- Heart failure

Not infrequently, patients may limit their activity in ways that mask the presence of symptoms but indicate a progressive and premature decline in functional capacity. In the setting of severe AS, these patients should be viewed as symptomatic.

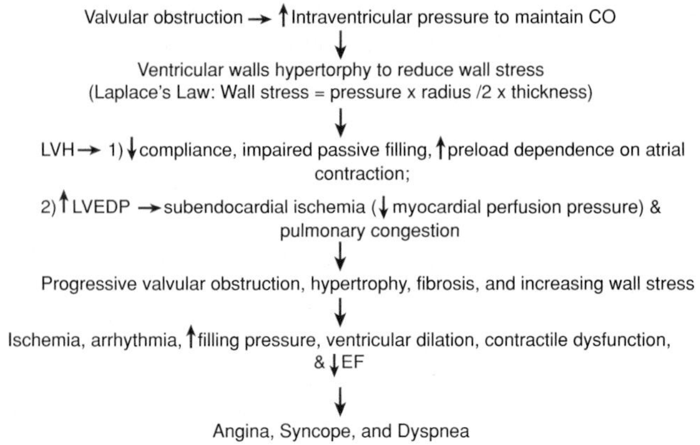

Valvular obstruction → ↑Intraventricular pressure to maintain CO

↓

Ventricular walls hypertorphy to reduce wall stress
(Laplace's Law: Wall stress = pressure x radius /2 x thickness)

↓

LVH→ 1)↓compliance, impaired passive filling,↑preload dependence on atrial contraction;

2)↑LVEDP →subendocardial ischemia (↓myocardial perfusion pressure) & pulmonary congestion

↓

Progressive valvular obstruction, hypertrophy, fibrosis, and increasing wall stress

↓

Ischemia, arrhythmia,↑filling pressure, ventricular dilation, contractile dysfunction, &↓EF

↓

Angina, Syncope, and Dyspnea

FIGURE 16-1. Pathophysiology of aortic stenosis. CO, cardiac output; LVH, left ventricular hypertrophy; LVEDP, left ventricular end diastolic pressure; EF, ejection fraction.

Physical Exam

- Harsh systolic crescendo–decrescendo murmur heard best at the right upper sternal border and radiating to both carotids; time to peak intensity correlates with severity (later peak = more severe).
- Diminished or absent A2 (soft S2) suggests severe AS.
- An opening snap suggests bicuspid AV.
- S4 reflects atrial contraction on a poorly compliant ventricle.
- Point of maximum impact (PMI) is sustained and diffuse and not displaced (unless the ventricle has dilated).
- Pulsus parvus et tardus: late-peaking and diminished carotid upstroke in severe AS.
- Gallavardin phenomenon is an AS murmur in which the musical element of the murmur is heard best at the apex (easily confused with MR).
- Between extremes, it is often difficult to assess AS severity on exam.

Diagnostic Testing

- Standard evaluation (Table 16-1)
- Severe AS (Table 16-2)
- Further evaluation in selected patients (Table 16-3)

Treatment

- **Surgery.** Therapeutic decisions are primarily based on the presence or absence of symptoms (Fig. 16-2). The treatment of severe AS is almost exclusively surgical AVR (see the end of this chapter for a discussion of valve prostheses). **Symptomatic severe AS is a deadly disease and deserves prompt surgical intervention**. Certain associated high-risk features or the need for another cardiac surgical intervention may lead to the recommendation for an AVR even when the patient is asymptomatic or has less than severe stenosis. Operative mortality varies significantly depending on age, comorbidities, and concurrent surgical procedures to be performed.
- **Medical therapy.** Severe symptomatic AS is a surgical disease. There are currently **no medical treatments proven to decrease mortality or delay surgery**. Nevertheless,

TABLE 16-1   STANDARD EVALUATION

ECG	• LAE and LVH
CXR	• LVH, cardiomegaly, and calcification of the aorta, AV, or coronaries • Rib notching suggests coarctation and BAV
TTE	• Leaflet number, morphology, and calcification • Calculate valve area using continuity equation [$Area_{AV} \times Velocity_{AV} = Area_{LVOT} \times Velocity_{LVOT}$] • The continuity equation is based on the principle that flow (velocity × area) is equal both proximal to and at the level of the obstruction • Transvalvular mean and peak gradients

LAE, left atrial enlargement; LVH, left ventricular hypertrophy; AV, aortic valve; BAV, bicuspid aortic valve; LVOT, left ventricular outflow tract.

TABLE 16-2   SEVERE AORTIC STENOSIS

Jet velocity (m/sec)	>4.0
Mean gradient (mm Hg)	>40
Valve area (cm^2)	<1.0

Source: From Bonow RO, Carabello BA, Chatterjee K, et al. ACC/AHA 2006 guidelines for the management of patients with valvular heart disease. *JACC* 2006;48(3):e1–e148, with permission.

TABLE 16-3   FURTHER EVALUATION IN SELECTED PATIENTS

TEE	• Clarify whether there is a bicuspid valve if unclear on TTE • Occasionally needed to evaluate for other or additional causes of LVOT obstruction
Exercise testing	• Evaluate for exercise capacity, abnormal blood pressure response (<20 mm Hg increase with exercise), or exercise-induced symptoms
Dobutamine stress echo	• Useful to assess the patient with LV dysfunction with a small valve area (suggesting severe AS) but a low (<30 mm Hg) mean transvalvular gradient (suggesting less severe AS) • Can help distinguish truly severe AS from aortic pseudostenosis • Assess for the presence of contractile reserve
Cath	• In patients undergoing AVR who are at risk for CAD • Evaluate for CAD in patients with moderate AS and symptoms of angina • Hemodynamic assessment of the severity of AS in patients in whom noninvasive tests are inconclusive or when there is a discrepancy between noninvasive tests and clinical findings regarding AS severity (utilizes the Gorlin formula)
CTA	• CTA may be an alternative to cath to evaluate coronary anatomy prior to valve surgery (the role and accuracy of CTA is still being investigated)

TEE, transesophageal echo; TTE, transthoracic echo; CTA, computed tomographic angiography.

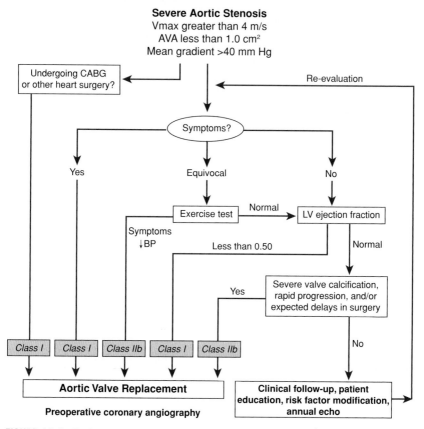

FIGURE 16-2. Evaluation and treatment of severe aortic stenosis. $\dot{V}_{max}$, maximum velocity; AVA, aortic valve area. (From Bonow RO, Carabello BA, Chatterjee K, et al. ACC/AHA 2006 guidelines for the management of patients with valvular heart disease. *JACC* 2006;48(3):e1–e148, with permission.)

there are some guidelines for medical therapy in nonsurgical candidates, asymptomatic patients, or those with less severe stenosis.

- Hypertension: treat with appropriate antihypertensive agents cautiously to avoid hypotension.
- Angiotensin converting enzyme (ACE) inhibitors: some data suggest that ACE inhibition may interfere with the valvular biology that leads to valve calcification.
- Statins: some clinical evidence suggests statins may slow progression of AS.
- Avoid overdiuresis and loss of preload, which may precipitate hypotension.
- Use vasodilators, particularly nitroglycerin, very cautiously so as to avoid hypotension.
- **Severe AS with decompensated heart failure.** Patients with severe AS and LV dysfunction may experience decompensated heart failure. Depending on the clinical scenario, several options may help bridge the patient to definitive surgical management (i.e., AVR).
  - Intraaortic balloon pump (IABP) (contraindicated in patients with moderate–severe AR).

- Sodium nitroprusside.
- Percutaneous valvuloplasty—AV area increases very modestly and restenosis occurs in weeks to months; may be used as a bridge to AVR, palliative measure in non-operative candidates, or if urgent noncardiac surgery is needed in patients with severe AS.

  Each of the above measures provides some degree of afterload reduction, either at the level of the valve (valvuloplasty) or by reduction in systemic vascular resistance (IABP, nipride); this afterload reduction can facilitate forward flow. The rationale is that as heart failure improves and transient end-organ damage is reversed (i.e., renal failure, respiratory failure), operative mortality decreases.
- **Percutaneous valve replacement.** In very high risk patients, **percutaneous aortic valves** may provide superior outcomes to percutaneous valvuloplasty and less morbidity and mortality than surgical AVR (clinical trials are currently under way). This may become a good option for an aging population with numerous comorbidities accompanying severe AS.

Challenging Clinical Scenarios

- *Asymptomatic severe AS—are they really asymptomatic?* Consider exercise testing to elicit symptoms. When done with appropriate supervision, this can be a very helpful means to determine the true impact of the stenotic valve.
- *Concomitant CAD and moderate AS in a patient with angina—what is causing the angina?* Incorporate all the data (including Doppler assessment of the coronary lesion in the cath lab, perfusion imaging, and severity of AS) to guide management. If AS is moderate and the coronary lesion appears obstructive, consider percutaneous coronary intervention to relieve angina; if there is no relief, then consider AVR.
- *Combined AS/AR—what if symptoms develop when the lesion(s) are only moderate?* Generally, surgical timing is still determined by the guidelines for isolated AS or AR. However, patients with combined moderate AS and AR may develop symptoms and/or LV dysfunction before either lesion is severe. It is reasonable to pursue AVR in combined moderate AS/AR when symptoms are present, LV function is reduced, or at the time of other cardiac surgery.
- *Aortic root disease—how does aortic root dilation influence the timing and extent of surgery?* Almost 50% of patients with severe AS have a bicuspid aortic valve (BAV). This is associated with aortic pathology that may predispose these patients to aortic dilation and dissection. It is critical to evaluate the aortic dimensions in patients with BAV, as significant enlargement may indicate a need for surgery even before valve stenosis is severe. Regardless of which drives the timing of surgery (aortic dimension or AV disease), both may need to be repaired or replaced at the time of surgery. All patients identified with a BAV should have imaging—computed tomography (CT) or magnetic resonance imaging (MRI)—to evaluate for thoracic aortic pathology.
- *LV dysfunction—should surgery be done when the valve area suggests severe AS but the gradient is low?* Dobutamine stress echo can be used to distinguish true severe AS from aortic pseudostenosis as well as to evaluate for the presence of contractile reserve. BNP may play a role in predicting outcome in these patients and may help management decisions. Surgery may be more beneficial and have the lowest mortality and morbidity in those patients with LV dysfunction, a truly stenotic aortic valve, lower BNP, and demonstrable contractile reserve. The role of surgery in patients with aortic pseudostenosis, a very elevated BNP, and/or a lack of contractile reserve is still unclear.

Aortic Regurgitation

Etiology

Aortic regurgitation (AR) results from pathology of the aortic valve with or without involvement of the aortic root. Several potential causes for AR variably affect the valve and aortic root. AR usually develops insidiously, but may be acute.

- **More common**
  - BAV
  - Rheumatic disease
  - Calcific degeneration
  - Infective endocarditis
  - Idiopathic dilatation of the aorta
  - Myxomatous degeneration
  - Systemic hypertension
  - Dissection of the ascending aorta
  - Marfan syndrome
- **Less common**
  - Traumatic injury to the aortic valve
  - Collagen vascular diseases (ankylosing spondylitis, rheumatoid arthritis, Reiter syndrome, giant-cell aortitis, and Whipple disease)
  - Syphilitic aortitis
  - Osteogenesis imperfecta
  - Ehlers–Danlos syndrome
  - Discrete subaortic stenosis
  - Ventricular septal defect (VSD) with prolapse of an aortic cusp
  - Anorectic drugs
- **Acute**
  - Infective endocarditis
  - Dissection of the ascending aorta
  - Trauma

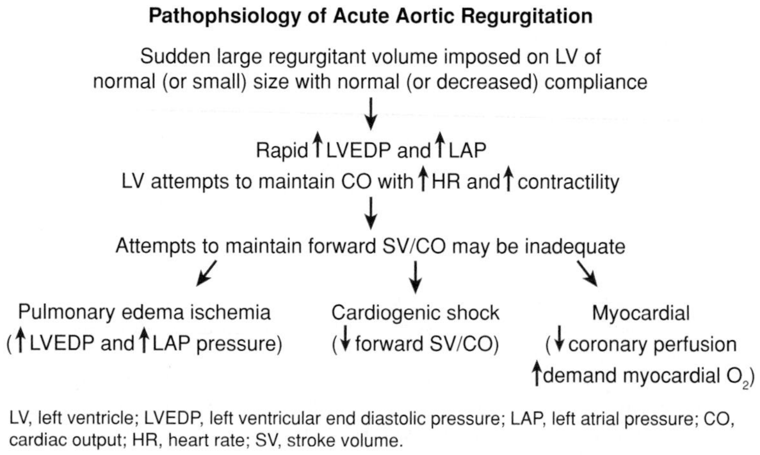

Pathophsiology of Acute Aortic Regurgitation

Sudden large regurgitant volume imposed on LV of normal (or small) size with normal (or decreased) compliance

↓

Rapid ↑LVEDP and ↑LAP
LV attempts to maintain CO with ↑HR and ↑contractility

↓

Attempts to maintain forward SV/CO may be inadequate

↙   ↓   ↘

| Pulmonary edema ischemia (↑LVEDP and ↑LAP pressure) | Cardiogenic shock (↓forward SV/CO) | Myocardial (↓coronary perfusion ↑demand myocardial O₂) |

LV, left ventricle; LVEDP, left ventricular end diastolic pressure; LAP, left atrial pressure; CO, cardiac output; HR, heart rate; SV, stroke volume.

FIGURE 16-3. Pathophysiology of acute aortic regurgitation.

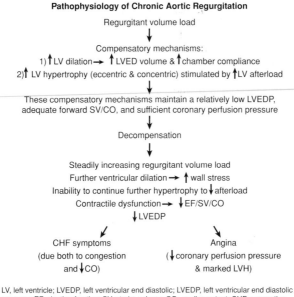

Pathophysiology of Chronic Aortic Regurgitation

Regurgitant volume load

↓

Compensatory mechanisms:
1) ↑LV dilation → ↑LVED volume & ↑chamber compliance
2) ↑ LV hypertrophy (eccentric & concentric) stimulated by ↑LV afterload

↓

These compensatory mechanisms maintain a relatively low LVEDP,
adequate forward SV/CO, and sufficient coronary perfusion pressure

↓

Decompensation

↓

Steadily increasing regurgitant volume load
Further ventricular dilation → ↑ wall stress
Inability to continue further hypertrophy to ↓afterload
Contractile dysfunction → ↓EF/SV/CO
↓LVEDP

CHF symptoms   Angina
(due both to congestion   (↓coronary perfusion pressure
and ↓CO)   & marked LVH)

LV, left ventricle; LVEDP, left ventricular end diastolic; LVEDP, left ventricular end diastolic
pressure; EF, ejection fraction; SV, stroke volume; CO, cardiac output; CHF, congestive
heart failure.

FIGURE 16-4. Pathophysiology of chronic aortic regurgitation.

Pathophysiology

- Acute aortic regurgitation (Fig. 16-3).
- Chronic aortic regurgitation (Fig. 16-4)

History
For the natural history of AR, see Table 16-4.

- **Acute:** Patients with acute AR typically present with **pulmonary edema manifested by severe dyspnea.** Other presenting symptoms may be related to the causes of acute AR listed under "Etiology," above.
- **Chronic:** Symptoms depend on the presence of LV dysfunction and whether the patient is in the **compensated versus decompensated stage.** Compensated patients are typically asymptomatic, whereas those in the decompensated stage may note decreased exercise tolerance, dyspnea, fatigue, and/or angina.

Physical Exam

- **Acute**
  - Tachycardia
  - Wide pulse pressure may be present but often is not because forward stroke volume (and therefore systolic blood pressure) is reduced.
  - A brief soft diastolic murmur heard best at the third left intercostal space (often not heard).

TABLE 16-4	NATURAL HISTORY OF AORTIC REGURGITATION	
Asymptomatic patients with normal LV systolic function		
Progression to symptoms and/or LV dysfunction		<6% per year
Progression to asymptomatic LV dysfunction		<3.5% per year
Sudden death		<0.2% per year
Asymptomatic patients with LV dysfunction		
Progression to cardiac symptoms		>25% per year
Symptomatic patients		
Mortality rate		>10% per year

Source: From Bonow RO, Carabello BA, Chatterjee K, et al. ACC/AHA 2006 guidelines for the management of patients with valvular heart disease. *JACC* 2006;48(3):e1–e148, with permission.

- Systolic flow murmur (due to volume overload and hyperdynamic LV).
- Diminished S1 due to increased LV end-diastolic pressure ($\uparrow$LVEDP) and premature mitral valve (MV) closure.
- LV heave.
- Pulsus paradoxus (may suggest cardiac tamponade secondary to aortic dissection).
- Measure blood pressure in both arms (a significant difference suggests aortic dissection).
- Look for evidence of infective endocarditis.
- Look for Marfanoid characteristics.
- **Chronic**
  - LV heave.
  - PMI is laterally displaced.
  - Diastolic decrescendo murmur heard best at lower sternal border (LSB) leaning forward at end-expiration (severity of AR correlates with duration, not intensity, of the murmur).
  - Systolic flow murmur (due mostly to volume overload; concomitant AS may also be present).
  - Austin Flint murmur—low-pitched diastolic murmur, heard best at the apex, caused by antegrade flow through a mitral orifice narrowed by severe AR, which restricts the motion of the anterior MV leaflet.
  - S3 is often heard as a manifestation of the volume overload and is not necessarily a sign of congestive heart failure (CHF).
  - Widened pulse pressure (often >100 mm Hg) with a low diastolic pressure.
  - Characteristic signs related to wide pulse pressure:
    - Musset sign: head bobbing with each cardiac cycle
    - Corrigan pulse: rapid carotid upstroke followed by arterial collapse
    - Müller sign: pulsation of the uvula
    - Traube sign: pistol-shot murmur heard on the femoral artery
    - Duroziez sign: to-and-fro murmur over the femoral artery when partially compressed
    - Quincke pulse: visible capillary pulsation in the nail bed after holding the tip of the nail

Diagnostic Testing

The diagnostic evaluation will depend somewhat on the acuity of the presentation but will likely include the following:

TABLE 16-5 **SEVERE AORTIC REGURGITATION**

Qualitative

Angiographic grade	3–4+
Color Doppler jet width	>65% of LVOT
Doppler vena contracta width (cm)	>0.6
PHT of AR jet (ms)	<200

Quantitative (cath or echo)

Regurgitant volume (mL/beat)	≥60
Regurgitant fraction (%)	≥50
Regurgitant orifice area (cm^2) (ERO)	≥0.30

Additional essential criteria

LV size	Increased*

AR, aortic regurgitation; LV, left ventricular; LVOT, left ventricular outflow tract; PHT, pressure half-time; ERO, effective regurgitant orifice.

*Except in acute AR in which the ventricle has not had time to dilate.

Adapted from Zoghbi WA, Enriquez-Sarano M, Foster E, et al. Recommendations for evaluation of the severity of native valvular regurgitation with two-dimensional and Doppler echocardiography. *J Am Soc Echocardiogr* 2003;16:777–802, with permission.

- **ECG**
  - Tachycardia
  - LV hypertrophy (LVH) and left atrial enlargement (LAE) (more common in chronic AR)
  - New heart block may suggest an aortic root abscess.
- **Chest x-ray (CXR)**
  - Look for pulmonary edema, widened mediastinum, and cardiomegaly.
- **Transthoracic echo**
  - LV systolic function
  - LV dimensions at end systole and end diastole
  - Leaflet number and morphology
  - Assessment of the severity of AR (see Table 16-5)
  - Look for evidence of endocarditis or aortic dissection
  - Dimension of aortic root
- **Transesophageal echo (TEE)**
  - Clarify whether there is a bicuspid valve if unclear on transthoracic echo
  - Better sensitivity and specificity for aortic dissection than transthoracic echo
  - Clarify whether there is endocarditis ± root abscess if unclear on transthoracic echo
  - Better visualization of aortic valve in patients with a prosthetic aortic valve
- **MRI/CT**
  - Depending on the institution, either of these may be the imaging modality of choice for evaluating aortic dimensions and/or aortic dissection.
  - If echo assessment of the severity of AR is inadequate, MRI is useful for assessing the severity of AR.
  - CT angiography (CTA) may be an alternative to cath to evaluate coronary anatomy prior to valve surgery (the role and accuracy of CTA are still being investigated).
- **Cath**
  - In patients undergoing AVR who are at risk for CAD

• Assessment of LV pressure, LV function, and severity of AR (via aortic root angiography) is indicated in symptomatic patients in whom the severity of AR is unclear on noninvasive imaging or discordant with clinical findings.

Treatment

• **Surgical. Surgery is indicated for any symptomatic patient with severe AR regardless of LV systolic function** (see Fig. 16-5 and Table 16-6). Acute, severe AR is almost always symptomatic. Valve repair may be feasible in a small subset of

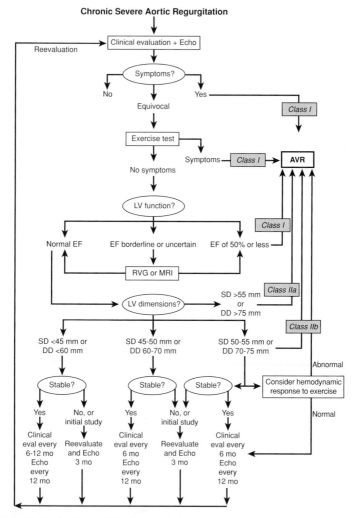

FIGURE 16-5. Evaluation and treatment of chronic severe aortic regurgitation. RVG, right ventriculogram; SD, systolic dimension, DD, diastolic dimension. (From From Bonow RO, Carabello BA, Chatterjee K, et al. ACC/AHA 2006 guidelines for the management of patients with valvular heart disease. *JACC* 2006;48(3):e1–e148, with permission.)

TABLE 16-6	ACC/AHA GUIDELINES—CLASS I INDICATIONS FOR AORTIC VALVE REPLACEMENT FOR AORTIC REGURGITATION

- Symptomatic with severe AR irrespective of LV systolic function
- Asymptomatic with chronic severe AR and LV systolic dysfunction (EF ≤50%)
- Chronic severe AR while undergoing CABG, surgery on the aorta, or other valve surgery

AR, aortic regurgitation; CABG, coronary artery bypass grafting; EF, ejection fraction; LV, left ventricular.
Source: From Bonow RO, Carabello BA, Chatterjee K, et al. ACC/AHA 2006 guidelines for the management of patients with valvular heart disease. *JACC* 2006;48(3):e1–e148, with permission.

patients, usually those in whom aortic dissection is the cause of the AR. If the aortic root is dilated, it may be repaired or replaced at the time of AVR (see Chapter 23). Although worse NYHA functional class, LV dysfunction, and the chronicity of these abnormalities are predictors of higher operative and postoperative mortality, AVR is usually a better alternative than medical therapy in improving overall mortality and morbidity. If a patient is in decompensated heart failure, short-term treatment with vasodilator therapy (i.e., nitroprusside) is reasonable to improve hemodynamics prior to surgery.

- **Medical.** The role of medical therapy in patients with AR is limited. There are no randomized, placebo-controlled data showing that vasodilator therapy delays the development of symptoms or LV dysfunction warranting surgery. Vasodilator therapy (i.e., nifedipine, ACE inhibitor, hydralazine) has a potential role in three situations: (1) used as chronic therapy in patients with severe AR who have symptoms or LV dysfunction but are *not* surgical candidates; (2) used as a short-term therapy to improve hemodynamics in patients with severe heart failure and severe LV dysfunction prior to surgery; and (3) may be considered for long-term therapy in asymptomatic patients with severe AR who have some degree of LV dilatation but normal systolic function. In general, vasodilator therapy is indicated to reduce systolic blood pressure in hypertensive patients with AR. In the absence of hypertension, it is not indicated for those who are asymptomatic, with mild or moderate AR, normal LV function, and normal LV cavity size. Aside from vasodilator therapy, medical therapy is important with respect to appropriate antibiotic usage when endocarditis is suspected.

MITRAL VALVE

The mitral valve permits unidirectional flow from the left atrium (LA) to the LV. The mitral apparatus is composed of an annulus, two leaflets, posteromedial and anterolateral papillary muscles, and chordae tendineae. The latter two are considered part of the mitral subvalvular apparatus. Together with the LV, the proper interaction between these various parts is necessary for the adequate function of the mitral valve.

Mitral stenosis (MS) is characterized by incomplete opening of the mitral valve during diastole, which limits anterograde flow and yields a sustained diastolic pressure gradient between the LA and LV. Mitral regurgitation (MR) is caused by inadequate coaptation of the valve leaflets, allowing blood to flow backward from the LV into the LA during systole.

Mitral Stenosis

Etiology

- **Rheumatic**
  - Predominant cause of MS.
  - Two-thirds of patients are female.
  - May be associated with MR.
  - Stenotic orifice often shaped like a "fish mouth."
  - Rheumatic fever can cause fibrosis, thickening, and calcification, leading to fusion of the commissures, cusps, chordae, or some combination.
- **Other causes (fairly rare)**
  - Congenital
  - Mucopolysaccharidoses
  - Malignant carcinoid
  - Systemic lupus erythematosus
  - Rheumatoid arthritis
  - Mitral annular calcification (MAC)
  - "Functional MS" may occur with obstruction of left atrial outflow due to:
    - Tumor, particularly myxoma
    - LA thrombus
    - Endocarditis with a large vegetation
    - Congenital membrane of the LA (i.e., cor triatriatum)
    - MV prosthesis dysfunction
    - Oversewn mitral annuloplasty ring

Pathophysiology

Physiologic states that either increase the transvalvular flow (enhance cardiac output) or decrease diastolic filling time (via tachycardia) can increase symptoms at any given valve area. Pregnancy, exercise, hyperthyroidism, atrial fibrillation with rapid ventricular response, and fever are examples in which either or both of these conditions occur. Symptoms are often first noticed at these times. (Fig. 16-6).

Natural History

MS usually progresses slowly, with a long latent period (several decades) between rheumatic fever and the development of stenosis severe enough to cause symptoms (usually $<2–2.5$ cm^2 with exercise or <1.5 cm^2 at rest). Ten-year survival of untreated patients with MS depends on the severity of symptoms at presentation: asymptomatic or minimally symptomatic patients have an 80% survival of 10 years, whereas those with significant limiting symptoms have a 10-year survival of 0 to 15%. Once severe pulmonary hypertension develops, mean survival is 3 years. Mortality in untreated patients is due mostly to progressive pulmonary and systemic congestion, systemic embolism, pulmonary embolism, and infection (in order of frequency).

History

After a prolonged asymptomatic period, patients may present with any of the following symptoms:

- Dyspnea
- Reduced functional capacity

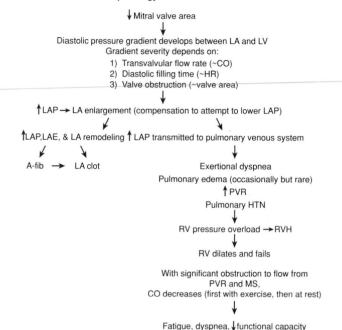

FIGURE 16-6. Pathophysiology of mitral stenosis. LA, left atrium; LV, left ventricle; CO, cardiac output; HR, heart rate; LAP, left atrial pressure; LAE, left atrial enlargement; PVR, pulmonary vascular resistance; RV, right ventricle; RVH, right ventricular hypertrophy.

- Orthopnea and/or paroxysmal nocturnal dyspnea
- Fatigue
- Palpitations—often due to atrial fibrillation
- Systemic embolism
- Hemoptysis
- Chest pain
- Signs and symptoms of infective endocarditis

Physical Exam

Findings on physical exam will depend on the severity of valve obstruction and the associated adaptations that have had time to develop in response to it.

- Accentuation of S1 may occur when the leaflets are flexible.
- Opening snap (OS)—caused by sudden tensing of the valve leaflets after they have completed their opening excursion; the A2–OS interval varies inversely with the severity of stenosis (shorter interval = more severe stenosis).
- Middiastolic rumble—low-pitched murmur heard best at the apex with the bell of the stethoscope; the severity of stenosis is related to the duration of the murmur, not intensity (more severe = longer duration).

- Irregularly irregular pulse due to atrial fibrillation (AF)
- MR murmur may be present
- Loud P2, tricuspid regurgitation (TR) murmur, pulmonary artery (PA) tap, and/or RV heave can indicate pulmonary hypertension.
- Increased jugular venous pressure (↑JVP), hepatic congestion, and peripheral edema can indicate varying degrees of right heart failure.

Diagnostic Testing

- **ECG**
  - P mitral (P wave duration in lead II ≥0.12 seconds, indicating LAE)
  - Atrial fibrillation
  - RVH
- **CXR**
  - LAE
  - Enlarged RA/RV and/or enlarged pulmonary arteries
  - Calcification of the MV and/or annulus
- **Transthoracic echo (TTE)**
  - Assess etiology of MS
  - Asseess severity of MS (see Table 16-7)
  - Leaflet mobility, leaflet thickening, subvalvular thickening, and leaflet calcification (these are determinants of the echo mitral valve score [Wilkins score]—ranging from 0–16—which is important in determining candidacy for percutaneous mitral balloon valvotomy [PMBV]).
  - Mean transmitral gradient.
  - Valve area can be measured by several methods (pressure half-time, continuity equation, direct planimetry).
  - Pulmonary artery systolic pressure (PASP) (utilizing the tricuspid regurgitation [TR] jet velocity).
  - RV size and function
- **Exercise testing with echo**
  - Helpful in clarifying functional capacity of those with an unclear history
  - Assess transmitral gradient and PASP with exercise when there is a discrepancy between resting doppler findings, clinical findings, signs and symptoms
- **TEE**
  - Assess presence or absence of clot and severity of MR in patients being considered for PMBV.
  - Evaluate MV morphology and hemodynamics in patients with MS for whom transthoracic echo was suboptimal.
- **Cath**
  - Indicated to determine severity of MS when clinical and echo assessments are discordant (see Fig. 16-7).
  - Reasonable to assess hemodynamic response of pulmonary artery and LA pressures to exercise when clinical symptoms and resting hemodynamics are discordant.
  - Reasonable in patients with MS to assess the cause of severe pulmonary hypertension when out of proportion to the severity of MS as determined by noninvasive testing.
  - Left heart cath when patients have risk factors for CAD and have chest pain of unclear etiology or are going for mitral valve replacement (MVR).

TABLE 16-7	SEVERE MITRAL STENOSIS
Mean gradient (mm Hg)	>10
PASP (mm Hg)	>50
Valve area (cm^2)	<1.0

Source: From Bonow RO, Carabello BA, Chatterjee K, et al. ACC/AHA 2006 guidelines for the management of patients with valvular heart disease. *JACC* 2006;48(3):e1–e148, with permission.

Treatment

Treatment of MS depends on the patient's symptoms, the severity of stenosis, the presence and severity of associated pulmonary hypertension, presence of an associated arrhythmia, and the risk of thromboembolism.

- **Medical.** Medical therapy is aimed at **slowing progression of pulmonary hypertension, preventing endocarditis, reducing the risk of thromboembolism, and reducing**

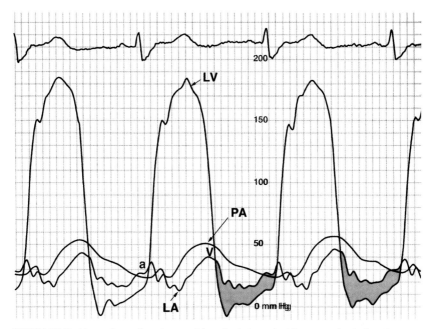

FIGURE 16-7. Hemodynamics observed in mitral stenosis. The gray-shaded region corresponds to the diastolic filling gradient between the left atrium (LA) and left ventricle (LV). PA, pulmonary artery. (From Murphy JG. *Mayo Clinic Cardiology Review*, 2nd ed. Philadelphia: Lippincott Williams & Wilkins; 2000, with permission.)

heart failure symptoms. For heart failure, intermittent diuretics and a low-salt diet are often adequate if there is evidence of pulmonary congestion. For patients who develop symptoms only with exercise (likely associated with tachycardia), negative chronotropic agents such as beta blockers or nondihydropyridine calcium channel blockers may be of benefit. Since almost all MS is rheumatic in origin, prophylaxis against rheumatic fever may be appropriate.

- *Atrial fibrillation:* Patients with MS are particularly prone to develop atrial fibrillation (AF) and/or flutter (30%–40% of patients with MS). AF can exacerbate and worsen symptoms (particularly in the setting of a rapid ventricular response) due to a shortened diastolic filling period and loss of atrial kick → increased LA pressure → increased pulmonary congestion. Therapy is mostly aimed at rate control and prevention of thromboembolism. For rate control, particularly tachycardia associated with exertion, beta blockers or nondihydropyridine calcium channel blockers tend to be more effective than digoxin. Efforts to maintain sinus rhythm (through direct current cardioversion, ablation, or with drugs) are focused on those patients with symptoms from their AF and can be particularly challenging in patients with MS. Anticoagulation for patients with MS and AF is routine (Table 16-8).

- **Percutaneous mitral balloon valvotomy (PMBV).** PMBV is generally performed via a transseptal approach. After transseptal puncture of the interatrial septum, a catheter with a balloon is passed across the interatrial septum and the balloon is positioned across the mitral valve. Balloon inflation separates the commissures and fractures some of the nodular calcium in the leaflets, yielding an increased valve area. Usually, the transmitral pressure gradient decreases by 50% to 60%, cardiac output increases 10% to 20%, and valve area increases from 1.0 to 2.0 cm^2. Contraindications to PMBV include LA thrombus, moderate–severe MR (>2+), and an echo score >8 (the latter is a relative contraindication). Complications include death (~1%), stroke, cardiac perforation, severe MR requiring surgical correction, and residual atrial septal defect requiring closure. When done in those with favorable MV morphology, event-free survival (freedom from death, repeat valvotomy, or MV replacement) is 80% to 90% at 3 to 7 years. This approach compares favorably with surgical mitral commissurotomy (open or closed) and is the procedure of choice in experienced centers for patients without contraindications (Table 16-9).

TABLE 16-8	ACC/AHA GUIDELINES—CLASS I INDICATIONS FOR PREVENTION OF SYSTEMIC EMBOLIZATION IN PATIENTS WITH MITRAL STENOSIS

- Anticoagulation is indicated in patients with MS and AF (paroxysmal, persistent, or permanent)
- Anticoagulation is indicated in patients with MS and a prior embolic event, even in sinus rhythm
- Anticoagulation is indicated in patients with MS with left atrial thrombus

AF, atrial fibrillation; MS, mitral stenosis.

Source: From Bonow RO, Carabello BA, Chatterjee K, et al. ACC/AHA 2006 guidelines for the management of patients with valvular heart disease. *JACC* 2006;48(3):e1–e148, with permission.

TABLE 16-9	ACC/AHA GUIDELINES—CLASS I INDICATIONS FOR PERCUTANEOUS MITRAL BALLOON VALVOTOMY

- Symptomatic (NYHA functional class II, III, or IV) with moderate or severe MS and valve morphology favorable for PMBV in the absence of LA thrombus or moderate–severe MR
- Asymptomatic with moderate or severe MS and valve morphology favorable for PMBV who have pulmonary hypertension (PASP >50 mm Hg at rest or >60 mm Hg with exercise) in the absence of LA thrombus or moderate–severe MR

LA, left atrial; MR, mitral regurgitation; PMBV, percutaneous mitral balloon valvotomy.

Source: From Bonow RO, Carabello BA, Chatterjee K, et al. ACC/AHA 2006 guidelines for the management of patients with valvular heart disease. *JACC* 2006;48(3):e1–e148, with permission.

- **Surgery.** Surgical treatment is usually reserved for those who are not candidates for PMBV because of the presence of one or more contraindications to PMBV or because the percutaneous option is unavailable. Surgical valvotomy can be done either closed (bypass unnecessary) or open (done under direct visualization on bypass). Open valvotomy yields better outcomes and is the preferred approach in developed countries; closed valvotomy continues to be used in some developing countries without access to open heart surgery or percutaneous approaches. When the valve cannot be repaired, valve replacement is required (see Table 16-10).

Mitral Regurgitation

Prevention of MR is dependent on the integrated and proper function of the mitral valve (annulus and leaflets), subvalvular apparatus (chordae tendineae and papillary muscles),

TABLE 16-10	ACC/AHA GUIDELINES—CLASS I INDICATIONS FOR SURGERY FOR MITRAL STENOSIS

- MV surgery (repair if possible) is indicated in symptomatic patients (NYHA functional class III or IV) with moderate or severe MS in a patient with acceptable operative risk when:
  - PMBV is unavailable
  - PMBV is contraindicated because:
    - Presence of LA thrombus despite anticoagulation or
    - Concomitant moderate–severe MR is present, or
    - Valve morphology is not favorable for PMBV
- Symptomatic with moderate or severe MS who also have moderate–severe MR should receive MV replacement unless valve repair is possible at the time of surgery

MR, mitral regurgitation; MS, mitral stenosis; MV, mitral valve; PMBV, percutaneous mitral balloon valvotomy.

Source: From Bonow RO, Carabello BA, Chatterjee K, et al. ACC/AHA 2006 guidelines for the management of patients with valvular heart disease. *JACC* 2006;48(3):e1–e148, with permission.

left atrium, and the ventricle. Abnormal function of any one of these components can lead to MR. Given the complexity of this interaction, the terminology to describe MR (the final common pathway of all abnormalities of the valve apparatus or ventricle that lead to MR) is often confusing. **Organic MR** is MR caused *primarily* by abnormalities of the valve leaflets and/or chordae tendinae (e.g., myxomatous degeneration, endocarditis, and rheumatic). **Functional MR** refers to MR caused *primarily* by ventricular dysfunction usually with accompanying annular dilatation (e.g., cardiomyopathy and ischemic MR).

Etiology

- **Degenerative** (essentially analogous to **mitral valve prolapse syndrome**)
- Usually occurs as a primary condition (Barlow disease or fibroelastic deficiency) but has also been associated with heritable diseases affecting the connective tissue, including Marfan syndrome, Ehlers–Danlos syndrome, osteogenesis imperfecta, etc.
  - May be familial or nonfamilial
  - Occurs in 1% to 2.5% of the population (based on stricter echo criteria)
  - Female-to-male ratio is 2:1
  - Either or both leaflets may prolapse
  - Most common reason for MV surgery
  - Myxomatous proliferation and cartilage formation can occur in the leaflets, chordae tendineae, and/or annulus
- **Dilated cardiomyopathy (DCM)**
  - Mechanism of MR due to both:
    - Annular dilatation from ventricular enlargement
    - Papillary muscle displacement due to ventricular enlargement and remodeling, which prevents adequate leaflet coaptation
  - May occur in the setting of nonischemic DCM or ischemic DCM (there is often an overlap of mechanism for MR in the setting of previous infarction)
- **Ischemic**
  - Ischemic MR is mostly a misnomer, as this is primarily postinfarction MR, not MR caused by active ischemia
  - The MR is due primarily to ventricular dysfunction, not papillary muscle dysfunction
  - The mechanism of MR usually involves one or both of the following:
    - Annular dilatation from ventricular enlargement
    - Local LV remodeling with papillary muscle displacement (both the dilatation of the ventricle and the akinesis/dyskinesis of the wall to which the papillary muscle is attached can prevent adequate leaflet coaptation)
  - Rarely, MR may develop acutely from papillary muscle rupture (more commonly of the posteromedial papillary muscle)
- **Rheumatic**
  - May be pure MR or combined MR/MS
  - Caused by thickening and/or calcification of the leaflets and chords
- **Infective endocarditis**
  - Usually caused by destruction of the leaflet tissue (i.e., perforation)
- **Other causes**
  - Congenital (cleft, parachute, or fenestrated mitral valves)
  - Infiltrative diseases (i.e., amyloid)
  - Systemic lupus erythematosus (Libman-Sacks lesion)
  - Hypertrophic cardiomyopathy with obstruction
  - Mitral annular calcification

- Paravalvular prosthetic leak
- Drug toxicity (e.g., phen-fen)
- **Acute causes**
  - Ruptured papillary muscle
  - Ruptured chordae tendineae
  - Infective endocarditis

Pathophysiology

For acute mitral regurgitation, see Figure 16-8A; for chronic mitral regurgitation, see Figure 16-8B.

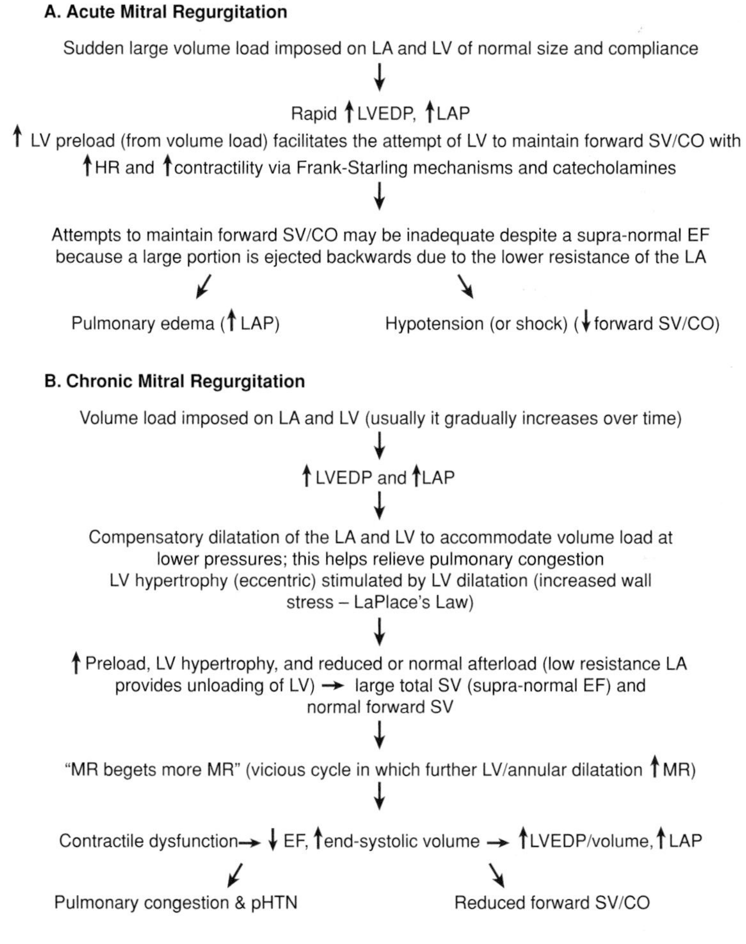

A. Acute Mitral Regurgitation

Sudden large volume load imposed on LA and LV of normal size and compliance

↓

Rapid ↑LVEDP, ↑LAP

↑ LV preload (from volume load) facilitates the attempt of LV to maintain forward SV/CO with ↑HR and ↑contractility via Frank-Starling mechanisms and catecholamines

↓

Attempts to maintain forward SV/CO may be inadequate despite a supra-normal EF because a large portion is ejected backwards due to the lower resistance of the LA

Pulmonary edema (↑LAP)   Hypotension (or shock) (↓forward SV/CO)

B. Chronic Mitral Regurgitation

Volume load imposed on LA and LV (usually it gradually increases over time)

↓

↑LVEDP and ↑LAP

↓

Compensatory dilatation of the LA and LV to accommodate volume load at lower pressures; this helps relieve pulmonary congestion LV hypertrophy (eccentric) stimulated by LV dilatation (increased wall stress – LaPlace's Law)

↓

↑Preload, LV hypertrophy, and reduced or normal afterload (low resistance LA provides unloading of LV) → large total SV (supra-normal EF) and normal forward SV

↓

"MR begets more MR" (vicious cycle in which further LV/annular dilatation ↑MR)

↓

Contractile dysfunction → ↓EF, ↑end-systolic volume → ↑LVEDP/volume, ↑LAP

Pulmonary congestion & pHTN   Reduced forward SV/CO

LA, left atrium; LV, left ventricle; LVEDP, left ventricular end diastolic pressure; LAP, left atrial pressure; SV, stroke volume; CO, cardiac output; EF, ejection fraction; pHTN, pulmonary hypertension.

FIGURE 16-8. Pathophysiology of **(A)** acute mitral regurgitation and **(B)** chronic mitral regurgitation.

Natural History

The natural history and progression of MR depends on etiology, associated LV dysfunction, and severity of MR at the time of diagnosis. MVP with little or no MR is most often associated with a benign prognosis and normal life expectancy; a minority of these patients (10%–15%) will go on to develop severe MR. The compensated asymptomatic phase of patients with severe organic MR (mostly degenerative but also due to rheumatic fever and endocarditis) with normal LV function is variable but may last several years. Two studies involving patients with severe asymptomatic MR showed an event-free survival (free of death or an indication for surgery) of 10% at 10 years and 55% at 8 years. Factors independently associated with increased mortality after surgery include preoperative ejection fraction (EF) <60%, NYHA functional class III–IV symptoms, age, associated CAD, AF, and effective regurgitant orifice (ERO) >40 mm^2. Several of these factors and others are also associated with postoperative LV dysfunction and CHF.

The natural history of ischemic MR and MR due to DCM (these populations overlap) is generally worse than for degenerative MR because of the associated comorbidities in these patients, namely CAD and LV dysfunction with or without CHF. Ischemic MR is independently associated with increased mortality after myocardial infarction (MI), in chronic CHF, and after revascularization. Its impact on mortality increases with the severity of regurgitation. Moreover, ischemic MR is an important predictor of future CHF. The presence of MR in the setting of DCM is common (up to 60% of patients) and independently associated with increased mortality. In both ischemic MR and MR due to DCM, because "MR begets MR," the ventricles of these patients dilate further and their CHF symptoms worsen.

History

- **Acute MR:** The most prominent symptom is relatively rapid onset of significant dyspnea, which may progress quickly to respiratory failure. Symptoms of reduced forward flow may also be present, depending on the patient's ability to compensate for the regurgitant volume.
- **Chronic MR:** The etiology of the MR and the time at which the patient presents will influence symptoms. In degenerative MR that has progressed gradually, the patient may be asymptomatic even when the MR is severe. As compensatory mechanisms begin to fail, patients may develop dyspnea on exertion (which may be due to pulmonary hypertension and/or pulmonary edema exacerbated by increased regurgitant volume during exercise), palpitations (from AF), fatigue, volume overload, and other symptoms of CHF. Patients with ischemic MR and MR due to DCM may report similar symptoms. In general, these patients will tend to be more symptomatic because of associated LV dysfunction.

Physical Exam

- **Acute**
  - Tachypnea with respiratory distress
  - Tachycardia
  - Systolic murmur, usually at the apex—may not be holosystolic and may be absent
  - S3 and/or early diastolic flow rumble may be present due to rapid early filling of LV during diastole because of large regurgitant volume load in the LA.
  - Apical impulse may be hyperdynamic
  - Crackles on lung exam
  - Relative hypotension (even shock)

- **Chronic**
  - Apical holosystolic murmur that radiates to the axilla
  - The murmur may radiate to the anterior chest wall if the posterior leaflet is prolapsed or toward the back if the anterior leaflet is prolapsed.
  - In mitral valve prolapse, a midsystolic click is heard before the murmur.
  - The LV apical impulse is displaced laterally.
  - S3 and/or early diastolic flow rumble may be present due to significant early antegrade flow over the MV during diastole; this does not necessarily indicate LV dysfunction.
  - Irregularly irregular rhythm (AF)
  - Loud P2 indicates pulmonary hypertension
  - S2 may be widely split due to an early A2
  - Other signs of CHF (lower extremity edema, ↑central venous pressure, crackles, etc.)

Diagnostic Testing

- **ECG**
  - LAE, LVH/LVE
  - Atrial fibrillation
  - Pathologic Q waves from previous MI in ischemic MR
- **CXR**
  - LAE
  - Pulmonary edema
  - Enlarged pulmonary arteries
  - Cardiomegaly
- **Transthoracic echocardiography (TTE)**
  - Assess etiology of MR
  - MVP is defined by valve prolapse of 2 mm or more above the mitral annulus in certain echo views
  - LA size (should be increased in chronic, severe MR)
  - LV dimensions at end-systole and end-diastole (should be dilated in chronic, severe MR of any etiology)
  - EF (LV dysfunction is present if EF ≤60%)
  - Qualitative and quantitative measures of MR severity (see Table 16-11)
- **TEE**
  - Provides better visualization of the valve to help define prolapsing leaflet(s)/scallop(s), presence of endocarditis, and feasibility of repair
  - May help determine severity of MR when TTE is nondiagnostic, particularly in the setting of an eccentric jet
  - Intraoperative TEE is indicated to guide repair and assess success
- **3D echo**
  - May provide additional and more accurate anatomic insights that can guide repair
- **Exercise testing with echo**
  - Helpful in clarifying functional capacity of those with an unclear history
  - Assess severity of MR with exercise in patients with exertional symptoms that seem discordant with the assessment of MR severity at rest
  - Assess PASP with exercise
  - Assess contractile reserve (change in EF with exercise)—may indicate onset of contractile dysfunction
- **MRI**
  - Assess EF in patients with severe MR, but with an inadequate assessment of EF by echo

- Assess quantitative measures of MR severity when echo is nondiagnostic
- Viability assessment may play a role in considering therapeutic strategy in ischemic MR
- **Nuclear**
  - Assess EF in patients with severe MR, but with an inadequate assessment of EF by echo
  - Viability assessment may play a role in considering therapeutic strategy in ischemic MR
- **Cath**
  - Right heart cath to evaluate:
    - Pulmonary hypertension in patients with chronic severe MR
    - LA filling pressure in patients with unclear symptoms
    - Giant *v* waves on pulmonary capillary wedge pressure (PCWP) tracing may suggest severe MR
  - Left heart cath:
    - May influence therapeutic strategy in ischemic MR
    - Evaluation of CAD in patients with risk factors undergoing MV surgery
    - Left ventriculogram can evaluate LV function and severity of MR
- **CTA**
  - CTA may be an alternative to left heart catheterization (LHC) to evaluate coronary anatomy prior to valve surgery (the role and accuracy of CTA is still being investigated).

Treatment
See Figure 16-9.

TABLE 16-11 SEVERE MITRAL REGURGITATION

Qualitative	
Angiographic grade	3–4+
Color Doppler jet area	>40% LA area*
Doppler vena contracta width (cm)	≥0.7
Quantitative (cath or echo)	
Regurgitant volume (mL/beat)	≥60
Regurgitant fraction (%)	≥50
Regurgitant orifice area (cm^2) (ERO)	≥0.40[†]
Additional essential criteria	
LA size	Enlarged[‡]
LV size	Enlarged[‡]

ERO, effective regurgitant orifice; LA, left atrial; LV, left ventricular.

*Or with a wall-impinging jet of any size swirling in the LA.

[†]Severe ischemic MR is defined by ERO ≥ 0.20.

[‡]Enlargement should be present with chronic severe MR but often is not present with acute severe MR.

Source: Adapted from Zoghbi WA, Enriquez-Sarano M, Foster E, et al. Recommendations for evaluation of the severity of native valvular regurgitation with two-dimensional and Doppler echocardiography. *J Am Soc Echocardiogr* 2003;16:777–802, with permission.

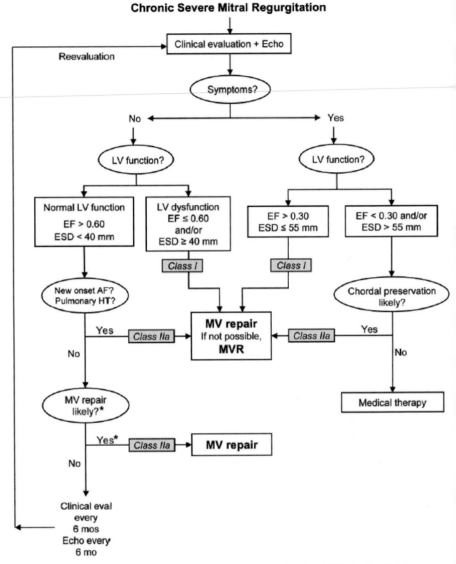

FIGURE 16-9. Treatment of chronic severe mitral regurgitation. *Mitral valve (MV) repair may be performed in asymptomatic patients with normal left ventricular (LV) function if performed by an experienced surgical team and if the likelihood of successful MV repair is greater than 90%. ESD, end-systolic dimension. (From Bonow RO, Carabello BA, Chatterjee K, et al. ACC/AHA 2006 guidelines for the management of patients with valvular heart disease. *JACC* 2006;48(3):e1–e148, with permission.)

- **Surgery.** Surgery for MR is most commonly performed in patients with degenerative mitral valve disease. With advances in surgical technique (including more frequent and better repairs instead of replacements) and lower operative mortality, there is a push in some centers to operate earlier on patients with severe MR, even when they are still asymptomatic. **A move toward earlier surgery, however, particularly in asymptomatic patients, requires that all efforts be made to repair the valve and that the surgery be done by surgeons experienced in valve repair.** Operative mortality is ~2%, even <1% in some centers for the best operative candidates. Preoperative factors that increase operative and/or postoperative mortality include worse NYHA functional class, LV dysfunction (EF <60%), age, associated CAD, and AF. **Compared with valve replacement, valve repair yields improved operative survival, long-term survival, and improved postoperative LV function** (see Table 16-12).

Surgery for **organic mitral disease** generally involves repair of the valve (with triangular or quadrangular resection) and ring annuloplasty. Long-term results at high-volume centers are excellent, with reoperation rates of 5% to 10% at 10 years and about 20% at 20 years. If repair cannot be performed, replacement should be performed with preservation of the subvalvular chordal structures. See the end of the chapter for a discussion of valve prostheses.

Surgery for patients with **ischemic MR and MR due to DCM** is more controversial and more complex. Since the MR is due primarily to a ventricular problem, isolated annuloplasty likely will not solve the problem. Revascularization alone—coronary artery bypass grafting (CABG) or percutaneous intervention (PCI)—for chronic ischemic MR can decrease the severity of MR in some cases. Adding annuloplasty to CABG can help reduce the presence and severity of postoperative MR, but the rate of persistent and recurrent significant MR is high, often >30%, even in experienced centers. Moreover, adding annuloplasty to CABG does not seem to improve postoperative mortality or decrease heart failure symptoms even if it does not add to the mortality of the surgery. Perhaps this is because of the high persistence/recurrence rate of MR. If so, surgical treatment for ischemic MR will need to address the ventricular aspect of problem. Various approaches are currently under investigation.

A similar quandary exists in patients with severe LV dysfunction and moderate to severe MR. Even though surgical mortality in experienced centers is lower (~5%) than previously assumed, mitral valve annuloplasty is not associated with improved long-term survival. Nevertheless, annuloplasty has been shown to improve heart failure symptoms, EF, and ventricular size. As with ischemic MR, the optimal surgical solution will likely incorporate more than just an annuloplasty ring that addresses the dilated annulus. The contribution of the dysfunctional ventricle (dilated, spherical, and with poor contractile function) will need to be therapeutically targeted as well.

Certain patients with AF should be considered for a concomitant **surgical maze procedure** to restore sinus rhythm, which may prevent future thromboembolic events, eliminate the need for anticoagulation, and prevent future heart failure.

- **Medical**
  - *Acute:* In the setting of severe acute MR, surgical treatment is indicated, often urgently or emergently. While awaiting surgery, aggressive afterload reduction with IV nitroprusside or an IABP can diminish the amount of MR and stabilize the patient by promoting forward flow and reducing pulmonary edema. These patients are usually tachycardic, but attempts to slow their heart rate should be avoided, as cardiac output is heart rate-dependent in these patients with reduced stroke volume.

TABLE 16-12	ACC/AHA GUIDELINES—CLASS I INDICATIONS FOR SURGERY IN MITRAL REGURGITATION

- Symptomatic acute severe MR
- Chronic severe MR and NYHA functional class II, III, or IV symptoms in the absence of severe LV dysfunction (EF <30%) and/or ESD >55 mm
- Asymptomatic with chronic severe MR and mild–moderate LV dysfunction (EF 30%–60%), and/or ESD ≥40 mm
- MV repair is recommended over MV replacement in the majority of patients with severe chronic MR who require surgery, and patients should be referred to surgical centers experienced in MV repair

EF, ejection fraction; ESD, end-systolic dimension; LV, left ventricular; MR, mitral regurgitation; MV, mitral valve.

Source: From Bonow RO, Carabello BA, Chatterjee K, et al. ACC/AHA 2006 guidelines for the management of patients with valvular heart disease. *JACC* 2006;48(3):e1–e148, with permission.

- *Chronic:* Given that chronic MR may have different etiologies, the role of medical therapy may differ in each setting. In the asymptomatic patient with normal LV function and chronic severe MR due to leaflet prolapse, there is no generally accepted medical therapy. In the absence of systemic hypertension, there is no known indication for vasodilating drugs. Whether ACE inhibitors or beta blockers delay ventricular remodeling and the need for surgery is being investigated in prospective studies. In contrast, patients with functional MR (ischemic MR and MR due to DCM) should be treated as other patients with LV dysfunction. ACE inhibitors and beta blockers are indicated and have been shown to reduce mortality and the severity of MR. Some patients may also qualify for cardiac resynchronization therapy, which has also been shown to reduce the severity of MR.
- **Percutaneous.** An ever-expanding number of percutaneous approaches are being considered for the treatment of MR, some of which are quite complex. Various approaches target each of the interrelated components that can contribute to MR: annular dilatation, lack of leaflet coaptation, and ventricular remodeling causing papillary muscle displacement. Currently, the most developed technique enhances coaptation with a clip that pinches the leaflets together at the central scallops. The clip is placed under TEE guidance by a catheter using a transseptal approach. Trials for this approach and others are currently under way.

TRICUSPID VALVE (TV)

The tricuspid valve lies between the right atrium and ventricle. It has three leaflets: anterior, posterior, and septal. Primary tricuspid valve disease is relatively uncommon.

Tricuspid Stenosis (TS)

Etiology

- Rheumatic heart disease (most common cause)
- Carcinoid

- Congenital abnormalities (see Chapter 15)
- Infective endocarditis (with bulky vegetations)
- Endocardial fibroelastosis
- Fabry disease
- Methysergide toxicity
- Loeffler's syndrome
- Right atrial mass may cause functional obstruction of the valve

History

Patients typically note symptoms consistent with right heart failure, including peripheral edema, increased abdominal girth, fatigue, and palpitations (if there are associated arrhythmias).

Physical Exam

- Elevated JVP with a giant *a* wave and diminished rate of *y* descent
- Hepatomegaly with a pulsatile liver
- Middiastolic murmur (low-pitched) that increases with inspiration
- Opening snap
- Edema in lower extremities, often anasarca

Diagnostic Testing

- **ECG**
  - Right atrial enlargement (RAE)
  - Atrial fibrillation
- **CXR**
  - Enlarged right heart border
- **Transthoracic echo (TTE)**
  - Evaluate morphology of valve
  - RAE
  - Associated congenital abnormalities
  - TV gradient
  - Calculate valve area (<1.0 cm^2 is severe)
- **TEE**
  - Better visualization of valve leaflets, right atrium, and subvalvular apparatus
- **Cath**
  - Evaluate diastolic gradient between RA and RV

Treatment

Medical treatment consists mostly of **diuretic therapy** for volume overload. Further medical management depends on other comorbidities. The most common cause of tricuspid stenosis is rheumatic valve disease, which inevitably will involve the mitral ± aortic valves. Timing of surgical intervention is usually driven by the severity of the left-sided valvular lesions. Tricuspid valvuloplasty or tricuspid valve (TV) replacement (preferably bioprosthetic) is indicated for severe TS. For congenital TS, there may be other associated abnormalities that influence management and therapeutic decisions (see Chapter 15).

Tricuspid Regurgitation (TR)

Mild TR is found in up to 70% of normal patients. It is clinically unremarkable in the majority of patients.

Etiology

Secondary TR is caused by RV and annular dilatation and RV failure, most commonly secondary to LV failure ± valvular disease which causes pulmonary hypertension or pulmonary hypertension independent of left-sided cardiac disease. Abnormalities of the TV itself leading to TR can be caused by:

- Infective endocarditis is the most common etiology and frequently associated with IV drug abuse
- Carcinoid heart disease, commonly presenting as TR but also associated with tricuspid stenosis
- Right-sided MI, causing papillary muscle dysfunction
- Trauma (e.g., from pacemaker/implanted cardiac defibrillator (ICD) lead or repeated RV biopsy after transplant)
- Rheumatoid arthritis
- Rheumatic heart disease, indicating severe aortic or MV disease
- Marfan syndrome
- Radiation-induced valvulitis

History

Generally, TR is clinically insignificant and well tolerated. Patients may complain of fatigue, lower extremity edema, increased abdominal girth, early satiety, or loss of appetite, depending on the degree of hepatic congestion, bowel wall edema, and ascites.

Physical Exam

- Examination of JVP may reveal prominent v waves
- Systolic murmur (usually holosystolic) heard best at the left lower sternal border that increases with inspiration (Carvallo sign)
- Right-sided S3 or increased P2 intensity may be present
- Pulsatile liver, hepatomegaly, lower extremity edema, and ascites may be present

Diagnostic Studies

- **ECG**
  - RAE
  - Atrial fibrillation
  - Incomplete or complete right bundle-branch block (RBBB)
  - RVH
- **CXR**
  - Enlarged right heart border
- **TTE**
  - Evaluate morphology and motion of valve leaflets
  - Right atrial enlargement, RV function, annular dilatation
  - Signs of RV volume overload (paradoxical septal motion)
  - Signs of RV pressure overload (flattened septum, D-shaped LV)
  - **PASP**
    - Calculated using the Bernoulli equation (assuming no pulmonary stenosis): PASP = $4 V^2$ + RAP, where V is the TR jet velocity and RAP (RA pressure) is estimated by IVC size and collapsibility
  - Severity of TR → severe TR diagnosed when:
    - Vena contracta width >0.7 cm; and
    - Systolic flow reversal in hepatic veins
- **TEE**
  - Better visualization of valve leaflets, RA, and subvalvular apparatus

- **Cath**
  - Prominent *v* waves in the RA
  - Direct measurement of RA, RV, and PA pressures which may help in diagnosing etiology of TR

Treatment

Medical therapy is limited to **diuretics and afterload reduction** to decrease the severity of right-sided heart failure. Usually TR is secondary to some other process—pulmonary hypertension, left-sided heart failure, or other valvular abnormality—that is the primary focus of treatment. When surgery is indicated for TR, repair with annuloplasty ring is preferred to replacement. If replacement is necessary, bioprosthetic valves are preferred to mechanical valves owing to the risk of thrombosis (lower pressure on the right side of the heart predisposes to thrombosis of mechanical valves). Increasing evidence suggests the value of a **TV annuloplasty for secondary TR (particularly with a dilated annulus) at the time of mitral valve surgery,** even if the TR is not severe.

PULMONARY VALVE

Clinically significant pulmonic valve disease is usually congenital in etiology. Pulmonary regurgitation due to pulmonary hypertension is common but usually not more than mild and rarely clinically significant (see Chapter 15).

VALVE PROSTHESES

The choice of valve prosthesis depends on many factors including the patient, surgeon, cardiologist, and clinical scenario. With improvements in bioprosthetic valves, the recommendation for a mechanical valve in patients <65 years of age is no longer as firm. As patient preference changes, the use of bioprosthetic valves in younger patients has increased.

- **Mechanical**
  - Ball-and-cage (Starr–Edwards) – rarely if ever used today
  - Bileaflet (i.e., St. Jude, Carbomedics) – most commonly used
  - Single tilting disc (i.e., Björk–Shiley, Medtronic Hall, Omnicarbon)
  - *Advantages:* structurally stable, long-lasting, relatively hemodynamically efficient (particularly bileaflet)
  - *Disadvantages:* need for anticoagulation, risk of bleeding, risk of thrombosis/embolism despite anticoagulation, severe hemodynamic compromise if disc thrombosis or immobility occurs (single tilting disc), risk of endocarditis
- **Bioprosthetic**
  - Porcine aortic valve tissue (i.e., Hancock, Carpentier–Edwards)
  - Bovine pericardial tissue (i.e., Carpentier–Edwards Perimount)
  - Stented or stentless
  - *Advantages:* no need for anticoagulation, low thromboembolism risk, low risk of catastrophic valve failure
  - *Disadvantages:* structural valve deterioration, imperfect hemodynamic efficiency, risk of endocarditis, still a small risk (0.7% per year) of thromboembolism without anticoagulation

- **Homograft** (cadaveric)
  - Rarely used for AV surgery; the only remaining use for aortic valve/root homograft may be in the setting AV endocarditis, particularly complex aortic root endocarditis
  - Most commonly used to replace the pulmonic valve

ACUTE RHEUMATIC FEVER

The incidence of **rheumatic fever** in the developed world has declined substantially, but it still remains the most common cause of acquired heart disease in children and young adults worldwide. Rheumatic fever can affect the heart, skin, joints, connective tissue, and nervous system. **Rheumatic carditis** is a pancarditis affecting the endocardium, myocardium, and pericardium to varying degrees. Beyond the morbidity and mortality of the acute illness, **valvulitis** with the initial illness predisposes to fibrosis of the heart valves (particularly of the mitral but also the aortic valve) and subsequent valve disease in a significant portion of individuals affected. An untreated **group A streptococcus tonsillopharyngitis** infection is the antecedent event in rheumatic fever, which develops in ~3% of such individuals. Diagnosis is based on the **Jones criteria** (Table 16-13). Treatment of acute rheumatic fever consists of antibiotics (penicillin or erythromycin), support for heart failure, and high doses of salicylates (aspirin at 75 mg/kg per day) or, for those who do not respond to salicylates or those with severe symptoms, corticosteroids (prednisone 1–2 mg/kg per day). Primary and secondary prevention are important to minimize the risk of the disease; particularly note the duration of secondary prevention.

Prevention of Rheumatic Fever
See Table 16-14.

TABLE 16-13 RHEUMATIC FEVER—JONES CRITERIA*

Supportive Evidence of Antecedent Group A Streptococcal Infection
- Positive throat culture or rapid streptococcal antigen test
- Elevated or rising streptococcal antibody titer

Major Criteria	Minor Criteria
• Carditis	• Clinical findings
• Polyarthritis	• Arthralgia
• Chorea	• Fever
• Erythema marginatum	• Laboratory findings
• Subcutaneous nodules	• ↑Acute phase reactants (ESR, CRP)
	• Prolonged PR interval

CRP, C-reactive protein; ESR, erythrocyte sedimentation rate.

*Supportive evidence for a diagnosis of acute rheumatic fever includes (1) evidence of preceding group A strep infection *and* (2) the presence of two major *or* one major and two minor criteria.

Source: From Dajani AS, Ayoub EM, Bierman FZ, et al. Guidelines for the diagnosis of rheumatic fever: Jones criteria, 1992 update. *JAMA* 1992;268:2069–2073, with permission.

TABLE 16-14	PREVENTION OF RHEUMATIC FEVER
Primary prevention	• Penicillin G IM once • Penicillin V PO for 10 days • Erythromycin PO for 10 days (for patients allergic to penicillin)
Secondary prevention	• Penicillin G IM every 3–4 weeks • Penicillin V PO bid • Sulfadiazine PO daily • Erythromycin PO bid (for patients allergic to penicillin and sulfadiazine)

Duration of Secondary Prophylaxis

Rheumatic fever with carditis and residual valvular disease	• At least 10 years after last episode and at least until age 40 • Sometimes lifelong prophylaxis
Rheumatic fever with carditis but no residual valvular disease	• 10 years or well into adulthood, whichever is longer
Rheumatic fever without carditis	• 5 years or until age 21, whichever is longer

Source: From Dajani AS, Taubert K, Ferrieri P, et al. Treatment of streptococcal pharyngitis and prevention of rheumatic fever. *Pediatrics* 1995;96:758, with permission.

KEY POINTS TO REMEMBER

- Assessment of valvular heart disease requires careful attention to history and physical exam findings. Take care not to be misled by a patient who minimizes limitations, thus seeming to be "asymptomatic." In uncertain cases, strongly consider exercise testing to clarify functional status.
- With advances in surgical management and lower operative mortality, consideration should be given to operating on some "higher-risk" asymptomatic patients to avoid irreversible LV dysfunction, atrial arrhythmias, pulmonary hypertension, and other sequelae that may portend a worse long-term outcome.
- AS is a chronic, progressive disease characterized by angina, syncope, and CHF. Symptomatic, severe AS requires prompt surgery.
- Aortic regurgitation is either an acute or chronic process. In acute settings when AR is severe and CHF is present, surgery should be done promptly; use of an IABP is contraindicated as a bridge to surgery. In chronic AR, vasodilators are generally indicated only in the setting of hypertension.
- Mitral stenosis is usually due to rheumatic fever. Treatment depends on the patient's symptoms, valve area, gradient, and pulmonary pressures. If no contraindications are present, PMBV can usually be performed with good short- and long-term results.
- In chronic severe degenerative MR, if surgery is not done for the presence of severe MR alone, it should be pursued at the first sign of symptoms, LV dysfunction (EF ≤60%), LV enlargement (left ventricular end-diastolic dimension [LVEDD] >40 mm), atrial fibrillation, or pulmonary hypertension.

KEY POINTS TO REMEMBER *(Continued)*

- Outcomes, including mortality, are better for MV repair than replacement. Surgery should be done in high-volume centers by operators skilled in valve repair.
- For ischemic MR and MR due to DCM, an annuloplasty does not decrease mortality and only helps symptoms in MR due to DCM. Greater success may be achieved as the ventricular component of the regurgitant lesion is more adequately addressed.

REFERENCES AND SUGGESTED READINGS

Bolling SF, Pagani FD, Deeb GM, et al. Intermediate-term outcome of mitral reconstruction in cardiomyopathy. *J Thorac Cardiovasc Surg* 1998;115:381–6.

Bonow RO, Braunwald E. Valvular heart disease. In: Zipes DP, Libby P, Bonow RO, et al, eds. *Braunwald's Heart Disease: A Textbook of Cardiovascular Medicine,* 7th ed. Philadelphia: Elsevier Saunders; 2005:1553–1632.

Bonow RO, Carabello BA, Chatterjee K, et al. ACC/AHA 2006 guidelines for the management of patients with valvular heart disease. *J Am Coll Cardiol* 2006;48(3): e1–e148.

Borer JS, Bonow RO. Contemporary approach to aortic and mitral regurgitation. *Circulation* 2003;108:2432–2438.

Carabello B, Crawford F. Valvular heart disease. *N Engl J Med* 1997;337:32–41.

Carpentier A. Cardiac valve surgery—the "French correction." *J Thorac Cardiovasc Surg* 1983;86(3):323–337.

Dajani AS. Rheumatic Fever. In: Zipes DP, Libby P, Bonow RO, Braunwald E, eds. *Braunwald's Heart Disease: A Textbook of Cardiovascular Medicine,* 7th ed. Philadelphia: Elsevier Saunders; 2005:2093–2099.

Diodato MD, Moon MR, Pasque MK, et al. Repair of ischemic mitral regurgitation does not increase mortality or improve long-term survival in patients undergoing coronary artery revascularization: a propensity analysis. *Ann Thorac Surg* 2004;78:794–799.

Dreyfus GD, Corbi PJ, Chan KM, et al. Secondary tricuspid regurgitation or dilatation: which should be the criteria for surgical repair? *Ann Thorac Surg* 2005;79:127–132.

Enriquez-Sarano M, Avierinos J-F, et al. Quantitative determinants of the outcome of asymptomatic mitral regurgitation. *N Engl J Med* 2005;352:875–883.

Enriquez-Sarano M, Schaff HV, et al. Valve repair improves the outcome of surgery for mitral regurgitation: a multivariate analysis. *Circulation* 1995;91:1022–1028.

Enriquez-Sarano M. Timing of mitral valve surgery. *Heart* 2003;87:79–85.

Evangelista A, Tornos P, Sambola A, et al. Long-term vasodilator therapy in patients with severe aortic regurgitation. *N Engl J Med* 2005;353:1342–1349.

Gillinov AM, Cosgrove DS, et al. Durability of mitral valve repair for degenerative disease. *J Thorac Cardiovasc Surg* 1998;116:734–743.

Grigioni F, Enriquez-Sarano M, Zehr KJ, et al. Ischemic mitral regurgitation: Long-term outcome and prognostic implications with quantitative Doppler assessment. *Circulation* 2001;103(13):1759–1764.

Ling LH, Enriquez-Sarano M, Seward JB, et al. Clinical outcome of mitral regurgitation due to flail leaflet. *N Engl J Med* 1996;335:1417–423.

Mihaljevic T, Lam B-K, Rajeswaran J, et al. Impact of mitral valve annuloplasty combined with revascularization in patients with functional ischemic mitral regurgitation. *J Am Coll Cardiol* 2007;49:2191–2201.

Mohty D, Orszulak TA, Schaff HV, et al. Very long-term survival and durability of mitral valve repair for mitral valve prolapse. *Circulation* 2001;104(Suppl I):I1–I7.

Moura LM, Ramos SF, Zamorano JL, et al. Rosuvastatin Affecting Aortic Valve Endothelium to slow the progression of aortic stenosis (RAAVE). *J Am Coll Cardiol* 2007;49: 554–561.

Multicenter experience with balloon mitral commissurotomy: NHLBI Balloon Valvuloplasty Registry Report on immediate and 30-day follow-up results: the National Heart, Lung, and Blood Institute Balloon Valvuloplasty Registry Participants. *Circulation* 1992;85:448–461.

Otto CM, Lind BK, Kitzman DW, et al. Association of aortic valve sclerosis with cardiovascular morbidity and mortality in the elderly. *N Engl J Med* 1999;341;142–147.

Otto CM. Evaluation and management of chronic mitral regurgitation. *N Engl J Med* 2001;345(10):740–746.

Otto CM. Valvular aortic stenosis: disease severity and timing of intervention. *J Am Coll Cardiol* 2006;47:2141–2151.

Otto CM. *Valvular Heart Disease*, 2nd ed. Philadelphia: Saunders; 2003.

Rajamannan NM, Subramaniam M, Springett, M, et al. Atorvastatin inhibits hypercholesterolemia-induced cellular proliferation and bone matrix production in the rabbit aortic valve. *Circulation* 2002;105:2260–2265.

Roberts WC, Ko JM. Frequency by decades of unicuspid, bicuspid, and tricuspid aortic valves in adults having isolated aortic valve replacement for aortic stenosis, with or without associated aortic regurgitation. *Circulation* 2005;111:920–925.

Rosenhek R, Klaar U, Schemper M, et al. Mild and moderate aortic stenosis – natural history and risk stratification by echocardiography. *Eur Heart J* 2004;25:199–205.

Rosenhek R, Binder T, Parenta G, et al. Predictors or outcome in severe, asymptomatic aortic stenosis. *N Engl J Med* 2000;343:611–617.

Rosenhek R, Rader F, Klaar U, et al. Outcome of watchful waiting in asymptomatic severe mitral regurgitation. *Circulation* 2006;113:2238–2244.

Stewart BF, Siscovick DS, Lind BK, et al. Clinical factors associated with calcific aortic valve disease. *J Am Coll Cardiol* 1997;29:630–644.

Trichon BH, Felker M, Shaw LK, et al. Relation of frequency and severity of mitral regurgitation to survival among patients with left ventricular systolic dysfunction and heart failure. *Am J Cardiol* 2003;91:538–543.

Wu AH, Aaronson KD, Bolling SF, et al. Impact of mitral valve annuloplasty on mortality risk in patients with mitral regurgitation and left ventricular systolic dysfunction. *J Am Coll Cardiol* 2005;45:381–387.

Infective Endocarditis

Brian R. Lindman and Michael Yeung

INTRODUCTION

Background

Infective endocarditis (IE) is a microbial infection involving the endothelial surface of the heart. It is predominantly characterized by the presence of vegetations consisting of microorganisms, inflammatory cells. and platelet-fibrin deposits. Valves are the most common location, although IE can also occur at ventricular/atrial septal defects (VSDs/ASDs), chordae tendineae, or damaged mural endocardium. Multiple organisms can cause IE (Table 17-1).

The annual incidence of infective endocarditis is about 1 to 5 cases per 100,000 patient-years, with mortality rates of up to 25% or more. In developed countries, the proportion of IE cases in patients with underlying rheumatic heart disease has markedly decreased. There has been a shift toward an older population (with degenerative valve disease) with a median age in the fifth to seventh decades. A higher incidence of IE is seen in the setting of IV drug use, cardiac and vascular prostheses, and nosocomial infections (often with resistant organisms).

Classification

IE may be categorized according to the following (see Table 17-2):

- Type of presentation
- Underlying valve characteristics
- Predisposing factors

Causes

The pathophysiology of infective endocarditis is outlined in Figure 17-1.

PRESENTATION

Risk Factors

The major risk factor for the development of IE is a structural abnormality of a heart valve, often causing a stenotic or regurgitant lesion (i.e., bicuspid aortic valve, myxomatous mitral disease). Predisposing risk factors for native valve endocarditis (NVE) include degenerative valve disease, age, IV drug use, poor dental hygiene, long-term hemodialysis, and diabetes mellitus.

TABLE 17-1	FREQUENCY OF VARIOUS ORGANISMS CAUSING INFECTIVE ENDOCARDITIS			
Organism	NVE (%)	IV Drug Abusers (%)	Early PVE (%)	Late PVE (%)
Streptococci	60	15–25	5	35
Viridans	35	5–10	<5	25
Bovis	10	<5	<5	<5
Enterococcus faecalis	10	10	<5	<5
Staphylococci	25	50	50	30
Coagulase-positive	23	50	20	10
Coagulase-negative	<5	<5	30	20
Gram-negative aerobic bacilli	<5	5	20	10
Fungi	<5	<5	10	5
Culture-negative endocarditis	5–10	<5	<5	<5

NVE, native valve endocarditis; PVE, prosthetic valve endocarditis.
Source: From O'Rourke RA, Fuster V, Alexander RW, eds. *Hurst's the Heart*, 10th ed. New York: McGraw-Hill; 2000:596; with permission.

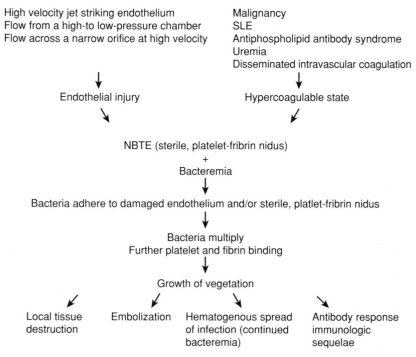

FIGURE 17-1. Pathophysiology of infective endocarditis.

TABLE 17-2   CLASSIFICATION OF ENDOCARDITIS

Acute bacterial endocarditis (ABE)	• Highly infective and particularly toxic
	• Develops within 1–2 days
	• Can cause significant valvular destruction and embolic infections
	• Most commonly caused by *S. aureus*
Subacute bacterial endocarditis (SBE)	• More indolent course than ABE
	• Develops within weeks to months
	• More often associated with immunologic phenomena
	• Often caused by streptococcal organisms, particularly *Streptococcus viridans;* also *HACEK* organisms and other gram-negative bacilli
	• *Streptococcus bovis* is often associated with colon cancer and polyps
Native valve endocarditis (NVE)	• Often predisposed by an abnormal native heart valve (e.g., mitral valve prolapse, bicuspid aortic valve)
	• Common organisms: *S. viridans, S. aureus, S. bovis,* and *Enterococcus*
Prosthetic valve endocarditis (PVE)	• Increased incidence in recent decades accounting for 10–30% of all IE
	• *Early* if it occurs within 2 months of valve replacement
	• Early PVE often involves coagulase-negative staphylococci
	• *Late* if it occurs after 2 months
	• Late PVE involves the usual NVE pathogens such as *S. viridans, S. aureus, and Enterococcus*
	• Fungal endocarditis (*Candida* and *Aspergillus*) is more common in PVE than NVE
	• Greatest risk of IE within 6 months of valve replacement
	• Rates of infection appear to be similar between mechanical and bioprosthetic valves
Right-sided endocarditis	• Often seen in IV drug users; almost always involves the *tricuspid valve*
	• Most common pathogen is *S. aureus* (60%)

(continued)

TABLE 17-2   CLASSIFICATION OF ENDOCARDITIS (*Continued*)

Nonbacterial thrombotic endocarditis (NBTE)	• Requires endothelial injury and a hypercoagulable state:
	• *Marantic endocarditis*, when associated with cancer
	• *Libman–Sacks endocarditis*, often with lupus
	• Antiphospholipid antibody syndrome
Culture-negative endocarditis	• Often related to prior antibiotic treatment
	• Incidence may be as high as 5%–10%
	• Caused by fastidious or slow-growing organisms such as *HACEK, fungi, anaerobes, Legionella, Chlamydia psittaci, Coxiella, Brucella, Bartonella*
Pacemaker/defibrillator endocarditis	• Increased incidence due to increased indications for implantation
	• Often caused by *S. aureus* or coagulase-negative staphylococci
Fungal endocarditis	• Often involves *Candida* or *Aspergillus*
	• Due to prosthetic valves, indwelling intravascular devices, immunosuppression, or IV drug use
HIV-related endocarditis	• *S. aureus* is the most common pathogen
	• Usually related to IV drug use or indwelling IV catheters

HACEK, **H**aemophilus aphrophilus, H. parainfluenzae and H. paraphrophilus, **A**ctinobacillus actinomycetemcomitans, **C**ardiobacterium hominis, **E**ikenella corrodens, **K**ingella kingae.

History

A thorough history should take into account a detailed assessment of conditions that may predispose to IE.

Physical Exam and Clinical Presentation

The physical exam (see Table 17-3) is an important component of the evaluation of a patient with IE, and several organ systems may be involved. Particular emphasis should be placed on searching for immunologic and embolic findings that may support the diagnosis of IE.

The clinical spectrum can range from subtle, indolent manifestations of subacute infection—presenting as a fever of undetermined origin (FUO)—to extensive valve destruction and fulminant congestive heart failure (CHF). The most common clinical features of IE are fever and a new heart murmur. Fever may not be present in the elderly, the immunocompromised, patients with CHF, or those with chronic renal failure.

MANAGEMENT

Diagnosis
There are several proposed criteria for the diagnosis of IE. The Duke criteria are shown in Tables 17-4 and 17-5.

Diagnostic Testing
Multiple modalities are available to assist in the diagnosis of IE:

- **Lab tests**
  - Blood cultures: Be sure to draw multiple sets from different sites and over a period of time (i.e., at least 1 hour between the first and last set, ideally at least 24 hours) *before administering antibiotics;* get fungal isolator cultures if fungal endocarditis is suspected.
  - Complete blood count (CBC): Evaluate for leukocytosis, ↑platelets (acute-phase reactant), ↓platelets (sepsis), ↓hemaglobin/hematocrit—subacute bacterial endocarditis (SBE) can lead to anemia of chronic disease.
  - Blood urea nitrogen (BUN)/creatinine and urinalysis to evaluate for evidence of immune complex glomerulonephritis.
  - Erythrocyte sedimentation rate (ESR), C-reactive protein (CRP), and rheumatoid factor are usually elevated.
  - Serologic testing for *Brucella, Legionella, Bartonella, Coxiella burnetii, Mycoplasma,* or *Chlamydia* species as indicated for culture-negative endocarditis.
  - Occasionally polymerase chain reaction (PCR) testing of explanted valve tissue is needed to confirm the microbe.
- **Electrocardiography (ECG)**
  - Assess for conduction abnormalities—such as varying and progressive degrees of atrioventricular (AV) block—suggestive of abscess formation particularly associated with aortic valve endocarditis.
  - Ischemic/infarct changes suggestive of coronary emboli
- **Chest x-ray**
  - Evidence of heart failure (pulmonary edema)
  - Septic emboli, particularly in IV drug abusers with suspected right-sided endocarditis
- **Transthoracic echo (TTE)**
  - Generally utilized if:
    - Suspicion for IE is low
    - Images are anticipated to be adequate
    - Transesophageal echo (TEE) is not immediately or easily available
- **Transesophageal echo (TEE)**
  - Generally preferred over TTE as initial echo study if:
    - At least "possible IE" by clinical Duke criteria
    - Prosthetic valve
    - Difficult imaging candidate
  - High-risk features on transthoracic echo that should be further evaluated by TEE:
    - Large vegetation(s)

TABLE 17-3	PHYSICAL EXAM FINDINGS IN ENDOCARDITIS
Organ System	**Findings**
Neurologic	• Any neurologic finding is associated with increased mortality
	• Range of clinical presentations (confusion, decreased alertness, focal deficit)
	• Due to embolic stroke, hemorrhagic stroke (transformed embolic stroke or mycotic aneurysm rupture), cerebritis from microabscesses, and meningitis
Cardiac	• Assess for new or worsening murmur due to valvular destruction, ruptured chordae tendineae, or obstruction due to large vegetation
	• Congestive heart failure
	• Irregular and/or bradycardic rhythm may indicate the presence of heart block
Abdominal	• Abdominal pain due to emboli and subsequent intestinal, splenic, and/or renal ischemia/infarcts
	• Splenomegaly may be present, more commonly in subacute IE
Skin and extremities	• Assess for signs of IV drug use
	• Noteworthy peripheral manifestations are:
	• **Petechiae:** usually found on conjunctiva, buccal and palatal mucosa, and behind ears
	• **Osler nodes:** tender subcutaneous nodules often found at the pulp of the fingers
	• **Janeway lesions:** painless, blanchable, macular red spots at the palms and soles
	• **Splinter hemorrhages:** dark linear streaks seen at the nail bed
Ophthalmologic	• **Roth spots:** round retinal hemorrhages with a pale center

- Moderate to severe valvular regurgitation or stenosis
- Suggestion of perivalvular extension (i.e., abscess, pseudoaneurysm, fistula)
- Evidence of ventricular dysfunction
- **Catheterization**
  - Evaluate coronary anatomy in patients with risk factors for CAD needing valve surgery.
- **Computed tomography angiography (CTA)**
  - CTA may be a useful alternative to LHC to evaluate coronary anatomy, particularly in less stable patients and those with complicated AV endocarditis.
- **Brain CT/magnetic resonance imaging (MRI)**
  - Assess any new neurologic symptoms.
  - MRI may be needed to assess the severity of damage and presence of hemorrhage caused by emboli to the brain.
  - MR angiography (MRA) may be needed to evaluate for cerebral mycotic aneurysms.

TABLE 17-4	DEFINITION OF TERMS USED IN THE PROPOSED MODIFIED DUKE CRITERIA FOR THE DIAGNOSIS OF INFECTIVE ENDOCARDITIS (PROPOSED MODIFICATIONS ARE IN BOLDFACE)

Major criteria

Blood culture positive for IE

Typical microorganisms consistent with IE from 2 separate blood cultures; Viridans streptococci. *streptococcus bovis.* HACEK group. *staphylococcus aureus;* or

Community-acquired enterococci, in the absence of a primary focus; or

Microorganisms consistent with IE from persistently positive blood cultures, defined as follows:

At least 2 positive cultures of blood samples drawn >12 hours apart; or

All of 3 or a majority of ≥4 separate cultures of blood (with first and last sample drawn at least 1 hour apart)

Single positive blood culture for *Coxiella burnetii* or antiphase I IgG antibody titer >1: 800

Evidence of endocardial involvement

Echocardiogram positive for IE **(TEE recommended in patients with prosthetic valves, rated at least "possible IE" by clinical criteria, or complicated IE [paravalvular abscess]: TTE as first test in other patients)** defined as follows:

Oscillating intracardiac mass on valve or supporting structures, in the path of regurgitant jets, or on implanted material in the absence of an alternative anatomic explanation; or

Abscess; or

New partial dehiscence of prosthetic valve

New valvular regurgitation (worsening or changing of pre-existing murmur not sufficient)

Minor criteria

Predisposition, predisposing heart condition or injection drug use

Fever, temperature >38°C

Vascular phenomena, major arterial emboli, septic pulmonary infarcts, mycotic aneurysm, intracranial hemorrhage, conjunctival hemorrhages, and Janeway's lesions

Immunologic phenomena: glomerulonephritis, Osler's nodes, Roth's spots, and rheumatoid factor

Microbiological evidence: positive blood culture but does not meet a major criterion as noted above or serological evidence of active infection with organism consistent with IE

Echocardiographic minor criteria eliminated

Medical Treatment

Effective treatment involves a coordinated approach including cardiology, infectious diseases, and cardiac surgery. See Table 17-6 for recommended antibiotic regimens.

- For SBE, initiation of antibiotics can often wait until blood cultures identify a particular organism.

TABLE 17-5	DEFINITION OF INFECTIVE ENDOCARDITIS ACCORDING TO THE PROPOSED MODIFIED DUKE CRITERIA (PROPOSED MODIFICATIONS IN BOLDFACE)

Definite Infective Endocarditis

Pathologic criteria

(1) Microorganisms demonstrated by culture or histologic examination of a vegetation, a vegetation that has embolized, or an intracardiac abscess specimen; or

(2) Pathologic lesions: vegetation or intracardiac abscess confirmed by histologic examination showing active endocarditis

Clinical criteria[a]

(1) 2 major criteria; or

(2) 1 major criterion and 3 minor criteria; or

(3) 5 minor criteria

Possible Infective Endocarditis

(1) **1 major criterion and 1 minor criterion; or**

(2) **3 minor criteria**

Rejected

(1) Firm alternate diagnosis explaining evidence of infective endocarditis; or

(2) Resolution of infective endocarditis syndrome with antibiotic therapy for ≤4 days; or

(3) No pathologic evidence of infective endocarditis at surgery or autopsy, with antibiotic therapy for ≤4 days; or

(4) Does not meet criteria for possible infective endocarditis, as above

HACEK, *Haemophilus aphrophilus*, *H. parainfluenzae* and *H. paraphrophilus*, *Actinobacillus actinomycetemcomitans*, *Cardiobacterium hominis*, *Eikenella corrodens*, *Kingella kingae*; TEE, transesophageal echochardiography; TTE, transthoracic echocardiography.

[a]Excludes single positive cultures for coagulase-negative staphylococci and organisms that do not cause endocarditis.

Source: From Li JS. Proposed modifications to the Duke criteria for the diagnosis of infective endocarditis. *Clin Infect Dis* 2000;30:633–638.

- For acute bacterial endocarditis (ABE) with hemodynamic compromise, empiric antibiotic coverage for the most likely organisms (*Staphylococcus aureus*, gram-negative bacilli, and streptococci, including enterococcus) is appropriate once adequate samples for blood culture have been drawn.
  - Vancomycin is often recommended by infectious diseases consultants as initial empiric therapy for *Staph. aureus* while awaiting culture results due to the high prevalence of methicillin-resistant *Staph. aureus* (MRSA); it is dosed for weight and renal function with a goal trough level of 15 to 25 μg/mL.
  - Oxacillin or nafcillin 2 g IV every 4 hours (if MRSA not suspected).
  - Ampicillin 2 g IV every 4 hours (if MRSA not suspected).
  - Gentamicin 1 or 1.5 mg/kg IV every 8 hours.
  - Rifampin can be added to nafcillin or vancomycin plus gentamicin for prosthetic valves.
- There is no role for anti-platelet or anticoagulant agents in preventing thromboemboli.

TABLE 17-6	RECOMMENDED ANTIBIOTIC REGIMENS FOR INFECTIVE ENDOCARDITIS

Microbe	Regimen (options listed for each microbe)
S. viridans and S. bovis Highly PCN-susceptible	• IV PCN G or Ceftriaxone • IV PCN G or Ceftriaxone + Gentamicin • Vancomycin
S. viridans and S. bovis Relatively PCN-resistant	• IV PCN G or ceftriaxone + gentamicin • Vancomycin
Enterococcus Susceptible to PCN, gent, vanc	• Ampicillin or IV PCN G + gentamicin • Vancomycin + Gentamicin
Staphylococcus (native)	MSSA: • Nafcillin or oxacillin + gentamicin (optional) • Cefazolin + gentamicin (optional) MRSA: • Vancomycin
Staphylococcus (prosthetic)	MSSA: • Nafcillin or oxacillin + rifampin + gentamicin MRSA: • Vancomycin + rifampin + gentamicin
HACEK	• Ceftriaxone or ampicillin-sulbactam or ciprofloxacin
Culture-negative (native)	• Ampicillin + gentamicin • Vancomycin + gentamicin + ciprofloxacin
Culture-negative (prosthetic) <1 year	• Vancomycin + gentamicin + cefepime + rifampin
Culture-negative (prosthetic) >1 year	• Ampicillin + gentamicin • Vancomycin + gentamicin + ciprofloxacin
Culture-negative Bartonella suspected	• Ceftriaxone + gentamicin ± Doxycycline
Bartonella documented	• Doxycycline + gentamicin
Fungal IE	• Amphotericin B ± long-term suppressive therapy with an oral azole

IE, infective endocarditis; HACEK, *Haemophilus aphrophilus, H. parainfluenzae* and *H. paraphrophilus, Actinobacillus actinomycetemcomitans, Cardiobacterium hominis, Eikenella corrodens, Kingella kingae*; PCN, penicillin; MSSA, methicillin-sensitive *S. aureus*; MRSA, methicillin-resistant *S. aureus*.

Source: Adapted from Baddour LM, Wilson WR, Bayer AS, et al. AHA Guidelines—infective endocarditis: diagnosis, antimicrobial therapy, and management of complications. *Circulation* 2005;111:394–434. For details regarding length of treatment, dosing, and other commentary, refer to the full document.

• In patients with an indication for anticoagulation (e.g., mechanical valve), warfarin should be changed over to unfractionated heparin in anticipation of possible surgery and/or for easy reversal if neurologic symptoms develop.

Surgical Treatment

Early surgical involvement is crucial, owing to advances in surgical technique and a growing understanding that surgery may improve the natural history of the disease. In general, surgery is performed in any patient with hemodynamic instability, heart failure, complicated IE, or IE caused by a highly resistant organism (see Table 17-7 for details).

Prompt surgical intervention should be initiated for hemodynamic instability and/or heart failure. There should be no delays for "sterilization" of the surgical field with several days of preoperative antibiotic therapy. When an acute neurologic event occurs, timing of surgery is more difficult, as early surgery can worsen neurologic function and increase

TABLE 17-7	ACC/AHA GUIDELINES—INDICATIONS FOR SURGERY FOR ENDOCARDITIS
Class I—indicated	• Valve stenosis or regurgitation resulting in heart failure
	• Acute MR or AR with hemodynamic evidence of elevated LV or LA pressures
	• IE caused by fungal or other highly resistant organisms
	• IE complicated by heart block, annular or aortic abscess or destructive penetrating lesions
	• Dehiscence of prosthetic valve evidenced by cine fluoroscopy or echocardiography
Class IIa—reasonable	• IE presenting with recurrent emboli and persistent vegetations despite appropriate antibiotic therapy (native valve)
	• IE presenting with evidence of persistent bacteremia or recurrent emboli despite appropriate antibiotic treatment (prosthetic)
Class IIb—may be considered	• IE presenting with mobile vegetations in excess of 10 mm with or without emboli
Class III—not indicated	• Uncomplicated IE caused by first infection with a sensitive organism (prosthetic)

AR, aortic regurgitation; IE, infective endocarditis; LA, left atrium; LV, left ventricle; MR, mitral regurgitation.
Source: From Bonow RO, Carabello BA, Chatterjee K, et al. ACC/AHA 2006 guidelines for the management of patients with valvular heart disease. *JACC* 2006;48(3):e1–e148, with permission.

mortality. In this case, consider delaying surgery for 2 to 3 weeks after a significant embolic infarct or for at least 1 month after intracerebral hemorrhage.

Prognosis

Several factors have been shown to independently predict increased mortality, including advanced age, presence of CHF, prosthetic valve, type of organism (*S. aureus*), diabetes mellitus type 2, renal insufficiency, and larger vegetation size, among others. A risk classification for mortality has been developed for patients with complicated left-sided native valve endocarditis (see Table 17-8).

Complications significantly contribute to the morbidity and mortality of IE and can include valvular dysfunction and heart failure, abscess formation (which can lead to heart block or fistulas between various chambers of the heart), emboli, and uncontrolled infection.

TABLE 17-8	PROGNOSIS WITH COMPLICATED LEFT-SIDED ENDOCARDITIS			
Parameter	**Points**			
Mental status				
Alert	0			
Lethargy or disorientation	4			
Charlson comorbidity scale score				
0–1	0			
≥2	3			
Congestive heart failure*				
None or mild	0			
Moderate or severe	3			
Microbiology				
Viridans streptococci	0			
Staphylococcus aureus	6			
Other†	8			
Treatment				
Surgery	0			
Medical	5			
Points	≤6	7–11	12–15	>15
6-month mortality	9%	25%	39%	63%

*None or mild: absence of rales, no SOB at rest, and no pulmonary edema; moderate or severe: presence of at least one.

†Includes other streptococci, *Enterococcus*, coagulase-negative staphylococci, Enterobacteriaceae, other gram-negative bacilli, HACEK, fungi, and culture negative endocarditis.

Adapted from Hasbun R, Vikram HR, Barakat LA, Buenconsejo J, Quagliarello VJ. Complicated left-sided native valve endocarditis in adults—risk classification for mortality. *JAMA* 2003;289: 1933–1940.

TABLE 17-9	AHA GUIDELINES—CARDIAC CONDITIONS FOR WHICH INFECTIVE ENDOCARDITIS PROPHYLAXIS IS RECOMMENDED

- Prosthetic cardiac valve
- Previous IE
- Congenital heart disease (CHD)
  - Unrepaired cyanotic CHD, including palliative shunts and conduits
  - Completely repaired congenital heart defect with prosthetic material or device, whether placed by surgery or by catheter intervention, during the first 6 months after the procedure
  - Repaired CHD with residual defects at the site of or adjacent to the site of a prosthetic patch or prosthetic device (which inhibits endothelialization)
- Cardiac transplantation recipients who develop cardiac valvulopathy

From Wilson W, Taubert KA, Gewitz M, et al. Prevention of Infective Endocarditis—Guidelines from the American Heart Association. *Circulation* 2007; 116:1736–1754.

Special Topics

- Endocarditis prophylaxis

In 2007, the recommendations for endocarditis prophylaxis were revised and significantly abbreviated (Tables 17-9, 17-10, and 17-11).

TABLE 17-10	AHA GUIDELINES—SCENARIOS IN WHICH INFECTIVE ENDOCARDITIS PROPHYLAXIS IS RECOMMENDED

- The recommendations below only apply to patients with the cardiac conditions listed in Table 17-9.
- All dental procedures that involve manipulation of gingival tissues or periapical region of teeth or perforation of oral mucosa.
- Invasive procedure of the respiratory tract that involves incision or biopsy of the respiratory mucosa (i.e., tonsillectomy).
- Antibiotic prophylaxis solely to prevent IE is not recommended for GU or GI tract procedures (for patients with GI or GU tract infections receiving antibiotics to prevent wound infection or sepsis associated with a GI or GU tract procedure, it may be reasonable that the antibiotic regimen include a drug active against enterococci).
- Surgical procedures involving infected skin, skin structures, or musculoskeletal tissue—it is reasonable that the antibiotic regimen administered for treatment of the infection include activity against staphylococci and β-hemolytic streptococci.

From Wilson W, Taubert KA, Gewitz M, et al. Prevention of infective endocarditis—guidelines from the American Heart Association. *Circulation* 2007;116:1736–1754.

TABLE 17-11	AHA GUIDELINES—REGIMENS FOR A DENTAL PROCEDURE		
		Regimen: Single Dose 30–60 Minute Before Procedure	
Situation	Agent	Adults	Children
Oral	Amoxicillin	2 g	50 mg/kg
Unable to take oral medication	Ampicillin OR	2 g IM or IV	50 mg/kg IM or IV
	Cefazolin or ceftriaxone	1 g IM or IV	50 mg/kg IM or IV
Allergic to penicillins or ampicillin—oral	Cephalexin*,† OR	2 g	50 mg/kg
	Clindamycin OR	600 mg	20 mg/kg
	Azithromycin or clarithromycin	500 mg	15 mg/kg
Allergic to penicillins or ampicillin and unable to take oral medication	Cefazolin or ceftriaxone† OR	1 g IM or IV	50 mg/kg IM or IV
	Clindamycin	600 mg IM or IV	20 mg/kg IM or IV

IM indicates intramuscular; IV, intravenous.

*Or other first- or second-generation oral cephalosporin in equivalent adult or pediatric dosage.

†Cephalosporins should not be used in an individual with a history of anaphylaxis, angioedema, or urticaria with penicillins or ampicillin.

Source: From Wilson W, Taubert KA, Gewitz M, et al. Prevention of infective endocarditis—guidelines from the American Heart Association. *Circulation* 2007;116:1736–1754.

KEY POINTS TO REMEMBER

- IE should be high in the differential diagnosis for any patient presenting with fever of unclear etiology, especially if there is a new murmur.
- Several sets of blood cultures are essential *prior* to administration of antibiotics.
- TEE should be the initial echo test for patients with prosthetic valves, at least "possible IE" based on clinical Duke criteria, and anticipated poor TTE imaging windows. It should be done as a follow-up to TTE in patients with large vegetations, moderate–severe regurgitation or stenosis, suggestion of perivalvular extension, or evidence of secondary LV dysfunction.
- In complicated left-sided endocarditis, surgery is associated with a mortality benefit; early surgery may increase the chances for valve repair (instead of replacement) and may prevent embolization in patients at risk.
- Numerous complications can occur, both intracardiac and extracardiac, that can increase morbidity and mortality, including valve dysfunction, heart failure, perivalvular extension, AV block, emboli, and uncontrolled infection.
- Effective treatment for IE involves collaboration between cardiology, infectious diseases, and cardiac surgery.

REFERENCES AND SUGGESTED READINGS

Baddour LM, Wilson WR, Bayer AS, et al. AHA Guidelines—infective endocarditis: diagnosis, antimicrobial therapy, and management of complications. *Circulation* 2005;111:394–434.

Bonow RO, Carabello BA, Chatterjee K, et al. ACC/AHA 2006 guidelines for the management of patients with valvular heart disease. *JACC* 2006;48(3):e1–e148.

Chu VH, Cabell CH, Benjamin DK, et al. Early predictors of in-hospital death in infective endocarditis. *Circulation* 2004;109:1745–1749.

Hasbun R, Vikram HR, Barakat LA, et al. Complicated left-sided native valve endocarditis in adults—risk classification for mortality. *JAMA* 2003;289:1933–1940.

Karchner AW. Infective endocarditis. In: Zipes DP, Libby P, Bonow RO, et al, eds. *Braunwald's Heart Disease: A Textbook of Cardiovascular Medicine,* 7th ed. Philadelphia: Elsevier Saunders; 2005:1633–1658.

Li JS. Proposed modifications to the Duke criteria for the diagnosis of infective endocarditis. *Clin Infect Dis* 2000;30:633–638.

Thuny F, Disalvo G, Belliard O, et al. Risk of embolism and death in infective endocarditis: prognostic value of echocardiography—a prospective multicenter study. *Circulation* 2005;112:69–75.

Vikram HR, Buenconsejo J, Hasbun R, et al. Impact of valve surgery on 6-month mortality in adults with complicated, left-sided native valve endocarditis. *JAMA* 2003;290:3207–3214.

Wilson W, Taubert KA, Gewitz M, et al. Prevention of infective endocarditis guidelines from the American Heart Association. A guideline from the American Heart Association Rheumatic Fever, Endocarditis, and Kawasaki Disease Committee, Council on Cardiovascular Disease in the Young, and the Council on Clinical Cardiology, Council on Cardiovascular Surgery and Anesthesia, and the Quality of Care and Outcomes Research Interdisciplinary Working Group. *Circulation* 2007;116:1736–1754.

Xu X-F, Murphy M. Infective endocarditis. In Griffin BP, Topol EJ, eds. *Manual of Cardiovascular Medicine*. Philadelphia: Lippincott Williams & Wilkins; 2004:249–266.

Advanced Electrocardiogram Interpretation (ECG 201)

Phillip S. Cuculich

18

Building on the overriding principles of Chapter 2 (read the ECG the same way every time to avoid mistakes; practice, practice, practice; keep a file of interesting ECGs), this chapter highlights some of the common clinical situations where more subtle ECG findings help clinch the diagnosis.

MYOCARDIAL INFARCTION (MI)

ST-segment elevations found in consecutive anatomic ECG leads is the classic finding for MI (see Fig. 2-4). The diagnosis is further confirmed with **reciprocal changes,** or ST depressions, in the area of the heart opposite the infarct. Other subtle findings and clinical pearls associated with various coronary artery distributions are as follows:

- Inferior MI is usually caused by an occlusion of the right coronary artery (RCA). The RCA supplies the AV node in most people, so **PR prolongation or atrioventricular (AV) block** is often found with inferior MI.
- Additionally, the RCA supplies the right ventricle (RV) through RV marginal arteries. Occlusion of the RCA proximal to these branch arteries can cause an **RV infarct.** Clinically, this is important, because the RV systolic function is dependent on preload, and in the setting of an RV infarct, nitrates can cause precipitous drops in blood pressure. An RV infarct is suspected when **ST elevations are greater in lead III than in lead II or lead aVF.** Diagnosis can be made using right-sided ECG leads (Fig. 18-1), looking for **any ST elevation in right-sided V4.**
- In most people, the posterior aspect of the heart is supplied by the distal left circumflex artery (LCX). Unfortunately, the standard 12-lead ECG does not have leads near this area of the heart, so posterior MIs are often missed. The diagnosis of a posterior MI can be suspected by finding the reciprocal changes of a posterior ST elevation (i.e., **anterior ST depression**), particularly in lead V1. Diagnosis can be made by finding ST elevations on additional leads V7 to V9 (Fig. 18-1).
- The diagnosis of MI can also be made with a new or suspect new left-bundle-branch block (LBBB) pattern **in the correct clinical setting**. It is important to know that the left bundle is richly supplied, primarily by the left anterior descending (LAD) artery and several septal and diagonal branches. Thus, a new LBBB pattern would suggest a large anterior infarct from a proximal LAD occlusion. Many patients with a proximal LAD occlusion will present dramatically, with signs and symptoms of chest pain, hypotension, and/or new heart failure. In contrast, a LBBB pattern is often found on a screening ECG in an asymptomatic patient. It is unlikely that a clinically stable and asymptomatic patient is having an acute, large anterior MI to cause this LBBB pattern, so good clinical judgment is essential.

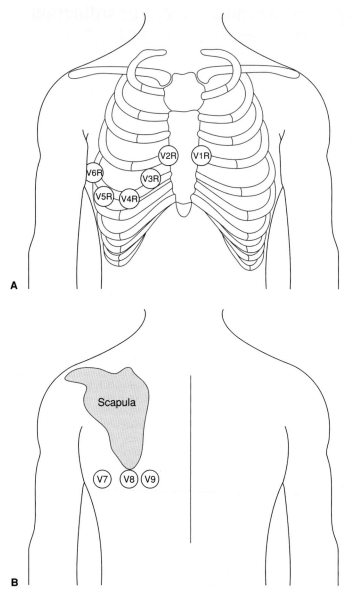

FIGURE 18-1. Alternate positions for ECG leads. **A:** Right-sided leads (V1R to V6R) for diagnosing an RV infarct. **B:** Posterior leads (V7 to V9) for diagnosing a posterior infarct.

- Patients presenting with chest pain and a known preexisting LBBB pattern can pose a diagnostic challenge. It is often incorrectly said that the diagnosis of acute MI cannot be made with an underlying LBBB pattern on the ECG. In fact, several ECG findings in this situation can be virtually diagnostic of an acute MI. Commonly cited criteria include:
  - ST elevation ≥1 mm and concordant with QRS.
  - ST depression ≥1 mm in V1, V2, or V3.
  - ST elevation ≥5 mm and discordant with QRS.
- There are many causes of ST elevations on the ECG that are not due to infarcting myocardium. Correct interpretation of the significance of ST-segment changes relies on an understanding of the clinical situation and a level of comfort with interpreting the shape and direction of the ST segment. **There is more to the ST segment than just elevation.** These causes range from benign to life-threatening. Many young adult men have an especially rapid ventricular repolarization, which causes concave ST elevations, usually largest in lead V2. An early repolarization pattern has been described with a notched J point (immediately after the QRS complex) and tall, upright T waves, most pronounced in lead V4. The LBBB pattern causes ST-segment deviation in the direction opposite the major QRS deflection. Hyperkalemia, pulmonary embolism, LV hypertrophy, and pericarditis (see below) can cause ST elevations in unique ways. Brugada syndrome can manifest with distinctive downsloping ST elevations in leads V1 and V2. Cardiac contusions and cardioversions can cause striking transient ST elevations as well.

Infarct Versus Pericarditis

A common mimic of MI is pericarditis. Patients with either disease can present with significant chest pain and have ST elevations on the ECG. Several important clinical and ECG distinctions are outlined in Table 18-1.

Common ECG Patterns

If you approach the ECG in the same way every time with a reasonable method of interpretation (see Chapter 2), it is unlikely that you will miss the following diagnoses. Nevertheless, these are common ECG patterns and buzzwords associated with some classic clinical situations:

- **Hyperkalemia:** Multiple ECG findings are seen as potassium levels rise, include peaked T waves, wide QRS, PR prolongation, loss of P wave, and finally a sine wave pattern.
- **Digitalis effect:** Downsloping, curved ST segments are seen with a characteristic "uptick" T wave.
- **Digitalis toxicity:** Because digitalis increases the automaticity of atrial and ventricular tissue while slowing the SA and AV nodes, two common ECG findings with digitalis toxicity are atrial tachycardia with AV block and bidirectional VT.
- **Wellens waves:** Described as deep, symmetric T-wave inversions in the precordial leads. Wellens waves can indicate a critical proximal LAD occlusion, a CNS catastrophe (subarachnoid hemorrhage, where they are known as Birch waves) or an apical variant of hypertrophic cardiomyopathy.
- **Osborne waves:** Also called J waves, these are seen as additional notching at the end of the QRS complex and are associated with profound hypothermia.
- **Left ventricular hypertrophy** (LVH): Many criteria have been studied to determine the presence of LVH by ECG (Table 18-2). These criteria have proven to be quite specific (>90%) but not very sensitive (<50%).

TABLE 18-1	FEATURES TO HELP DISTINGUISH PERICARDITIS FROM MYOCARDIAL INFARCTION	
	Myocardial Infarction	**Pericarditis**
History	Risk factors of prior coronary artery disease (CAD), advanced age, diabetes, hypertension, hypercholesterolemia, tobacco use, early family history of CAD.	Recent viral illness. History of chest radiation. History of cancer.
Chest pain characteristics	Variable, but classically "constant, severe squeezing" in the substernal area, with or without radiation to the left jaw and arm.	Variable, but worse with respiration and lying down. Improved with sitting forward.
Physical exam	Variable, but dyspnea, diaphoresis, rales more specific for MI.	Variable, but friction rub is specific for pericarditis.
ECG characteristics	ST elevations in an "anatomic" distribution. Reciprocal ST-segment depressions.	Diffuse ST elevations. PR depression.
Cardiac-specific biomarkers (troponin)	With large MI, markedly elevated biomarkers.	Mild to absent elevation of biomarkers.
Echocardiogram	Wall motion abnormalities in the distribution of the infarcting artery.	No wall motion abnormalities.

- **Ventricular preexcitation:** Known as Wolff–Parkinson–White (WPW) syndrome, this disease is characterized by an accessory connection between the atrium and the ventricle, which bypasses the AV node to activate the ventricle. ECG findings include a short PR interval (<120 ms), a slurring of the QRS complex (known as a delta wave), and ST-T-wave changes in the opposite direction of the QRS vector.
- **Pulmonary disease pattern:** Because of hyperinflated lungs, a more vertical heart, and elevated pulmonary artery pressures, patients with chronic obstructive pulmonary disease may have smaller QRS size, right axis deviation, incomplete right bundle branch (RBBB) in V1 (rSR' pattern), right atrial enlargement, and delayed R-wave transition in the precordial leads (QRS becomes more positive than negative in V5 or V6).
- **Pulmonary embolism** (PE): Acute elevation of pulmonary pressures, as seen with acute PE, can cause sinus tachycardia or atrial arrhythmias, incomplete RBBB pattern, and the classic S1Q3T3 pattern (S wave in lead I, Q wave in lead III, inverted T wave in lead III).

TABLE 18-2	VARIOUS ECG CRITERIA FOR DETERMINING THE PRESENCE OF LEFT VENTRICULAR HYPERTROPHY	

Criteria	Measurement	Points
Cornell voltage	S in V3 + R in aVL >28 mm (men)	
	S in V3 + R in aVL >20 mm (women)	
Framingham	R in aVL >11 mm, R in V4 to V6 >25 mm	
	S in V1 to V3 >25 mm	
	S in V1 or V2 + R in V5 or V6 >35 mm	
	R in I + S in III >25 mm	
Sokolow–Lyon index	S in V1 + R in V5 or V6 >35 mm	
Romhilt–Estes point score	Any limb lead R wave or S wave ≥20 mm Or S in V1/V2 ≥30 mm Or R in V5/V6 ≥30 mm	3 points
	ST-T wave abnormality (with or without digitalis)	1 or 3 points
	Left atrial abnormality	3 points
	Left axis deviation	2 points
	QRS duration ≥90 msec	1 point
	Intrinsicoid deflection in V5/V6 ≥50 msec	1 point
	Definite LVH = 5 or more points; probable LVH = 4 points	

Tachycardias

The interpretation of an ECG during a tachycardia can be invaluable to correctly diagnose and treat the arrhythmia. Management of patients with various tachycardias is outlined in Chapter 6.

Tachycardias can be classified as either narrow-complex or wide-complex, based on QRS duration of less than or greater than 120 msec, respectively. Narrow-complex tachycardias use the His–Purkinje system to activate the ventricles, and most of these arrhythmias are supraventricular in origin. Wide-complex tachycardias have some degree of aberrant conduction through the ventricles and can be found in one of three scenarios: **ventricular tachycardia (VT); supraventricular tachycardia (SVT) with aberrancy; or preexcited tachycardia.**

Determining the rhythm of an ECG with a wide-complex tachycardia has important prognostic and treatment implications, as each of the three situations on the differential diagnosis list is treated very differently. Clinical clues that favor VT or SVT with aberrancy are outlined in Table 18-3. In general, VT is less likely to use the rapidly conducting His–Purkinje system, so the ventricular activation is more bizarre, with

TABLE 18-3	CLINICAL CLUES TO DISTINGUISH BETWEEN VENTRICULAR AND SUPRAVENTRICULAR TACHYCARDIAS FOR A WIDE-COMPLEX TACHYCARDIA	

Clinical Clue	Ventricular Tachycardia	Supraventricular Tachycardia with Aberrancy
History	Structural heart disease present	No structural heart disease
Initiation	Ventricular premature depolarization (VPD) initiates	Atrial premature depolarization (APD) initates "Long–short" sequence prior to initiation
P-wave timing	AV dissociation	AV relationship
QRS morphology	Tachycardia QRS morphology similar to prior VPDs Fusion beats or capture beats Positive QRS concordance (positive QRS V1–V6) QRS duration >140 msec if RBBB QRS duration >160 msec if LBBB Extreme axis (−90–180 degrees)	Characteristic QRS morphology for aberrant conduction (V1, V6)
Response to vagal maneuvers	No change	Can slow or terminate with vagal maneuvers

notching and extremely wide QRS complexes. Often, the atria and ventricles are dissociated, and sinus P waves can be seen marching through the VT. Further tools, such as the Brugada criteria, are often needed to discriminate VT from SVT with aberrancy (Fig. 18-2A, B). Patients with WPW syndrome, a form of ventricular preexcitation, can develop life-threatening atrial fibrillation with rapid ventricular conduction. This should be suspected if the tachycardia is irregular or especially fast (ventricular rates 150–250 bpm).

Narrow-complex tachycardias are often supraventricular in origin. The differential diagnosis (in order of frequency) includes sinus tachycardia, atrial fibrillation, atrial flutter, AV nodal reentry tachycardia (AVNRT), accessory pathway-mediated tachycardia (atrioventricular reentrant tachycardia, or AVRT), ectopic atrial tachycardia (EAT), multifocal atrial tachycardia (MAT), and junctional tachycardia. A schematic of these tachycardia mechanisms and representative ECGs are shown in Figure 18-3A.

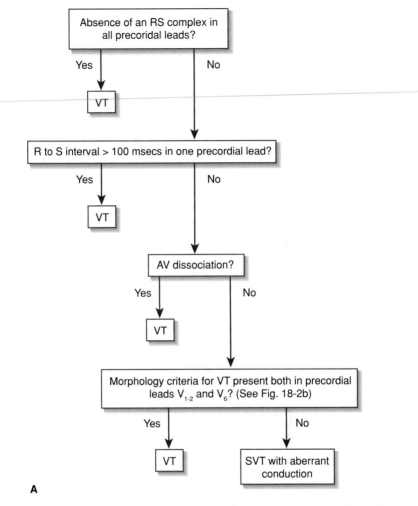

FIGURE 18-2. A and **B:** Brugada criteria for distinguishing ventricular tachycardia from supraventricular tachycardia with aberrancy in wide-complex tachycardias.

(continued)

Two keys to determine the underlying rhythm in narrow-complex tachycardias are analysis of the **P wave** (Fig. 18-3B) and the administration of **adenosine** or use of **vagal maneuvers** (Fig. 18-3C).

- P waves are absent or very irregular in atrial fibrillation.
- Flutter waves, which are regular, sawtooth atrial activations at ~300 bpm, can be seen in atrial flutter.

	LBBB		RBBB	
	VT	**SVT**	**VT**	**SVT**
Lead V1	In V1, V2 any of: (a) r≥0.04 sec (b) Notched S downstroke (c) Delayed S nadir >0.06 sec	In V1, V2 absence of: (a) r≥0.04 sec (b) Notched S downstroke (c) Delayed S nadir >0.06 sec	Taller left peak Biphasic RS or QR	Triphasic rsR' or rR'
	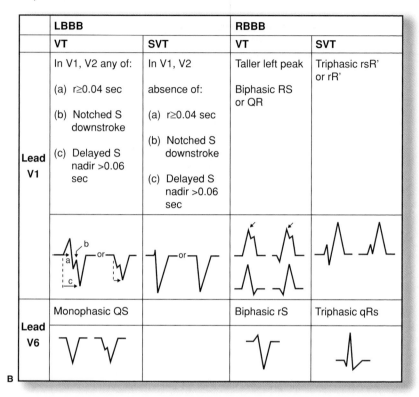			
Lead V6	Monophasic QS		Biphasic rS	Triphasic qRs

B

FIGURE 18-2. *Continued.*

- **Short-RP tachycardia:** P waves can be "buried" near the end of the QRS complex during typical AVNRT (activating the ventricle though the slow pathway, activating the atrium through the fast pathway of the AV node) or orthodromic AVRT (activating the ventricle through the AV node [slow], activating the atrium through the accessory pathway [fast]).
- **Long-RP tachycardia:** P waves are more visible, further away from the QRS complex. Causes include ectopic atrial tachycardia and atypical AVNRT (activation of the ventricle through the fast pathway, activating the atrium through the slow pathway of the AV node).

Vagal maneuvers and adenosine temporarily slow conduction through the AV node, which accomplishes two important functions: (1) it **reduces the ventricular rate** which allows the physician to see purely atrial tracings (atrial fibrillation, atrial flutter, EAT, MAT) and (2) it **terminates an arrhythmia that uses the AV node** as part of the circuit (AVNRT, AVRT).

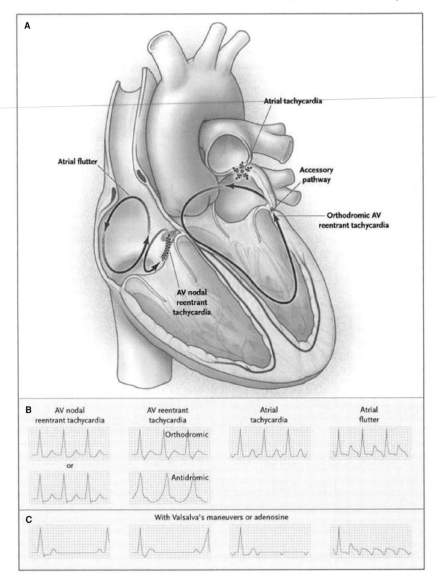

FIGURE 18-3. Main mechanisms and typical ECG recordings of supraventricular tachycardia. (Modified from Delacretaz E. Supraventricular tachycardia. *N Engl J Med* 2006;354:1039–1051, with permission.)

KEY POINTS TO REMEMBER

- In considering the diagnosis of MI, look for ST-segment changes in a consistent anatomic distribution and reciprocal changes in leads opposite the injured territory.
- It can be challenging to distinguish MI from pericarditis, but certain historical clues and physical findings can be helpful. The ECG findings favoring pericarditis include PR depressions and diffuse, non-anatomic ST elevations without reciprocal changes.
- Common ECG patterns can be found that signify specific diseases or conditions, including hyperkalemia, hypothermia, pulmonary disease, pulmonary embolism, digitalis use, and LV hypertrophy.
- Wide-complex tachycardias can be due to ventricular tachycardia, supraventricular tachycardia with aberrancy, or ventricular preexcitation. Clinical clues and ECG findings are essential to determine the appropriate rhythm.
- Narrow-complex tachycardias are usually supraventricular in origin, and the specific mechanism can often be determined by analysis of the P wave and the response to vagal stimulation or adenosine administration.
- Practice, practice, practice. This chapter concludes with several unknown ECG tracings (with interpretations, Figs. 18-4 through 18-8) to exercise your ECG analysis skills.

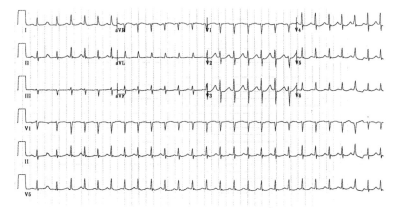

FIGURE 18-4. ECG tracing for interpretation.

Rate: 160 bpm.

Rhythm: Regular rhythm with a narrow QRS and **no P obvious waves**. This is a narrow-complex tachycardia. Differential diagnosis includes AV nodal reentry tachycardia (AVNRT), atrioventricular reentrant tachycardia, or (AVRT), automatic atrial tachycardia, atrial flutter, atrial fibrillation.

Axis: Up in lead I, up in lead II, so normal axis.

Intervals: Without a P wave there is no PR interval. QRS is narrow, and there is no LVH. QT interval is <400 ms.

Injury: No significant ST-segment elevation no depression. No significant Q waves.

Putting it all together: Narrow-complex tachycardia, likely due to **AVNRT**. Note that the retrograde P waves are likely buried within the QRS complex.

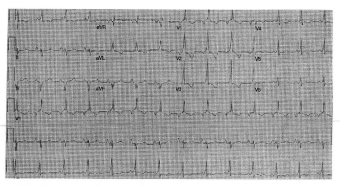

FIGURE 18-5. ECG tracing for interpretation.

Rate: 80 bpm.

Rhythm: Sinus rhythm.

Axis: Up in lead I, down in lead II, so left axis deviation.

Intervals: P waves are markedly negative in lead V1 (LAE) and markedly positive in lead II (RAE). **PR interval is <120 msec**, seen best in the precordial leads. QRS is wide, but only at the initial upstroke **(delta wave)**. No LVH. QT intervals are normal.

Injury: No significant ST-segment deviations nor Q waves, but **marked T-wave inversions V2 to V3**.

Putting it all together: With a short PR interval, a delta wave, and localized T-wave inversions, this patient has **ventricular preexcitation and Wolff–Parkinson–White syndrome**.

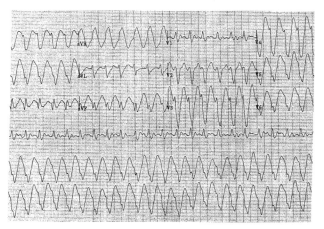

FIGURE 18-6. ECG tracing for interpretation.

Rate: 150 bpm.

Rhythm: No obvious P waves. Wide, regular QRS complex. This is a wide-complex tachycardia. Differential diagnosis includes ventricular tachycardia, SVT with aberrancy, ventricular preexcitation.

Axis: Down in lead I and down in lead II. This is **extreme left axis deviation**.

Intervals: No P waves, so no PR interval. **QRS is markedly wide (200 msec)**. It is neither a LBBB nor RBBB morphology, so it is termed **idioventricular conduction delay (IVCD)**. LVH and QT intervals cannot be assessed in this wide-complex tachycardia.

Injury: Difficult to assess in this wide-complex rhythm.

Putting it all together: Using the various tools available, including Brugada criteria, this is a ventricular tachycardia. Because the QRS is extremely wide and of IVCD morphology (not a true RBBB nor LBBB), suspect **hyperkalemia** as well.

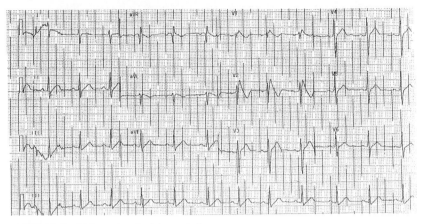

FIGURE 18-7. ECG tracing for interpretation.

Rate: 70 bpm.
Rhythm: Sinus.
Axis: Down in lead I, up in lead II. Right axis deviation.
Intervals: P-wave and PR intervals are normal. QRS is narrow without LVH. **QT interval is short** (QTc = 340 msec).
Injury: Large, rapidly downsloping ST-segment elevations in leads V1 and V2. No reciprocal changes or Q waves.
Putting it all together: This is a classic ECG of a patient with **Brugada syndrome**, with coved ST elevations in leads V1 to V2 and an incomplete RBBB pattern.

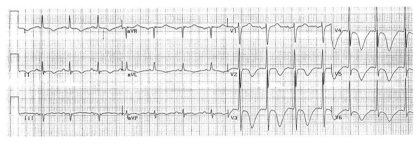

FIGURE 18-8. ECG tracing for interpretation.

Rate: 90 bpm.
Rhythm: Sinus.
Axis: Up in lead I, up in lead II. Normal axis.
Intervals: P wave and PR intervals are normal. QRS is narrow. LVH by Sokolow–Lyon criteria (S in lead I + R in V5 is >35 mm). **QT interval is long** (QTc >600 msec). Differential diagnosis includes: hypo's, anti's, congenital, cerebral or impending infarction (Wellens' waves).
Injury: No significant ST-segment deviations. Isolated Q wave in lead III is generally normal. **Large, deep, symmetric T-wave inversions, primarily in the precordial leads.**
Putting it all together: This is a classic ECG of a patient with **Wellens' waves** due to a critical proximal left anterior descending (LAD) artery lesion.

REFERENCES AND SUGGESTED READINGS

Delacretaz E. Supraventricular tachycardia. *N Engl J Med* 2006;354:1039–1051.

Miller JM, Hsia HH, Rothman SA, et al. Ventricular tachycardia versus supraventricular tachycardia with aberration: electrocardiographic distinctions. In Zipes DP, Jalife J, eds. *Cardiac Electrophysiology from Cell to Bedside*, 3rd ed. Philadelphia: Saunders; 2000:521–530.

Mirvis DM, Goldberger AL. Electrocardiography. In: Zipes DP, Libby P, Bonow RO, et al., eds. *Braunwald's Heart Disease: A Textbook of Cardiovascular Medicine*, 7th ed. Philadelphia: Elsevier Saunders; 2005:107–148.

Sgarbossa EB, Pinski SL, Barbagelata A, et al. Electrocardiographic diagnosis of evolving acute myocardial infarction in the presence of left-bundle branch block. *N Engl J Med* 1996;334:481–487.

Wang K, Asinger RW, Marriott HJL. ST-segment elevation in conditions other than acute myocardial infarction. *N Engl J Med* 2003;349:2128–2135.

Zimetbaum PJ, Josephson ME. Use of the electrocardiogram in acute myocardial infarction. *N Engl J Med* 2003;348:933–940.

Bradyarrhythmias and Permanent Pacemakers

19

Daniel H. Cooper

INTRODUCTION

Bradyarrhythmias are commonly encountered rhythms in the inpatient setting; they result in a ventricular rate of <60 bpm. Their presence may have prompted the admission or they may be discovered during the hospital course. As the cardiology consultant, the common inquiries you will receive specific to the management of bradyarrhythmias will include the following:

- Our patient was found to have a heart rate <60 bpm on telemetry. What should we do?
- Does my patient need a pacemaker?
- Is my patient's pacemaker functioning properly?

The aim of the following discussion is to give you the tools needed to answer these questions. Our approach attempts to highlight the "in the trenches" clinical approach to bradyarrhythmias, with particular emphasis on electrocardiographic (ECG) diagnosis and indications for therapies. The basic anatomy of the cardiac conduction system and clinical syndromes associated with bradycardia serve as the appropriate "bookends" of the discussion.

ANATOMY OF THE CARDIAC CONDUCTION SYSTEM

Bradycardias can be attributed to dysfunction somewhere within the native conduction system. Therefore a review of normal propagation of the wave of depolarization, the respective vascular supply to each section, and the intrinsic and extrinsic influences (Table 19-1) on the conduction system is useful.

The **sinus node** is a collection of specialized pacemaker cells located in the high right atrium. Under normal conditions, it initiates a wave of depolarization that spreads inferiorly and leftward via atrial myocardium and intranodal tracts, producing atrial systole.

- The typical resting rate of the sinus node, between 50 and 90 bpm, is inversely related to age, and is determined by the relative balance of sympathetic and parasympathetic inputs.
- Arterial blood is supplied to the sinus node via the sinus node artery, which has variable anatomic origins: right coronary artery (RCA), 65%; circumflex, 25%; or dual (RCA and circumflex), 10%.

The wave of depolarization then reaches another grouping of specialized cells, **the AV node**, located in the right atrial side of the intraatrial septum. Normally, the AV node should serve as the lone electrical connection between the atria and ventricles.

TABLE 19-1	CAUSES OF BRADYCARDIA

Intrinsic
Congenital disease (may present later in life)
Idiopathic degeneration (aging)
Infarction or ischemia
Cardiomyopathy
Infiltrative disease: sarcoidosis, amyloidosis, hemochromatosis
Collagen vascular diseases: systemic lupus erythematosus, rheumatoid
    arthritis, scleroderma
Surgical trauma: valve surgery, transplantation
Infectious disease: endocarditis, Lyme disease, Chagas' disease

Extrinsic
Autonomically mediated
Neurocardiogenic syncope
Carotid sinus hypersensitivity
Increased vagal tone: coughing, vomiting, micturition, defecation, intubation
Drugs: beta blockers, calcium channel blockers, digoxin, antiarrhythmic agents
Hypothyroidism
Hypothermia
Neurologic disorders: increased intracranial pressure
Electrolyte imbalances: hyperkalemia, hypermagnesemia
Hypercarbia/obstructive sleep apnea
Sepsis

- Conduction through the AV node is decremental, producing a delay typically in the range of 55 to 110 ms; this accounts for the majority of the PR interval measured on ECG.
- The AV node consists of slow-response fibers that, like the sinus node, possess inherent pacemaking properties and produce rates of 40 to 50 bpm. Because of its slower rate of depolarization, this becomes clinically relevant only in the setting of sinus node dysfunction.
- The ventricular response to atrial depolarization is modulated by the effects of the autonomic nervous system on the AV node.
- Blood supply to the AV node is primarily via the AV nodal artery, which typically originates from the proximal posterior descending artery (PDA) (80%), but can also come off the circumflex (10%) or both (10%). In addition, it receives collateral flow from the left anterior descending (LAD) artery. This gives the AV node relative protection from vascular compromise.

From the AV node, the wave of depolarization travels down the **His bundle**, located in the membranous septum, and into the **right and left bundle branches** before reaching the Purkinje fibers, which depolarize the rest of the ventricular myocardium.

- The His and right bundle receive blood via the AV nodal artery and from septal perforators off the LAD.
- The left bundle divides further into an anterior fascicle, supplied by septal perforators, and a posterior fascicle, which runs posterior and inferior to the anterior fascicle and is supplied by branches off the PDA and septal perforators off the LAD.

APPROACH TO BRADYARRHYTHMIAS

When consulted to evaluate a suspected bradyarrhythmia, the focus of the consultant should be to efficiently utilize the history, physical exam and available data to address the following "five S's" approach to a SSSSSlow heart rate:

- STABLE: Is the patient hemodynamically unstable?
- SYMPTOMS: Does the patient have symptoms and do the symptoms correlate with the bradycardia?
- SHORT-TERM: Are the circumstances surrounding the arrhythmia reversible or transient?
- SOURCE: Where in the conduction system is the dysfunction? Has the bradyarrhythmia been captured on ECG monitoring?
- SCHEDULE A PACEMAKER: Does the patient require a permanent pacemaker?

History and Physical Exam

The clinical manifestations of bradyarrhythmias are variable, ranging from asymptomatic to nonspecific (light-headedness, fatigue, weakness, exercise intolerance) to overt (syncope). Tolerance for bradyarrhythmias is largely dictated by the patient's ability to augment cardiac output in response to the decreased heart rate. Emphasis should be placed on delineating **whether the presenting symptoms have a direct temporal relationship to underlying bradycardia.** Other historical points of emphasis include the following:

- Ischemic heart disease, particularly involving the right-sided circulation, can precipitate a number of bradyarrhythmias. Therefore, **symptoms of acute coronary syndrome** should always be sought.
- **Precipitating circumstances** (micturition, coughing, defecation, noxious smells) surrounding episodes may help to identify a neurocardiogenic etiology.
- Tachyarrhythmias, particularly in patients with underlying sinus node dysfunction, can be followed by long pauses due to sinus node suppression during tachycardia. Therefore symptoms of palpitations may reveal the presence of an underlying **tachy–brady syndrome.** Given that the agents used to treat tachyarrhythmias are designed to promote decreased heart rates, this syndrome leads to management dilemmas.
- History of structural heart disease, hypothyroidism, obstructive sleep apnea, collagen vascular disease, infections (bacteremia, endocarditis, Lyme, Chagas'), infiltrative diseases (amyloid, hemochromatosis, sarcoid), neuromuscular diseases, and prior cardiac surgery (valve replacement, congenital repair) should be sought.
- **Medications** should be reviewed, with particular emphasis on those that affect the sinus and AV nodes (i.e., calcium channel blockers, beta blockers, digoxin).

If the bradycardia is ongoing, the initial history and physical examination should be truncated, focusing on assessing the hemodynamic stability of the arrhythmia. If the patient is demonstrating signs of poor perfusion (hypotension, confusion, decreased consciousness, cyanosis, etc.), **immediate management per the acute cardiac life support (ACLS) protocol** should be initiated. If the patient is stable, a more thorough examination can be obtained, with particular emphasis on the cardiovascular exam and any findings consistent with the aforementioned comorbidities (Fig. 19-1).

Diagnostic Evaluation

The **12-lead ECG** is the cornerstone diagnostic tool in any workup where arrhythmia is suspected. Rhythm strips from leads that provide the best view of atrial activity (II, III,

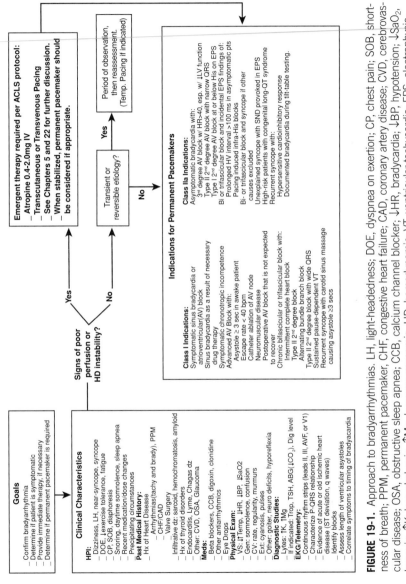

Goals
- Confirm bradyarrhythmia
- Determine if patient is symptomatic
- Provide immediate therapy, if necessary
- Determine if permanent pacemaker is required

Clinical Characteristics

HPI:
- Dizziness, LH, near-fainting, syncope
- DOE, ↓exercise tolerance, fatigue
- CP, SOB, diaphoresis
- Snoring, daytime somnolence, sleep apnea
- Recent medication/dose changes
- Precipitating circumstances

Past Medical History:
- Hx of Heart Disease
  - Arrhythmias (tachy and brady), PPM
  - CHF/CAD
  - Valve Surgery
- Infiltrative dz: sarcoid, hemochromatosis, amyloid
- Hx of thyroid disorders
- Endocarditis, Lyme, Chagas dz
- Other: CVD, OSA, Glaucoma

Meds:
- Beta blockers, CCB, digoxin, clonidine
- Other antiarrhythmics
- Eye Drops

Physical Exam:
- VS: ↕Temp, ↓HR, ↓BP, ↓SaO2
- Gen: somnolence, confusion
- CV: rate, regularity, murmurs
- Ext: cyanosis, pulses
- Other: goiter, neuro deficits, hyperreflexia

Diagnostic Studies:
- Lytes: ↑K, ↑Mg
- If indicated: Trop, TSH, ABG (↓CO₂), Dig level

EKG/Telemetry:
- Continuous rhythm strips (leads II, III, AVF, or V1)
- Characterize P-QRS relationship
- Evidence of acute or old ischemic heart disease (ST deviation, q waves)
- Identify blocks
- Assess length of ventricular asystoles
- Correlate symptoms to timing of bradycardia

Signs of poor perfusion or HD instability?

Yes →

Emergent therapy required per ACLS protocol:
- Atropine 0.4-2.0mg IV
- Transcutaneous or Transvenous Pacing
- See Chapters 5 and 22 for further discussion.
- When stabilized, permanent pacemaker should be considered if appropriate.

No ↓

Transient or reversible etiology?

Yes →

Period of observation, then reassessment. (Temp. Pacing if indicated)

No ↓

Indications for Permanent Pacemakers

Class I Indications:
Symptomatic sinus bradycardia or atrioventricular (AV) block
Sinus bradycardia as a result of necessary drug therapy
Symptomatic chronotropic incompetence
Advanced AV Block with:
- Asystole ≥ 3 sec in awake patient
- Escape rate < 40 bpm
- Catheter ablation of AV node
- Neuromuscular disease
- Postoperative AV block that is not expected to recover
Chronic bifascicular or trifascicular block with:
- Intermittent complete heart block
- Type II 2nd degree block
- Alternating bundle branch block
Type II 2nd degree block with wide QRS
Sustained pause-dependent VT
Recurrent syncope with carotid sinus massage causing asystole ≥3 secs

Class IIa Indications:
Asymptomatic bradycardia with:
- 3rd degree AV block w/ HR>40, esp. w/ ↓LV function
- Type II 2nd degree AV block with narrow QRS
- Type I 2nd degree AV block at or below His on EPS
Bi or trifascicular block and incidental EPS findings of pts:
- Prolonged HV interval >100 ms in asymptomatic pts
- Pacing induced infra-His blocks
Bi- or trifascicular block and syncope if other causes excluded
Unexplained syncope with SND provoked in EPS
High-risk patients with congenital long-QT syndrome
Recurrent syncope with:
- Hypersensitive cardioinhibitory response
- Documented bradycardia during tilt-table testing.

FIGURE 19-1. Approach to bradyarrhythmias. LH, light-headedness; DOE, dyspnea on exertion; CP, chest pain; SOB, shortness of breath; PPM, permanent pacemaker; CHF, congestive heart failure; CAD, coronary artery disease; CVD, cerebrovascular disease; OSA, obstructive sleep apnea; CCB, calcium channel blocker; ↓HR, bradycardia; ↓BP, hypotension; ↓SaO₂, hypoxia; ↑K, hyperkalemia; ↑Mg, hypermagnesemia; HD, hemodynamic; VT, ventricular tachycardia; EPS, electrophysiologic study; SND, sinus node dysfunction.

AVF, or V1) should be examined. Emphasis should be placed on identifying evidence of **sinus node dysfunction** (P-wave intervals) or **AV conduction abnormalities** (PR interval). Evidence of both old and acute manifestations of ischemic heart disease should be sought as well.

A baseline ECG, however, may not be sufficient if the arrhythmia is episodic and transient. In these circumstances, some form of continuous monitoring is indicated. In the inpatient setting, **continuous central telemetry monitoring** can be utilized. To evaluate the sinus node's response to exertion (chronotropic competence), walking the patient in the hallway or up a flight of stairs is easy and inexpensive. A formal **exercise ECG** can be ordered if necessary.

If the workup is continued on an outpatient basis, **24 to 72 hour Holter monitoring** can be used if the episodes occur daily. If they are less frequent, an **event recorder** or **implantable loop recorder** should be considered. Again, as it is vital to correlate symptoms to the rhythm disturbance, so the patients should be encouraged to maintain accurate symptom diaries.

Laboratory studies should include electrolytes and thyroid function tests in most patients. Digoxin levels and cardiac troponins should be checked when clinically appropriate.

ECG Analysis

The analysis of ECGs in the setting of bradycardia should focus on localizing the likely site of dysfunction along the conduction system. Along with correlating symptoms to the arrhythmia, localization of the block will help determine whether pacemaker implantation is necessary. See Figures 19-2 and 19-3 for some representative ECG strips of the rhythms described below.

Sinus Node Dysfunction

Sinus node dysfunction, or sick sinus syndrome, represents the most common reason for pacemaker implantation in the United States. On ECG monitoring, it can manifest in several ways:

- **Sinus bradycardia** is defined as a regular rhythm with QRS complexes preceded by "sinus" P waves (upright in II, III, AVF) at a rate <60 bpm. Young patients and athletes often have resting sinus bradycardia that is well tolerated. Nocturnal heart rates are lower in all patients, but the elderly tend to have higher resting heart rates and sinus bradycardia is a far less common normal variant.
- **Sinus arrest** and **sinus pauses** refer to failure of the sinus node to depolarize, which manifest as periods of atrial asystole (no P waves). This may be accompanied by ventricular asystole or escape beats from junctional tissue or ventricular myocardium. Pauses of 2 to 3 seconds can be found in healthy, asymptomatic people, especially during sleep. Pauses >3 seconds, particularly during daytime hours, raise concern for sinus node dysfunction.
- **Sinus exit block** represents the appropriate firing of the sinus node, but the wave of depolarization fails to traverse past the perinodal tissue. It is indistinguishable from sinus arrest on surface ECGs except that the R-R interval will be a multiple of the R-R preceding the bradycardia.
- **Tachy–brady syndrome** occurs when tachyarrhythmias alternate with bradyarrhythmias, especially atrial fibrillation. The rapid atrial rate suppresses sinus node output leading to sinus node dysfunction following termination of the tachyarrhythmia.
- **Chronotropic incompetence** is the inability to increase the heart rate appropriately in response to metabolic need.

Sinus Bradycardia

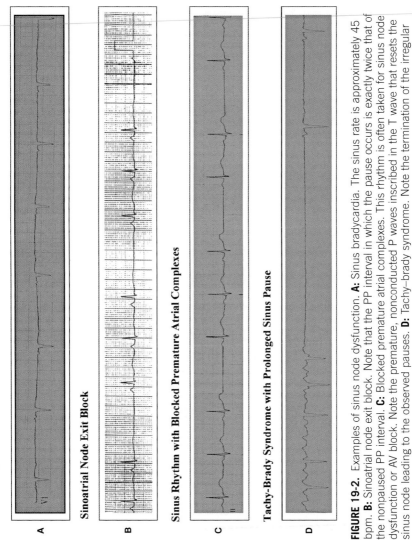

Sinoatrial Node Exit Block

Sinus Rhythm with Blocked Premature Atrial Complexes

Tachy-Brady Syndrome with Prolonged Sinus Pause

FIGURE 19-2. Examples of sinus node dysfunction. **A:** Sinus bradycardia. The sinus rate is approximately 45 bpm. **B:** Sinoatrial node exit block. Note that the PP interval in which the pause occurs is exactly twice that of the nonpaused PP interval. **C:** Blocked premature atrial complexes. This rhythm is often taken for sinus node dysfunction or AV block. Note the premature, nonconducted P waves inscribed in the T wave that resets the sinus node leading to the observed pauses. **D:** Tachy-brady syndrome. Note the termination of the irregular tachyarrhythmia followed by a prolonged 4.5-second pause prior to the first sinus beat.

First Degree AV Block

A
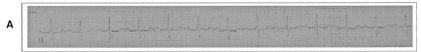

Second Degree AV Block- Mobitz type I (Wenckebach Block)

B
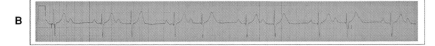

Second Degree AV Block- Mobitz type II

C

2:1 Second Degree AV Block

D
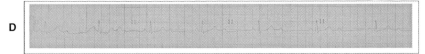

Third Degree (Complete) AV Block

E

FIGURE 19.3. Examples of atrioventricular block. **A:** First-degree AVB. There are no dropped beats and the PR interval is greater than 200 ms. **B:** 3:2 second-degree AVB–Mobitz I. Note the "group beating" and the prolonging PR interval prior to the dropped beat. The third P wave in the sequence is subtly inscribed in the T wave of the preceding beat. **C:** Second-degree AVB–Mobitz II. Note the abrupt AV conduction block without evidence of progressive conduction delay. **D:** 2:1 AVB. This pattern makes it difficult to distinguish between a Mobitz I versus a Mobitz II–type mechanisms of block. Note the narrow QRS complex, which supports a more proximal origin of block (type I mechanism). A wider QRS (concomitant bundle-branch or fascicular block) would suggest a type II mechanism. **E:** Complete heart block. Note the independent regularity of both the atrial and ventricular rhythms (junctional escape), which have no clear association with each other throughout the rhythm strip.

AV Conduction Disturbances

Atrioventricular conduction can be diverted (fascicular or bundle-branch blocks), delayed (first-degree AV block), occasionally interrupted (second-degree AV block), frequently but not always interrupted (advanced or high-degree AV block), or completely absent (third-degree AV block). Assignment of the bradyarrhythmia under investigation to one of these categories allows the consultant to better determine prognosis and therefore guide therapy.

- **First-degree AV block** describes a conduction delay, usually localized to the AV node, that results in a PR interval >200 ms on the surface ECG. "Block" is a misnomer because, by definition, there are no dropped beats (i.e., there is a P wave for every QRS complex).

- **Second-degree AV block** is present when there are periodic interruptions (i.e., "dropped beats") in atrioventricular conduction. Distinction between Mobitz I and Mobitz II is important because each has a different natural history of progression to higher degrees of heart block.
  - **Mobitz type I block (Wenckebach)** is represented by a progressive delay in AV conduction with successive atrial impulses until an impulse fails to conduct, followed by reiterations of the sequence. On surface ECG, classic Wenckebach block manifests as:
    - Progressive prolongation of the PR interval each beat before the dropped beat.
    - Shortening of each subsequent RR interval before the dropped beat. Therefore the RR interval of the dropped beat will equal less than twice the shortest RR on the tracing.
    - A regularly irregular grouping of QRS complexes (group beating). Type I block is usually within the AV node and portends a more benign natural history, with progression to complete heart block unlikely.
  - **Mobitz type II block** carries a less favorable prognosis and is characterized by abrupt AV conduction block without evidence of progressive conduction delay. On ECG, the PR intervals remained unchanged preceding the nonconducted P wave. The presence of type II block, particularly if a bundle-branch block is present, often antedates progression to complete heart block.
  - The presence of **AV 2:1 block** makes the differentiation between Mobitz type I or type II mechanisms difficult. Diagnostic clues to the site of block include the following:
    - Concomitant first-degree AV block, periodic AV Wenckebach, or improved conduction (1:1) with enhanced sinus rates or sympathetic input suggests a more proximal interruption of conduction (i.e., Mobitz type 1 mechanism).
    - Concomitant bundle-branch block, fascicular block, or worsened conduction (3:1, 4:1, etc.) with enhanced sympathetic input localizes the site of block more distally (Mobitz type II mechanism).
- **Third-degree (complete) AV block** is present when all atrial impulses fail to conduct to the ventricles. There is complete dissociation between the atria and ventricles.
- **Advanced or high-degree AV block** is present when more than one consecutive atrial depolarization fails to conduct to the ventricles (i.e., 3:1 block or greater). On ECG, consecutive P waves will be seen without associated QRS complexes. However, there will be demonstrable P:QRS conduction somewhere on the record to avoid a "third-degree" designation.

Management

Bradyarrhythmias that lead to significant symptoms and hemodynamic instability are considered cardiovascular emergencies and should be managed as outlined in ACLS guidelines. See Chapters 6 and 27 for a more in-depth discussion of temporary pacing and management of severe, hemodynamically unstable bradycardia. In emergent situations, there are a few points of emphasis worth reinforcing:

- Atropine, an anticholinergic agent given in doses of 0.5 to 2.0 mg intravenously, is the cornerstone pharmacologic agent for emergent treatment of bradycardia.
- Dysfunction localized more proximally in the conduction system (i.e., symptomatic sinus bradycardia, first-degree AV block, Mobitz I second-degree AV block) tends to be atropine-responsive. Distal disease is not responsive and can be worsened by atropine.

- Self-limited causes of bradyarrhythmias should be identified as previously described and any agents (digoxin, calcium channel blockers, beta blockers) that caused or exacerbated the underlying dysrhythmia should be withheld.
- For bradyarrhythmias that are unresponsive to pharmacologic interventions or that have irreversible etiologies, pacemaker therapy should be considered.
- Temporary pacing is indicated for symptomatic second- or third-degree heart block caused by transient drug intoxication or electrolyte imbalance and complete heart block or Mobitz II second-degree AV block in the setting of an acute myocardial infarction (MI).
- Sinus bradycardia, atrial fibrillation with a slow ventricular response, or Mobitz I second-degree AV block should be treated with temporary pacing only if significant symptoms or hemodynamic instability is present.
- Temporary pacing is achieved preferably via insertion of a transvenous pacemaker. Transthoracic external pacing can be utilized, although the lack of reliability of capture and patient discomfort clearly makes this a second-line modality.

For the consultant, once hemodynamic stability has been confirmed or reestablished as above, the focus turns to determining whether the patient's condition warrants permanent pacemaker placement. In symptomatic patients, key determinants include **potential reversibility of causative factors** and **temporal correlation of symptoms to the arrhythmia**. In asymptomatic patients, the key determinant is based on whether the **discovered conduction abnormality has a natural history of progression to higher degrees of heart block**.

Permanent Pacing

Permanent pacing involves the placement of anchored, intracardiac pacing leads for the purpose of maintaining a heart rate sufficient to avoid the aforementioned symptoms and hemodynamic consequences of certain bradyarrhythmias. In addition, advances in pacemaker technology allows contemporary pacers, through maintenance of atrioventricular (AV) synchrony and rate adaptive programming, to more closely mimic normal physiologic pacing.

- Class I (general agreement/evidence for benefit) and IIa (weight of conflicting opinion/evidence in favor of benefit) indications for permanent pacing are listed in Figure 19-1.
- Pacemakers are designed to provide an electrical stimulus to the heart whenever the rate drops below a preprogrammed **lower rate limit**. Therefore the ECG appearance of a permanent pacemaker (PPM) varies with the pacer's dependence of the individual heart rate.
- The pacing spikes produced by contemporary pacemakers are of low amplitude and sharp; they immediately precede the generated P wave or QRS complex, indicating capture of the chamber. Atrial leads are typically placed in the right atrial appendage and therefore generate P waves of normal (sinus) morphology. However, the QRS complexes generated by a typical right ventricular pacing lead are wide and typically assume a "LBBB-like" morphology. Figure 19-4 illustrates some common ECG appearances of normally and abnormally functioning pacemakers.
- The pacemaker generator is commonly placed subcutaneously in the pectoral region on the side of the nondominant arm. The electronic lead(s) are placed in their cardiac chamber(s) via central veins. Complications of placement include **pneumothorax, device infection, bleeding, and, rarely, cardiac perforation with tamponade**.
- Before implantation, the patient must be free of any active infections, and anticoagulation issues must be carefully considered. Hematomas in the pacemaker

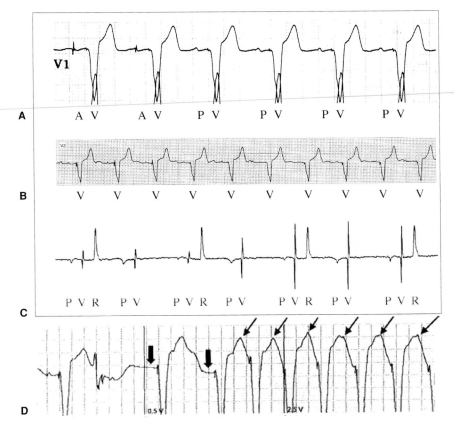

FIGURE 19-4. Pacemaker rhythms. **A:** Normal dual-chamber (DDD) pacing. First two complexes are atrioventricular (AV) sequential pacing, followed by sinus with atrial sensing and ventricular pacing. **B:** Normal single-chamber (VVI) pacing. The underlying rhythm is atrial fibrillation (no distinct P waves), with ventricular pacing at 60 bpm. **C:** Pacemaker malfunction. The underlying rhythm is sinus (P) at 80 bpm with 2:1 heart block and first-degree AV block (long PR). Ventricular pacing spikes are seen (V) after each P wave, demonstrating appropriate sensing and tracking of the P waves; however, there is failure to capture. **D:** Pacemaker mediated tachycardia. A, paced atrial events; V, paced ventricular events; P, sensed atrial events; R, sensed ventricular events. (A to C from Cooper DH, Faddis MN. Cardiac arrhythmias. In Cooper DH et al., eds. *The Washington Manual of Medical Therapeutics,* 32nd ed. Philadelphia: Lippincott Williams & Wilkins; 2007, with permission.)

pocket develop most commonly in patients who are receiving IV heparin or subcutaneous low-molecular-weight heparin. In severe cases, surgical evacuation is required.

- Following implantation, **posteroanterior and lateral chest x-rays** are obtained to confirm appropriate lead placement. The pacemaker is interrogated at appropriate intervals: typically, before discharge, 2 to 6 weeks following discharge, and every 6 to 12 months thereafter.

Pacing Modes

Pacing modes are classified by a sequence of 3 to 5 letters. **Position I denotes the chamber that is paced:** A for atria, V for ventricle, D for dual (A + V). **Position II refers to the chamber that is sensed:** A for atria, V for ventricle, D for dual (A + V), or O for none. **Position III denotes the type of response** the pacemaker will have to a sensed signal: I for inhibition, T for triggering, D for dual (I + T), or O for none. **Position IV is utilized to signify the presence of rate-adaptive pacing (R)** in response to increased metabolic need. Almost all contemporary pacers implanted have rate-modulating capabilities. **Position V identifies the presence or absence of multisite pacing:** O for none, A for multiple sites within the atria, V for multiple ventricular sites, or D for both (A + V). Biventricular pacing for resynchronization therapy in heart failure is the most common application of this position. Most often, a pacemaker will be referred to by the three-letter code alone.

- There are several variables to consider in choosing the most appropriate pacing system for your patient—**the primary indication for placement, the responsiveness of the SA node, the state of AV conduction, the presence of comorbid tachyarrhythmias, and the patient's activity level.** The 2002 guidelines from the American Heart Association/North American Society of Pacing and Electrophysiology (AHA/ NASPE) provide an algorithm to help guide pacing system decisions.
- The most common pacing systems utilized today include VVIR, DDDR, or AAIR devices.
- In general, AAI systems should be utilized only for sinus node dysfunction in the absence of any AV conduction abnormalities. The presence of AV nodal or His–Purkinje disease makes a dual chamber device (DDD) more appropriate. Patients in chronic atrial fibrillation (AF) warrant a single ventricular lead with VVI programming.
- Modern-day pacemakers also have the capability of **mode switching.** This is useful in patients with DDD pacers who have paroxysmal tachyarrhythmias. When such a patient develops tachycardia, the pacer will track atrial depolarizations and pace the ventricle up to a preprogrammed **upper rate limit**, at which time it will switch to a mode (i.e., VVI) that does not track atrial signals. It will return to DDD when the tachyarrhythmia resolves.

Pacemaker Malfunction

Pacemaker malfunction is a potentially life-threatening situation, particularly for patients who are pacemaker-dependent. The workup of suspected malfunction should begin with a 12-lead ECG. (Fig. 19-4).

- If no pacing activity is seen, one can place a magnet over the pacemaker to assess for output failure and ability to capture. **Application of the magnet switches the pacemaker to an asynchronous pacing mode.** For example, VVI mode becomes VOO (ventricular asynchronous pacing), and DDD mode becomes DOO (asynchronous AV pacing).
- If malfunction is obvious or if the ECG is unrevealing and malfunction is still suspected, then a formal interrogation of the device should be done. **Patients are given a card to carry upon implantation that will identify the make and model of the device.**
- **A chest radiograph (two views)** should also be obtained to assess for evidence of overt lead abnormalities (dislodgement, fracture, migration, etc.).

General categories of pacemaker malfunction include failure to pace (output failure), failure to capture, failure to sense (undersensing), and pacemaker-mediated dysrhythmias.

- **"Failure to pace"** refers to situations where a pacemaker does not deliver a stimulus when it should. **Oversensing** of skeletal muscle myopotentials is commonly at fault.

Also, atrial leads can misinterpret or oversense ventricular depolarizations as atrial activity leading to inhibition of atrial outputs. Lead fracture or dislodgment, battery failure, and generator failure are less common causes of output failure.

- **"Failure to capture"** refers to those situations where the pacing stimulus is delivered but fails to generate evidence of myocardial depolarization (i.e., P or QRS complex). Elevation in the threshold voltage required to initiate a wave of depolarization due to changes in the tissue surrounding the electrode is often at fault.
- **Undersensing** occurs when the preprogrammed amplitude and/or frequency thresholds for sensing are no longer sufficient to identify native cardiac activity. This may lead to pacing spikes being identified on top of native P, QRS, or T complexes.
- **Pacemaker-mediated tachycardias** are wide-complex tachyarrhythmias caused by ventricular pacing at a rapid rate, due either to device tracking of an atrial tachyarrhythmia or an "endless loop tachycardia" created by tracking of retrograde atrial impulses created by the previous ventricular paced beat. The rate of the arrhythmia provides a clue to diagnosis because it is typically at or below the programmed upper rate limit (URL). A rate exceeding the URL excludes the diagnosis. Similarly, pacemakers with rate-modulation programming can misinterpret febrile illness, external vibrations, hyperventilation, and other external stimuli and cause a **sensor-mediated, paced tachycardia.**

Clinical Syndromes Associated With Bradyarrhythmias

Acute MI and Conduction Abnormalities

Bradyarrhythmias and conduction abnormalities in the setting of MI are not uncommon. Although their incidence has diminished in the era of early reperfusion, these dysrhythmias, when present, have important prognostic connotations. **Careful consideration must be given to the artery involved, the extent of infarct, prior conduction disease, and success of reperfusion to best determine if the arrhythmia will be self-limiting or irreversible.**

- During inferior infarction, the site of block is typically at the level of the AV node. These dysrhythmias are often due to **heightened vagal tone (Bezold–Jarisch Reflex) during the first 24 hours post-MI** and are typically responsive to atropine. After 24 hours, persistent or worsening block may occur, which is less responsive to atropine. These later blocks may respond to a methylxanthine, such as theophylline or aminophylline. In most cases, conduction abnormalities resolve within 1 to 2 weeks and permanent pacing is not needed.
- Anterior MI, on the other hand, is more likely to cause conduction abnormalities due to ischemia and tissue necrosis. **The site of block is typically infranodal and is less likely to respond to atropine.** It is more likely to lead to symptomatic, irreversible bradyarrhythmias that require permanent pacing.

Cardiac Transplant and Bradyarrhythmias

Following cardiac transplant, denervation causes donor hearts to generate faster sinus rates due to loss of vagal input, particularly if the donor was young. However, bradyarrhythmias have been reported to occur in 8% to 28% of patients, with sinus node dysfunction being the most common presentation. Potential causes include surgical trauma, perioperative ischemia, pretransplant medications, and rejection. AV conduction abnormalities are much less common.

- Bicaval anastomosis, now more common than atrial anastomosis, decreases the likelihood of surgical trauma to the sinoatrial (SA) node or SA nodal artery and therefore decreases the incidence of postoperative bradyarrhythmias.

- If AV conduction blocks develop, suspicion for rejection or coronary vasculopathy should be high.
- Right bundle-branch block (RBBB) is a common conduction disturbance following transplant, often due to the need for periodic endomyocardial biopsy of the right ventricular (RV) septum to ensure appropriate immunosuppression.

Infection and Bradycardia

Although infections and febrile illness typically cause resting tachycardia, there are some infectious syndromes that can be complicated by bradyarrhythmias.

- In patients with suspected or known **endocarditis**, ECGs should be ordered and carefully reviewed daily for **prolongation of the PR interval or higher-degree AV block,** which can signal the presence of an underlying or developing aortic root abscess.
- **Lyme disease,** a tick-borne illness caused by *Borrelia burgdorferi* and endemic to the northeastern United States, can present with a constellation of findings that includes myocarditis, conduction abnormalities, and rarely, LV failure. AV conduction blocks are the most common. These dysrhythmias typically resolve spontaneously within days to weeks, rarely requiring permanent pacing. However, **symptomatic bradycardia and marked PR prolongation (>300 ms) seem to predict a more ominous prognosis with higher likelihood of progression to complete heart block.**
- **Chagas' disease,** a protozoan illness endemic to South America, presents with cardiac involvement in over 90% of cases. In addition to heart failure, **patients can present with all degrees of AV block.**

Increased Intracranial Pressure

The presence of **bradycardia, hypertension, and respiratory depression (Cushing's triad or reflex)** should raise significant suspicion for dangerously elevated intracranial pressure.

- Clinical situations that could lead to intracranial hypertension include hepatic failure, CNS tumors, trauma, and hydrocephalus.
- These are medical emergencies that require immediate treatment to avoid catastrophic neurologic compromise.

Drug Toxicity

Toxicity or overdose of medications with known cardiac conduction adverse effects should be considered in all patients that present with significant bradyarrhythmias.

- **Digoxin** toxicity should be suspected in any patient taking digoxin, particularly in the elderly, patients with renal insufficiency, or patients taking new medications such as amiodarone. Digoxin toxicity classically presents with **enhanced automaticity and increased AV block.**
  - In life-threatening situations, **Digibind,** the Fab fragments of digoxin antibodies, can be utilized. Digibind can precipitate heart failure and severe hypokalemia and carries significant expense. It should be reserved for situations where significant overdose (>10 mg) is suspected, extreme serum digoxin levels (>10 ng/mL) are discovered, or life-threatening bradyarrhythmias are present.
- If **beta-blocker** toxicity is suspected, atropine (up to 2 mg IV), IV fluids, and glucagon (50–150 μg/kg IV over 1 minute, followed by 1–5 mg/hour in 5% dextrose) can be used to bypass the beta-adrenergic receptor blockade and act downstream to improve contractility and heart rate.
  - If bradycardia and hypotension persist, escalation of management would sequentially include IV insulin/glucose, calcium, isoproterenol, and vasopressors (norepinephrine or milrinone).

- Hemodialysis may be useful with sotalol, atenolol, acebutolol, and nadolol but not metoprolol, propranolol, or timolol. Transvenous pacing can be utilized for high-grade AV block unresponsive to initial management.
- If **calcium channel blocker** (CCB) overdose is suspected, **glucagon and calcium** should be administered. Transvenous pacing can be utilized for heart block refractory to noninvasive management.
  - The nondihydropyridines (diltiazem and verapramil) are more likely to cause severe bradycardia, sinus pauses, and high-grade AV block. Dihydropyridines (amlodipine, nifedipine, nicardipine) will cause hypotension and, more commonly, a reflex *tachycardia*.
  - CCB toxicity tends to not be responsive to atropine.
  - If long-acting formulations were ingested, close monitoring must be maintained for a longer duration depending on the total dose and pharmacokinetics of the medication in question.

KEY POINTS TO REMEMBER

- Use the "SSSSSlow heart rate" mnemonic to address the questions of the consultation: Stable patient? Symptoms related to bradycardia? Short-term or reversible causes? Source of the bradycardia? Schedule a pacemaker?
- Hemodynamic tolerance of slow heart rate and conduction disturbance is the first and only concern during initial evaluation of these patients, and unstable rhythms should be managed as outlined in the ACLS protocol.
- There are a number of intrinsic and extrinsic causes of bradycardia. Determining the likely etiology and the reversibility of the bradyarrhythmia is key to determining management.
- ECG analysis of bradyarrhythmias should focus on localizing the site of block to help differentiate arrhythmias with benign natural histories from those likely to progress to worsening block.
- Correlating the presence of a bradyarrhythmia on monitoring to the onset of symptoms is of paramount importance to management decisions regarding pacemaker placement.

REFERENCES AND SUGGESTED READINGS

Antman, EM, Wenger, TL, Butler, VP, et al. Treatment of 150 cases of life-threatening digitalis intoxication with digoxin-specific Fab antibody fragments. Final report of a multicenter study. *Circulation* 1990;81:1744–1752.

Bernstein AD, Daubert JC, Fletcher RD, et al. The revised NASPE/BPEG generic code for antibradycardia, adaptive-rate, and multisite pacing. *Pacing Clin Electrophysiol* 2002;25:260–264.

Cooper DH, Faddis MN. Cardiac arrhythmias. In: Cooper DH, Krainik AJ, Lubner SJ, et al, eds. *Washington Manual of Medical Therapeutics.* 32nd ed. Philadelphia: Lippincott Williams & Wilkins; 2007:193–223.

Gregoratos G, Abrams J, Epstein AE, et al. ACC/AHA/NASPE 2002 Guideline update for implantation of cardiac pacemakers and antiarrhythmia devices. Summary article:

a Report of the American College of Cardiology/American Heart Association Task Force on Practice Guidelines(ACC/AHA/NASPE Committee to Update the 1998. Pacemaker Guidelines. *Circulation* 2002;106:2145–2161.

Lamas GA, Ellenbogen KA. Evidence base for pacemaker mode selection: from physiology to randomized trials. *Circulation* 2004;109:443–451.

Mangrum JM, Dimarco JP. The evaluation and management of bradycardia. *N Engl J Med* 2000;342:703–709.

Zimetbaum PJ, Josephson ME. Use of the electrocardiogram in acute myocardial infarction. *N Engl J Med* 2003;348:933–940.

Sudden Cardiac Death

Anthony Hart and Phillip S. Cuculich

INTRODUCTION

Sudden cardiac death (SCD) is broadly defined as an unexpected, abrupt natural death from cardiac causes within 1 hour of symptom onset. Most SCD events are due to ventricular arrhythmias, specifically ventricular fibrillation (VF) and ventricular tachycardia (VT).

The toll of SCD is substantial. Estimates within the United States range widely, but an oft-quoted figure reports 300,000 to 350,000 SCDs per year. With 2.4 million total deaths and 650,000 cardiac deaths in the United States each year, **SCD accounts for roughly 15% of all deaths and 50% of cardiac-related deaths.**

The overall incidence of SCD is 1 to 2 per 1000 people each year (0.1%–0.2%) (Fig. 20-1). However, in selected high-risk groups, the yearly incidence of SCD has been reported as high as 100 to 120 per 1000 per year (10%–12%). While these high-risk groups are the most identifiable targets for prevention of SCD, **more than two-thirds of patients who die from SCD either do not have an obvious cardiac risk factor or have "low risk" coronary artery disease (CAD)** according to current risk-stratification methods.

Etiology

Eighty percent of SCDs are associated with CAD, and 10% to 15% are caused by various cardiomyopathies. The remainder are due to ion channelopathies, valvular or inflammatory causes (Fig. 20-2).

Electrically, the mechanism of SCD can be separated into tachyarrhythmias (including monomorphic VT, polymorphic VT, or VF) and bradyarrhythmias (asystole or pulseless electrical activity [PEA]). Overall, bradyarrhythmias are less common causes but are associated with multiple organ failure, while tachyarrhythmias are thought to be more closely associated with the various effects of myocardial ischemia and inherited ion channel diseases.

Biologically, a "perfect storm" of structural abnormalities, biochemical alterations, and electrical instability conspires to bring about the arrhythmia that causes SCD (Table 20-1 and Fig. 20-3).

Risk Factors

Because most SCD events are related to CAD, risk factors for SCD closely mirror those of atherosclerosis.

- Age—1 in 100,000 per year for adolescents; 1 in 1000 per year for middle-aged adults, 1 in 500 per year for older adults.
- Gender—In younger people, SCD is much more likely among men. This risk is nearly even between genders after age 65.

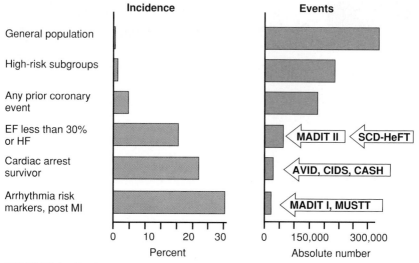

FIGURE 20-1. Absolute numbers of events and event rates of sudden cardiac death in the general population and in specific subpopulations over 1 year. "General population" refers to an unselected population of age ≥35 years and high-risk subgroups of those with multiple risk factors for a first coronary event. Clinical trials that include specific subpopulations of patients are shown at the right side of the figure. AVID, Antiarrhythmics Versus Implantable Defibrillators; CASH, Cardiac Arrest Study Hamburg; CIDS, Canadian Implantable Defibrillator Study; EF, ejection fraction; HF, heart failure; MADIT, Multicenter Automatic Defibrillator Implantation Trial; MI, myocardial infarction; MUSTT, Multicenter UnSustained Tachycardia Trial; SCD-HeFT, Sudden Cardiac Death in Heart Failure Trial. (Modified with permission from Myerburg RJ, Kessler KM, Castellanos A. SCD. Structure, function, and time-dependence of risk. *Circulation* 1992;85:I2–10.)

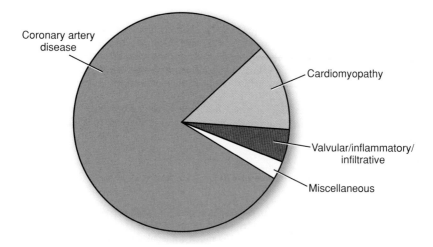

FIGURE 20-2. Etiology of sudden cardiac death.

TABLE 20-1	ABNORMALITIES ASSOCIATED WITH SUDDEN CARDIAC DEATH

Coronary Artery
- Coronary atherosclerosis
- Congenital coronary abnormalities
- Coronary artery embolism and other mechanical obstructions (e.g., dissection)
- Coronary arteritis

Hypertrophic states
- Left ventricular hypertrophy
- Hypertensive heart disease
- Obstructive and nonobstructive hypertrophic cardiomyopathy
- Pulmonary hypertension

Myocardial disease
- Ischemic cardiomyopathy, chronic and acute myocardial infarction
- Nonischemic cardiomyopathy—dilated, alcoholic, postpartum

Inflammatory, infiltrative, neoplastic, and degenerative processes
- Viral myocarditis
- Sarcoidosis
- Amyloidosis
- Hemochromatosis
- Chagas' disease
- Arrhythmogenic right ventricular dysplasia
- Neuromuscular disorders – muscular dystrophy, Friedreich's ataxia

Valvular abnormalities
- Aortic regurgitation/stenosis
- Endocarditis
- Prosthetic valve dysfunction

Congenital heart disease
- Congenital aortic and pulmonic stenosis
- Right-to-left shunts
- Postsurgical repair

Electrophysiologic abnormalities
- Conduction system abnormalities—His–Purkinje fibrosis, Wolff–Parkinson–White syndrome
- Repolarization abnormalities—congenital and acquired long-QT syndromes, Brugada syndrome

CNS and neurohormonally mediated abnormalities

Sudden infant death syndrome

Commotio cordis

Drug-induced—antiarrhythmic (Class Ia, Ic, III), psychotropics (Haloperidol, tricyclics)

Toxin/metabolic disturbances—hypomagenesemia, hypo/hyperkalemia, hypocalcemia

Source: Zipes DP, Libby P, Bonow RO, et al., eds. *Braunwald's Heart Disease: A Textbook of Cardiovascular Medicine*, 7th ed. Philadelphia: Elsevier Saunders; 2005.

Biological model of sudden cardiac death

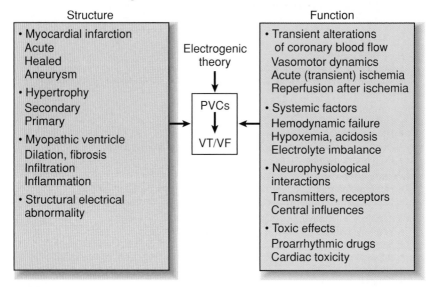

FIGURE 20-3. Biological model of sudden cardiac death (SCD). Structural cardiac abnormalities are commonly defined as the causative basis for SCD. However, functional alterations of the abnormal anatomic substrate are usually required to alter stability of the myocardium, permitting a potentially fatal arrhythmia to be initiated. In this conceptual model, short- or long-term structural abnormalities interact with functional modulations to influence the probability that premature ventricular contractions (PVCs) initiate ventricular tachycardia or fibrillation (VT/VF). (From Myerburg RJ, Kessler KM, Bassett AL, et al. A biological approach to sudden cardiac death: Structure, function, and cause. *Am J Cardiol* 1989;63:1512, with permission.)

- Hypertension, hypercholesterolemia—these are strong risk factors for SCD as both increase likelihood of CAD. Left ventricular (LV) hypertrophy (as a consequence of hypertension) increases SCD risk beyond that of CAD effects alone.
- Cigarette smoking, obesity—these carry higher than expected rates of SCD when adjusted for the risk related to CAD.
- Interestingly, large population studies have also demonstrated modestly increased SCD risk in the morning hours, on Mondays, during the winter months, and with acute psychosocial stressors.

Specifically among patients with chronic ischemic heart disease and other select cardiomyopathies, a **significantly reduced left ventricular ejection fraction (LVEF) is the single most powerful independent predictor for SCD**, although its specificity for predicting SCD is remarkably low. Electrical instability, manifested by frequent premature ventricular contractions (PVCs) or runs of nonsustained VT, is a marker for increased risk of SCD in patients with reduced ejection fraction, but this finding is not specific enough to be clinically useful at this time.

Clinical Presentation

Despite the unexpected and abrupt nature of SCD, a time-related sequence has been described that includes the following:

- Prodrome—nearly one-quarter of patients have chest pain, palpitations, dyspnea, or fatigue in the days or months leading up to the SCD event.
- Onset of terminal event—change in clinical status from seconds to an hour in duration.
- Cardiac arrest—abrupt loss of consciousness due to lack of cerebral blood flow. Successful resuscitation will depend on type of arrhythmia (VF/VT survival is better than PEA/asystole), setting of the arrest (access to a defibrillator, personnel trained in cardiopulmonary resuscitation [CPR]), and underlying clinical status.
- Biological death—failure of resuscitation or progression of irreversible organ dysfunction after resuscitation.

TREATMENT

Management of SCD involves rapid recovery efforts, as the time between onset and resuscitation has a dramatic effect on the rate of success. Irreversible brain damage begins within 5 minutes of the arrest.

A five-step approach to managing SCD includes the following:

- **Initial assessment**—Witnesses to the arrest should assess for loss of consciousness and pulse. If SCD is suspected, immediate activation of the emergency medical system (EMS) is the first priority.
- **Basic Life Support (BLS)**—Using the ABC mnemonic (airway, breathing, and circulation), trained rescuers can clear the airway, establish ventilation, and begin chest compressions. Because timely defibrillation of VF/VT is the most effective treatment for SCD, requesting a defibrillator is an important early step.
- **Advanced Cardiac Life Support (ACLS)**—Goals of ACLS are to establish a perfusing cardiac rhythm, maintain ventilation, and support circulation. Algorithms for various cardiac rhythms can be found in Chapter 6. The importance of early defibrillation for VT/VF cannot be overstated.
- **Stabilization**—Further stabilization and a search for reversible underlying cause for the arrest should take place in an intensive care unit setting. Appropriate tests include **electrocardiography** (ECG) (for ischemia, infarction, or long-QT syndrome); **blood work** (particularly potassium, magnesium, and cardiac biomarkers); **evaluation of LV structure and function** with either 2D echocardiography, radionuclide testing, and/or cardiac magnetic resonance imaging (MRI). Noncardiac causes, such as pulmonary embolus, should be excluded when appropriate. Because of the high prevalence of CAD, most treatment plans include an urgent **evaluation for cardiac ischemia with coronary angiography**. For most episodes of resuscitated SCD, an IV **antiarrhythmic drug** is given.
    - Amiodarone (Pacerone, Corderone) may be given during the early resuscitation (150 mg IV over 10 minutes) and continued as an IV infusion (1 mg/kg for 6 hours, 0.5 mg/kg for the next 18 hours).
    - Lidocaine (Xylocaine) or procainamide (Procanbid, Pronestyl) are alternative IV drugs that are occasionally used.
    - Beta blocker therapy is reasonable for most patients with VT. However, patients with bradycardia-induced VT/VF should not be given beta blockers; rather, these patients benefit from an increase in heart rate with atropine, isoproterenol (Isuprel), or pacing.
    - IV magnesium is useful in the setting of polymorphic VT and long-QT intervals.
- **Long-term management**—Patients who survive a cardiac arrest due to an arrhythmia are at high risk for recurrence. In addition to correcting reversible causes, prevention of a second event usually involves the use of implantable cardioverter-defibrillator

therapy (ICD), antiarrhythmic drug (AAD) therapy, and/or percutaneous endocardial catheter ablation.

The ICD is an implantable device that is programmed to recognize life-threatening arrhythmias and deliver therapies to restore sinus rhythm. Most ICDs are implanted subcutaneously in the upper chest with leads placed transvenously into the right heart chambers. In rare cases, an ICD can be implanted in the abdomen and leads can be placed on the epicardium surgically. ICDs can have one lead (single-chamber system), two leads (dual-chamber system), or three leads in the heart (biventricular cardiac resynchronization system). The device can be programmed to perform various therapies (rapid antitachycardia pacing [ATP] or electrical shocks) at specific heart rates (zones). The success rates of terminating VT and VF exceed 95%.

Several randomized studies have compared antiarrhythmic drug (AAD) therapy to ICD therapy to prevent recurrent cardiac arrests. In summary, compared with AAD alone, an ICD confers a 28% relative risk reduction in mortality and a 51% relative risk reduction in arrhythmic death. (Secondary prevention trials: AVID, CIDS, CASH. See Table 20-2.) Therefore, **ICD therapy has become the standard of care for most survivors of cardiac arrest.**

AADs are generally used to reduce arrhythmia burden for patients with recurring tachyarrhythmias. Commonly used oral AADs for secondary prevention of VT include amiodarone, sotalol (Betapace), mexiletine (Mexitil), and beta blockers such as metoprolol (Lopressor, Toprol XL), atenolol (Tenormin), and acebutolol (Sectral). Endocardial catheter ablation serves an adjuvant role for patients who experience recurring VT despite AAD therapy.

PREVENTION

While survivors of cardiac arrest represent a high-risk population, the number of patients who are at risk for SCD but have not yet suffered an arrest is substantially higher (Fig. 20-1). The mean survival rate of out-of-hospital cardiac arrest is <10% to 20%. Therefore the prevention of SCD in at-risk patients (primary prevention) is a more ambitious and challenging goal. Specific at-risk patient populations are discussed below.

Ischemic Cardiomyopathy (ICM)
The landscape of ICD use in primary prevention is strongly influenced by six recent trials in post-MI patients with reduced LV ejection fraction (MADIT I, CABG-PATCH, MUSTT, MADIT II, DINAMIT, SCD-HeFT; see Table 20-2). Several important conclusions and observations from these trials are as follows:

- **The risk of SCD in this high-risk group is ~2% to 5% per year.** This is considerably lower than earlier studies, likely due to the success of contemporary aggressive medical regimens.
- The estimated **number of ICDs needed to prevent one SCD in patients with ICM is 18.**
- With the possible exception of beta blockers, **antiarrhythmic drug therapy does not prevent SCD.**
- In an effort to identify the highest-risk patients, early studies enrolled patients with background arrhythmias (NSVT) who had inducible arrhythmia during electrophysiologic (EP) study (MADIT I, MUSTT). This likely explains the large benefit of ICD in these trials (54%–60% RRR in all-cause mortality).
- The two largest trials (MADIT II, SCD-HeFT) enrolled patients based on reduced LV ejection fraction alone and found a 23% to 31% RRR in all-cause mortality with an ICD.

TABLE 20-2			THE TEN MOST CITED ICD TRIALS ORGANIZED BY TYPE OF CARDIOMYOPATHY AND TYPE OF SCD PREVENTION	
Combined ICM and NICM	Secondary Prevention	AVID (Antiarrhythmic Drug Versus Defibrillator)	1016 patients resuscitated from VF or sustained VT with syncope or other serious cardiac symptoms and an LVEF ≤40%. ICD (75.4%) vs. antiarrhythmic drugs (64.1%) alive at 3 years.	31% RRR mortality ($P = 0.02$)
		CASH (Cardiac Arrest Survival in Hamburg)	288 survivors of cardiac arrest due to ventricular arrhythmias. ICD (65.4%) vs. amiodarone or metoprolol (55.6%) alive average 57 months.	23% RRR mortality ($P =$ NS, 0.08)
		CIDS (Canadian Implantable Defibrillator Study)	659 survivors of cardiac arrest or syncope secondary to arrhythmia. ICD (76.7%) vs. amiodarone (73.0%) alive at 3 years.	20% RRR mortality ($P =$ NS, 0.142)
ICM	Primary Prevention	SCD-HeFT (Sudden Cardiac Death in Heart Failure Trial)	2521 patients with NYHA class 2–3 HF and LVEF ≤35%. ICD (78%) vs. amiodarone (72%) vs. placebo (71%) alive average 45 months.	23% RRR mortality ($P = 0.007$)
		CABG-PATCH (Coronary Artery Bypass Graft Patch Trial)	900 patients undergoing elective CABG, LVEF <35%, abnormal SAECG. ICD (77.4%) vs. conventional therapy (79.1%) alive average 32 months.	7% RRI mortality ($P =$ NS, 0.64)
		DINAMIT (Defibrillator in Acute Myocardial Infarction Trial)	674 patients with a recent MI (6–40 days), LVEF ≤35%, NYHA class 1–3 HF, abnormal HRV, or elevated average heart rate. ICD (81.3%) vs. conventional therapy (83%) alive average 30 months. Death from arrhythmia reduced 58% ($P = 0.009$)	8% RRI mortality ($P =$ NS, 0.66)
		MUSTT (Multicenter Unsustained Tachycardia Trial)	704 patients with prior MI, LVEF ≤40%, NSVT, and inducible VT on EPS. ICD +AAD (76%) vs. AAD (45%) vs. conventional therapy (52%) alive at 5 years.	55%–60% RRR mortality ($P = <0.001$)

(*continued*)

TABLE 20-2	THE TEN MOST CITED ICD TRIALS ORGANIZED BY TYPE OF CARDIOMYOPATHY AND TYPE OF SCD PREVENTION *(Continued)*		
ICM — **Primary Prevention**	**MADIT-I (Multicenter Automatic Defibrillator Implantation Trial)**	196 patients with prior MI, LVEF ≤0.35%, NYHA class 1–3 HF, NSVT and inducible VT on EPS. ICD (84.2%) vs. conventional therapy (61.4%) alive average 27 months.	54% RRR mortality (*P* = 0.009)
	MADIT-II (Multicenter Automatic Defibrillator Implantation Trial)	1232 patients with a prior MI and LVEF ≤30%. ICD (85.8%) vs. conventional therapy (80.2%) alive average 20 months.	31% RRR mortality (*P* = 0.016)
NICM	**DEFINITE (Defibrillators in Non-Ischemic Cardiomyopathy Treatment Evaluation)**	458 patients with NICM, a LVEF ≤35%, and PVCs or NSVT. ICD (87.8%) vs. standard therapy (82.5%) alive at 2 years. ICD reduced the risk of sudden death from arrhythmia specifically.	35% RRR mortality (*P* = NS, 0.08)

AAD, antiarrhythmic drug; ICD, implantable cardioverter-defibrillator; ICM, ischemic cardiomyopathy; NICM, Nonischemic cardiomyopathy; VF, ventricular fibrillation; VT, ventricular tachycardia; LVEF, left ventricular ejection fraction; NYHA, New York Heart Association; HF, heart failure; SAECG, signal-averaged ECG; MI, myocardial infarction; HRV, heart rate variability; NSVT, nonsustained ventricular tachycardia; EPS, electrophysiologic study; RRR, relative risk reduction; RRI, relative risk increase.

- The recommendation regarding the timing of ICD implantation for ischemic cardiomyopathy is **>1 month post-MI or >3 months postrevascularization**. This reflects the complex natural history of arrhythmia in the setting of an MI. First, although patients are at the highest risk of arrhythmic death at the time of the MI, many of the arrhythmias that occur around the time of an MI are not predictive of long-term mortality. Second, the mortality benefit of ICD for patients in MADIT II was greatest for those with more remote MI. Third, ICD trials enrolling patients who had recent coronary revascularization or recent MI (CABG-PATCH, DINAMIT) did not demonstrate a mortality benefit for early ICD placement.

The current recommendations for primary prevention of SCD specify that patients with ICM should be treated with **appropriate heart failure medications** (beta blocker, angiotensin converting enzyme [ACE] inhibitor, angiotensin receptor blocker [ARB], aldosterone antagonist), **antiplatelet medications** (aspirin), and **atherosclerotic medications** (statins). **Viable ischemic myocardium should be revascularized** if indicated. After that, an ICD is indicated for patients with severe LV dysfunction who have an expected survival with good functional status of >1 year.

Identification of those who will benefit from treatment is important, as ICD therapy has substantial cost in addition to risk of adverse events and inappropriate discharge. If 2%–5% of patients with ICDs experience SCD each year, this means that 95% to 98% of these patients do not, and they have assumed the risk and cost of an ICD without benefit. For these reasons, "risk stratification" is a popular topic of research. Much focus has surrounded the role of a reduced LVEF as an indication for treatment, but this cutoff misses a significant proportion of patients dying from SCD. Other factors that have been linked to increased risk for SCD after MI include NSVT, symptomatic heart failure, and sustained monomorphic VT inducible by EP testing. However, the relatively low sensitivity and specificity of these markers limit their use in clinical practice.

Rather than identifying the highest-risk patients, microvolt T-wave alternans (TWA) seems to identify low-risk patients who are unlikely to benefit from an ICD. This test measures beat-to-beat variations in the shape, amplitude, or timing of the electrocardiographic T wave. Its negative predictive value appears to be independent of LVEF and is probably more robust in patients with ischemic rather than nonischemic cardiomyopathy.

Nonischemic Cardiomyopathy (NICM)

Although NICM is less common than ICM (Fig. 20-2), patients with NICM are also at risk for SCD. Two major trials have examined the use of ICDs in this patient population (Table 20-2), with conclusions summarized below:

- A meta-analysis of all NICM primary prevention trials revealed a **26% RRR in all-cause mortality with an ICD.**
- The estimated **number needed to treat to prevent one SCD in patients with NICM is 25.**
- The SCD-HeFT trial reported a 23% RRR in all-cause mortality, which was similar among its patients with ICM and NICM.
- The largest study of exclusively NICM patients (DEFINITE) demonstrated a non-significant trend toward reduction in mortality and a significant 80% reduction in arrhythmic death with an ICD.
- Because some nonischemic cardiomyopathies resolve with treatment over time, the Centers for Medicare and Medicaid Services approved **ICD implantation for patients with reduced LVEF after a minimum of 3 months of medical treatment.**

Risk factors for SCD and overall mortality in NICM mirror those that indicate the severity of the disease (LVEF, end-diastolic volume, older age, hyponatremia, pulmonary capillary wedge pressure, systemic hypotension, AF). Despite the use of these factors to stratify for mortality, they do not appear applicable in predicting SCD, nor are they useful in mild disease. It does appear that syncope, regardless of etiology, confers a higher risk of SCD in patients with NICM. Induction of VT during an EP study has positive predictive value for future SCD, but the negative predictive value is poor. Microvolt TWA has also been proposed as a method for identifying patients with NICM at low risk for SCD.

The management of patients with NICM at risk for SCD starts with **appropriate heart failure therapy** (see Chapter 11). **Reassessment of LV function with noninvasive cardiac imaging** after 3 to 9 months of treatment determines whether an ICD is to be recommended.

Hypertrophic Cardiomyopathy

Patients with hypertrophic cardiomyopathy (HCM) are also at an increased risk of SCD (see Chapter 12). The first presentation of HCM can be SCD, often in adolescents or young adults. However, because of the low prevalence of this disease compared with ICM or NICM, prospective randomized prevention ICD trials in this population have not been performed. Observational studies have identified proposed risk factors for SCD in patients with HCM:

- Previous SCD or ventricular arrhythmias
- Family history of SCD
- Unexplained syncope
- LV thickness >30 mm
- Abnormal exercise blood pressure response
- Nonsustained VT

Patients who received an ICD for secondary prevention have appropriate ICD therapy at a reported rate of 10.6% per year. Thus **it is the standard of care to provide survivors of SCD with HCM with an ICD.**

Use of ICDs for primary prevention in high-risk HCM patients is evolving, though widely accepted, especially in those with risk factors for SCD, as listed above. The yearly rate of appropriate ICD therapy in patients with one or more risk factors has been reported as 3.6%. However, the rate of inappropriate ICD therapy was ~7% per year.

Arrhythmogenic Right Ventricular Cardiomyopathy (ARVC)

ARVC has been implicated as a cause of SCD in both young and old patients. The classic pathology is a fibrofatty replacement of right ventricular myocardium, although it can occur in either ventricle. Genetic and molecular studies have demonstrated ARVC to be a disease of the desmosome cardiac structural complex. Overt structural abnormalities are not always present, and the disease often presents with syncope, tachycardia (monomorphic or polymorphic VT, often LBBB pattern), or SCD. ARVC, like HCM, is associated with SCD in young athletes. In fact, evidence suggests that strenuous cardiopulmonary exercise contributes to an accelerated disease process. The incidence of SCD in patients varies, with reported values ranging from 0.8% to 9%. Observational studies have identified clinical risk factors that may predict an increased risk of SCD: a family of history of SCD, history of unexplained syncope, and left heart failure. **An ICD is generally recommended in patients with ARVC for primary prevention of SCD if these risk factors are present as well as for secondary prevention regardless of risk factors.**

Inflammatory and Infiltrative Cardiomyopathies

Inflammatory and infectious cardiomyopathies can induce SCD via complete heart block or ventricular tachyarrhythmias. The most common inciting agents are thought to be viral, but many other infective agents have been implicated, including bacterial, fungal, protozoal, parasitic, spirochetal, and rickettsial. Noninfective agents have been implicated as well, including toxins, radiation, and chemotherapeutics. The management of SCD in the acute setting is largely supportive, but drug therapy, catheter ablation, or device placement may be necessary in the face of persistent arrhythmias. Immunomodulation with steroids does not appear to alter outcome.

Infiltrative cardiomyopathy encompasses a heterogenous mix of diseases, including sarcoidosis, amyloidosis, hemochromatosis, and Fabry's disease. SCD may be the first manifestation of sarcoidosis. **One-quarter of patients with cardiac sarcoidosis will develop complete heart block and up to 70% will have SCD as the terminal event.** Corticosteroids may reduce the burden of granuloma formation and subsequent arrhythmias as well as attenuate but not completely obviate the incidence of SCD. Therefore the presence of spontaneous VT, severe LV dysfunction, and severe intraventricular conduction disturbance warrant therapy with an ICD and/or a pacemaker.

Cardiac amyloidosis is associated with a poor outcome. Several markers of mortality exist, including cardiac troponins. Detectable cardiac troponins carry a median survival of 6 to 8 months, versus 21 to 22 months in patients with undetectable levels. Regardless, an

ICD does not appear to affect long-term outcome with the exception of those with familial amyloidosis awaiting cardiac transplantation.

On the whole, the management of infiltrative and inflammatory diseases generally involves treatment of the underlying condition. The indication for an ICD in chronic cardiomyopathy secondary to inflammatory diseases is the same as it is in NICM.

Primary Electrical Abnormalities

There are several inherited arrhythmogenic diseases that predispose patients to SCD in the absence of any structural abnormalities. These include long-QT syndrome (LQTS), Brugada syndrome, right ventricular outflow tract (RVOT) VT, and idiopathic fascicular VT. Like many of the structural diseases above, incidence of these diseases is rare, and prospective randomized data are limited.

Congenital LQTS is a heterogenous group of genetic diseases characterized by prolonged ventricular repolarization ($QT_{corrected}$ interval) which can result in polymorphic VT (torsade de pointes) and SCD. It is estimated to affect one in 7000 to 10,000 people in the United States. Several genetic variants of LQTS have been described, with unique phenotypes and risks of SCD (Table 20-3). In particular, syncope with a long QTc interval portends a worse prognosis: ~20% die within 1 year and ~50% die within 10 years. Interestingly, carriers of LQTS mutations may have normal QTc intervals, but 10% of these patients have a cardiac event by age 40. Other contributors to QTc prolongation include hypomagnesemia, hypokalemia, hypothermia, and certain medications. The number of medications that prolong the QTc interval is constantly growing; an updated list can be found at www.torsades.org.

Management of LQTS begins with **avoidance and correction of triggers** known to prolong the QT interval. **Beta-blocker therapy** is recommended in all patients with LQT mutation, with or without a prolonged QT, particularly if syncope has occurred. An **ICD is recommended for survivors of SCD without an identifiable reversible cause of long QT.** ICD use for the primary prevention of SCD in LQTS is controversial. One evidence-based recommendation based on genotype and ECG data suggests primary prevention ICD for LQT1 with QTc >500 ms, male LQT2 with QTc >500 ms, female LQT2, and all LQT3.

Brugada syndrome is a rare cause of SCD associated with RBBB and persistent ST-segment elevation in the early precordial leads (V1, V2). It is largely due to alterations in sodium channel function (SCN5A). The risk appears to be higher in Asian populations and has been implicated as the cause of death in Lai Tai (death during sleep) in Thailand, Bangungut (to rise and moan in sleep followed by death) in the Philippines, and Pokkuri (unexpected sudden death at night) in Japan. Ninety percent of the patients are male. Risk factors for SCD include syncope and ST-segment elevation. ST elevation can be observed either spontaneously or induced by the administration of sodium channel blockers, such as flecainide, procainamide, or ajmaline. The role of EPS remains less well established in risk stratification. Treatment with quinidine or isoproterenol may be useful in patients with arrhythmia storm even in the presence of an ICD. Long-term prevention of SCD involves the placement of an ICD for patients with a history of syncope, sustained VT, or prior cardiac arrest.

The right ventricular outflow tract (RVOT) is an area that is particularly susceptible to arrhythmia. A tachycardia from this region is monomorphic with a LBBB pattern and inferior axis (QRS is positive in II, III, aVF) and leftward axis (QRS is positive in I). **RVOT-VT is classically worse with exercise and stress.** It is often self-terminating, but may be sustained. Patients may present with light-headedness and palpitations. In general, patients with RVOT VT have a low risk of sudden death. Treatment should start with beta blockers or calcium channel blockers, with catheter ablation reserved for patients with refractory symptoms. An ICD is almost never required.

Fascicular VT is an idiopathic VT that is thought to arise from and involve the fascicles of the left bundle branch in the left ventricle. The most common type manifests as a

TABLE 20-3	**GENETIC LONG-QT SYNDROMES**			

Type	Mutation (channel)	Frequency of LQT	Phenotype	Miscellaneous
LQT1	KCNQ1 (Kslow)	50%	During exercise, swimming Syndactyly Broad-based T waves	Beta blockers most effective
LQT2	KCNE2 (Krapid)	35%	Auditory stimuli Emotional stimuli Postpartum Low-amplitude notched T waves	Highest female risk (0.82%/year)
LQT3	SCN5A (Na)	5%–10%	During sleep, rest Long JT segment, normal T wave	Highest male risk (0.96%/year) Most common LQT found in sudden infant death syndrome Least responsive to beta blocker
LQT4	ANKB (anchors Na)	Rare	During exercise	
LQT5	KCNE1 (Kslow)	2%–3%		
LQT6	KCNE2 (Krapid)	Rare	Associated with QT-prolonging drug sensitivity	
LQT7	KCNJ2 (K)	Rare	Periodic paralysis Distinct facial features Often normal QT interval but long QU interval Bidirectional VT	Andersen–Tawil syndrome
LQT8	CACNA1C (Ca)	Rare	Long JT segment, normal T wave	Timothy syndrome (infants)
JLN1	KCNQ1 (Kslow)	Rare	Deafness	Autosomal recessive
JLN2	KCNE1 (Kslow)	Rare	Deafness	Autosomal recessive

monomorphic VT with a RBBB pattern and superior axis. Classically, it is responsive to calcium channel blockers. Catheter ablation can be performed for refractory symptoms. An ICD is almost never required.

Commotio Cordis

Low-impact trauma to the anterior chest at a specific time during ventricular repolarization (15–30 ms before the T-wave peak) can cause ventricular fibrillation and SCD. In the

United States, this occurs almost exclusively in young men playing sports involving a high-speed projectile (baseball, lacrosse, hockey). Witnesses to commotio cordis events typically report a seemingly inconsequential impact to the victim's chest. Some victims collapse immediately while others participate for several seconds before collapsing. Immediate CPR and defibrillation have been associated with improved survival. On-site automated external defibrillators (AED) have reduced the time to defibrillation and have been credited with dramatic survival stories. **Historically, out-of-hospital defibrillation within 3 minutes of a witnessed adult arrest produces survival rates of >50%. Every 1-minute delay in defibrillation beyond the first 3 minutes decreases the likelihood of survival by approximately 10%.** Most bystanders underestimate the severity of the trauma or believe that the wind has been knocked out of the person, which delays CPR efforts.

ACKNOWLEDGMENT

The authors are indebted to Dr. Marye Gleva, Associate Professor of Medicine, Washington University School of Medicine, for her enduring guidance, dedication to her patients, and considerate review of this chapter.

KEY POINTS TO REMEMBER

- The most common etiology of heart disease associated with SCD is atherosclerotic CAD (80%).
- The SCD paradox: patients with severe risk factors are more likely to have SCD, but two-thirds of people who have SCD have either no identifiable cardiac risk factors or have CAD and are considered to be at low risk.
- A significantly reduced LVEF is the single most powerful independent predictor for SCD, although its specificity for predicting SCD is remarkably low.
- Because it is not possible to identify people who will have SCD in the general population, current treatment goals can be summarized by "do the best for the highest-risk patients" (ICD for aborted SCD and patients with reduced LVEF) and "be ready for the rest" (AED availability, CPR training, coordinated rapid EMS response).
- Recommendation for ICD therapy is based on large clinical trials but should be individualized to each patient based on the natural history of the specific cause of the cardiomyopathy, clinical judgment, and patient comorbidities.

REFERENCES AND SUGGESTED READINGS

2005 American Heart Association guidelines for cardiopulmonary resuscitation and emergency cardiovascular care. *Circulation* 2005;112:IV-1–IV-203.

ACC/AHA/ESC 2006 guidelines for management of patients with ventricular arrhythmias and the prevention of sudden cardiac death: a report of the American College of Cardiology/American Heart Association Task Force and the European Society of Cardiology Committee for Practice Guidelines (Writing Committee to Develop Guidelines for Management of Patients With Ventricular Arrhythmias and the Prevention of Sudden Cardiac Death). *J Am Coll Cardiol* 2006;8:e247–e346.

Ali Z, Zafari AM. Narrative review: cardiopulmonary resuscitation and emergency cardiovascular care: review of the current guidelines. *Ann Intern Med* 2007;147:171–179.

Bardy GH, Lee KL, Mark DB, et al. Sudden Cardiac Death in Heart Failure Trial (SCD-HeFT) Investigators. Amiodarone or an implantable cardioverter-defibrillator for congestive heart failure. *N Engl J Med* 2005;352(3):225–237.

Bigger JT Jr. Prophylactic use of implanted cardiac defibrillators in patients at high risk for ventricular arrhythmias after coronary-artery bypass graft surgery. Coronary Artery Bypass Graft (CABG) Patch Trial Investigators. *N Engl J Med* 1997;337(22):1569–1575.

Bloomfield DM, Bigger, JT, Steinman RC, et al. Microvolt T-wave alternans and the risk of death or sustained ventricular arrhythmias in patients with left ventricular dysfunction. *J Am Coll Cardiol* 2006;47:456–463.

Brugada P, Brugada J. Right bundle branch block, persistent ST segment elevation and sudden cardiac death: a distinct clinical and electrocardiographic syndrome. A multicenter report. *J Am Coll Cardiol* 1992;20:1391–1396.

Buxton AE, Lee KL, Fisher JD, et al. A randomized study of the prevention of sudden death in patients with coronary artery disease. Multicenter Unsustained Tachycardia Trial Investigators. *N Engl J Med* 1999;341:1882–1890.

Collins KK, Van Hare GF. Advances in congenital long QT syndrome. *Curr Opin Pediatr* 2006;18:497–502.

Connolly SJ, Gent M, Roberts RS, et al. Canadian Implantable Defibrillator Study (CIDS): a randomized trial of the implantable cardioverter defibrillator against amiodarone. *Circulation* 2000;101:1297–1302.

Corrado D, Leoni L, Link MS, et al. Implantable cardioverter-defibrillator therapy for prevention of sudden death in patients with arrhythmogenic right ventricular cardiomyopathy/dysplasia. *Circulation* 2003;108:3084–3091.

Dispenzieri A, Kyle RA, Gertz MA, et al. Survival in patients with primary systemic amyloidosis and raised serum cardiac troponins. *Lancet* 2003;361:1787–1789.

Domanski M, Exner D, Borkowf C, et al. Effect of angiotensin converting enzyme inhibition on sudden cardiac death in patients following a myocardial infarction: a meta-analysis of randomized clinical trials. *J Am Coll Cardiol* 1999;33:598–604.

Gemayel C, Pelliccia A, Thompson PD. Arrhythmogenic right ventricular cardiomyopathy. *J Am Coll Cardiol* 2001;38:1773–1781.

Hobbs JB, Peterson DR, Moss AJ, et al. Risk of aborted cardiac arrest or sudden cardiac death during adolescence in the long-QT syndrome. *JAMA* 2006;296:1249–1254.

Hohnloser SH, Kuck KH, Dorian P, et al, on behalf of the DINAMIT Investigators. Prophylactic use of an implantable cardioverter-defibrillator after acute myocardial infarction. *N Engl J Med* 2004;351:2481–2488.

Kadish A, Dyer A, Daubert JP, et al. Prophylactic defibrillator implantation in patients with nonischemic dilated cardiomyopathy. *N Engl J Med* 2004;350:2151–2158.

Kuck KH, Cappato R, Siebels J, et al. Randomized comparison of antiarrhythmic drug therapy with implantable defibrillators in patients resuscitated from cardiac arrest: the Cardiac Arrest Study Hamburg (CASH). *Circulation* 2000;102:748–754.

Link MS, Estes NA III. Mechanically induced ventricular fibrillation (commotio cordis). *Heart Rhythm* 2007;4:529–532.

Maron BJ. Hypertrophic cardiomyopathy: a systematic review. *JAMA* 2002;287:1308–1320.

Maron BJ, McKenna WJ, Danielson GK. American College of Cardiology/European Society of Cardiology Clinical Expert Consensus Document on Hypertrophic Cardiomyopathy. A Report of the American College of Cardiology Foundation Task Force on Clinical Expert Consensus Documents and the European Society of Cardiology Committee for Practice Guidelines. *JACC* 2003;42(9):1687–1713.

Maron BJ, Spirito P, Shen WK, et al. Implantable cardioverter-defibrillators and prevention of sudden cardiac death in hypertrophic cardiomyopathy. *JAMA* 2007;298(4):405–412.

Maron BJ, Zipes DP. 36th Bethesda Conference. Introduction: eligibility recommendations for competitive athletes with cardiovascular abnormalities—general considerations. *JACC* 2005;45:1318–1321.

Mitchell DN, du Bois RM, Oldershaw PJ. Cardiac sarcoidosis. *BMJ* 1997;314:320–321.

Moss AJ, Hall WJ, Cannom DS, et al. Improved survival with an implanted defibrillator in patients with coronary disease at high risk for ventricular arrhythmia. Multicenter Automatic Defibrillator Implantation Trial Investigators. *N Engl J Med* 1996;335: 1933–1940.

Moss AJ, Zareba W, Hall WJ, et al. Prophylactic implantation of a defibrillator in patients with myocardial infarction and reduced ejection fraction. *N Engl J Med* 2002;346: 877–883.

Myerburg RJ, Castellanos A. Cardiac arrest and sudden cardiac death. Zipes DP, Libby P, Bonow RO, et al, eds. *Braunwald's Heart Disease: A Textbook of Cardiovascular Medicine,* 7th ed. Philadelphia: Elsevier Saunders; 2005.

Pitt B, White H, Nicolau J, et al. Eplerenone reduces mortality 30 days after randomization following acute myocardial infarction in patients with left ventricular systolic dysfunction and heart failure. *J Am Coll Cardiol* 2005;46:425–431.

Priori SG, Napolitano C, Gasparini M, et al. Natural history of Brugada syndrome: insights for risk stratification and management. *Circulation* 2002;105:1342–1347.

Priori SG, Napolitano C, Memmi M, et al. Clinical and molecular characterization of patients with catecholaminergic polymorphic ventricular tachycardia. *Circulation* 2002;106:69–74.

Priori SG, Schwartz PJ, Napolitano C, et al. Risk stratification in the long-QT syndrome. *N Engl J Med* 2003;348(19):1866–1874.

The Antiarrhythmics versus Implantable Defibrillators (AVID) Investigators. A comparison of antiarrhythmic-drug therapy with implantable defibrillators in patients resuscitated from near-fatal ventricular arrhythmias. *N Engl J Med* 1997;337:1576–1583.

Theleman KP, Kuiper JJ, Roberts WC: Acute myocarditis (predominately lymphocytic) causing sudden death without heart failure. *Am J Cardiol* 2001;88:1078.

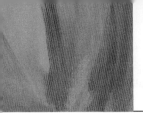

Atrial Fibrillation

21

Russell M. Canham

INTRODUCTION

Background

Atrial fibrillation (AF) is a supraventricular arrhythmia characterized by uncoordinated electrical activity and deterioration of proper atrial mechanical function, with an irregular ventricular response. AF is the most common sustained arrhythmia, accounting for over one-third of hospitalizations for cardiac arrhythmias. **AF is strongly associated with an increased risk of stroke.**

Epidemiology

AF afflicts over 2.3 million people in North America alone, but it is frequently asymptomatic and diagnosed only after a complication. It often coexists with other conditions, including hypertension, heart failure, coronary heart disease, and valvular/structural heart disease. It is strongly associated with increasing age. The estimated prevalence of AF is ~1% in the general population, with a wide range from 0.1% among adults <55 years to over 9% among octogenarians. The lifetime risk of developing AF is nearly 1 in 4.

Classification

- **Paroxysmal AF**—Several episodes, lasting ≤7 days, often self-terminating within 24 hours.
- **Persistent AF**—Lasts >7 days and fails to stop spontaneously. Persistent AF requires medical and/or electrical intervention to achieve sinus rhythm. Persistent AF may be the first presentation, the culmination of several episodes of paroxysmal AF, or **long-standing persistent AF** (>1 year).
- **Permanent AF**—Continuous AF where cardioversion has failed or has not been attempted, lasting >1 year.
- **Lone AF**—Paroxysmal, persistent, or permanent AF in younger patients (<60 years old) with a structurally normal heart.

Pathophysiology

The exact mechanisms of AF are not known, although it is likely due to a spectrum of mechanisms. Studies with holter monitoring have demonstrated that the majority of paroxysmal AF episodes are initiated by premature atrial beats. In most patients, these ectopic foci are commonly located around the pulmonary veins. The mechanism of AF is thought to involve a combination of multiple reentrant wavelets, mostly initiated by focal triggers at or near pulmonary veins and possibly maintained by high-frequency reentrant rotors in the posterior left atrium. The conduction properties of the atrium are influenced by underlying structural disease, which affects cardiac autonomic tone, the size of the atria, and the degree of atrial fibrosis.

TABLE 21-1	FACTORS THAT PREDISPOSE PATIENTS TO ATRIAL FIBRILLATION ("PIRATES" MNEMONIC)

- P—pericarditis, pulmonary disease, pulmonary embolism, postoperative state
- I—ischemia, infection
- R—rheumatic heart disease (particularly mitral valve disease)
- A—alcohol ("holiday heart"), atrial myxoma
- T—thyrotoxicosis, theophylline
- E—enlargement (particularly left atrial enlargement)
- S—systemic hypertension, sick sinus syndrome

Restoration of sinus rhythm has a higher success rate when it is achieved rapidly; there is increasing susceptibility to AF the longer the arrhythmia is present. The axiom "a-fib begets a-fib" relates to atrial electrical remodeling and delayed mechanical recovery of proper atrial contraction once sinus rhythm is restored.

PRESENTATION

Risk Factors

There are many common etiologies and risk factors that predispose to the development of atrial fibrillation, only some of which are reversible (Table 21-1). The **mnemonic PIRATES** can be a helpful way to remember the causes.

History

It is important to obtain the clinical pattern of AF, including time of onset, precipitating cause, and duration and frequency of symptoms, along with complications and coexisting disorders. In addition, a past medical history can assess for underlying cardiac disease, and social habits can be helpful to identify risk factors.

Common symptoms include **palpitations, fatigue, decreased exertional capacity, and chest discomfort.** Less commonly, orthopnea and edema from heart failure can occur. In the setting of sick sinus syndrome, patients may present with syncope. An embolic event can cause focal neurologic symptoms or organ/limb ischemia. **Many occurrences of AF are unaccompanied by symptoms.**

Physical Exam

Significant findings may be absent if AF is paroxysmal. If present, there can be an irregular pulse, tachycardia, or the absence of a venous *a* wave. For more severe cases, heart failure signs may be present. It is important to identify possible etiologies such as valvular murmurs or wheezing for underlying pulmonary disease. A goiter may be present, indicating hyperthyroidism. Other findings may include focal neurologic deficits demonstrating recent thromboembolism.

Diagnostic Testing

Initial diagnostic testing should include the following:

- **Electrocardiography (ECG)**—AF can be identified on ECG or rhythm strip with an **irregular ventricular rhythm that is void of P waves** (Fig. 21-1). The ventricular response will vary according to different properties of the AV node and conduction system, vagal and sympathetic tone, and the presence of accessory pathways. AF may

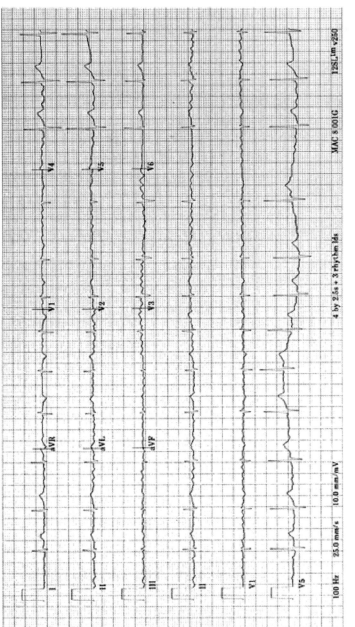

FIGURE 21-1. Typical ECG demonstrating AF. Note the irregular ventricular rhythm and lack of organized atrial contractions with P waves. (From Fuster V, Ryden LE, Cannom DS, et al. ACC/AHA/ESC 2006 Guidelines for the Management of Patients with Atrial Fibrillation. *J Am Coll Cardiol* 2006;48:e149, with permission.)

be associated and occur with additional arrhythmias, including atrial flutter and other atrial tachycardias. The **Ashman phenomenon** is aberrant ventricular conduction—usually right bundle-branch block (RBBB)—of the atrial impulses at varying cycle lengths, often preceded by a "long–short" interval.

- **Echocardiography**—The transthoracic echocardiogram (TTE) can evaluate the size of the atria and ventricles and detect valvular heart disease. Transesophageal echocardiography (TEE) is much more sensitive for identifying thrombi in the left atrium and is useful to assess if cardioversion can occur without the need for prior anticoagulation.
- **Thyroid function tests**
- **Ambulatory cardiac rhythm monitoring**—For outpatients in whom AF is suspected, this is helpful to identify the frequency and duration of paroxysmal AF.
- **Chest x-ray**—This can be helpful to identify intrinsic pulmonary pathology and assess cardiac borders.

MANAGEMENT

Treatment

Patients with new-onset AF do not always need admission to the hospital. Indications for admission include active ischemia, rapid heart rate, significant ST-segment changes, associated medical problems, elderly patients, underlying heart disease with hemodynamic compromise, or the need for initiation of certain antiarrhythmic medications in patients receiving cardioversion therapy.

The three main goals to be considered in the treatment of AF are **rate control, rhythm control, and anticoagulation to prevent thromboembolism.** The appropriate choice of therapy is tailored to each patient based on the type of AF, safety factors, symptoms, and patient preference. Refer to the management overview and algorithm for evaluating newly diagnosed AF, recurrent paroxysmal AF, recurrent persistent AF, and permanent AF (Figs. 21-2–21-4).

Rate Control

Ventricular rate control is important for avoiding hemodynamic instability associated with a rapid rate, relieving patient symptoms, and preventing a tachycardia-associated cardiomyopathy. Appropriate rate control allows time for proper ventricular filling in diastole, avoids rate-related ischemia, and generally improves hemodynamics. Correction of associated causes (hypoxia, hyperthyroidism infection) dramatically improves the success of rate control. Medically, rate control is accomplished by depressing AV nodal conduction with use of a beta blocker or nondihydropyridine calcium-channel blocker or with nodal blocking and vagal tone enhancement using digoxin. All classes are available in PO or IV formulation. A summary of pharmacologic agents for heart rate control with AF is presented in the Appendix of this book.

- **Beta blocker**—Preferred drug for AF associated with thyrotoxicosis, acute myocardial infarction, and high adrenergic tone in the postsurgical state. It is reasonable for most other causes of AF. Caution should be used in administering beta blockers to patients with acute decompensated heart failure or with reactive airways disease.
- Nondihydropyridine **calcium-channel blocker**—Reasonable for most causes of AF. These also should also be used cautiously in patients with heart failure or hypotension.
- **Digoxin**—Preferred in patients with AF and symptomatic heart failure with reduced left ventricular (LV) ejection fraction. Less effective for ambulatory, active patients. Digoxin should be avoided in the setting of acute renal failure or chronic kidney disease.
- **Amiodarone**—A class III antiarrhythmic that has AV-nodal-blocking properties along with sympatholytic and calcium channel–antagonist properties. It should be considered a secondary agent, used primarily for refractory rate control or in

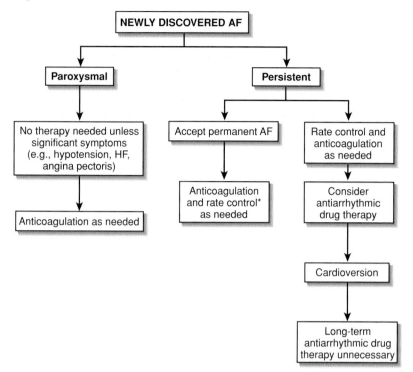

FIGURE 21-2. Management overview and algorithm with pharmacologic therapy for patients with newly diagnosed AF. (From Fuster V, Ryden LE, Cannom DS, et al. ACC/AHA/ESC 2006 Guidelines for the Management of Patients with Atrial Fibrillation. *J Am Coll Cardiol* 2006;48:e149, with permission.)

hypotensive patients. It may convert a patient to sinus rhythm, thus increasing the risk of thromboembolism in those with prolonged AF who are not anticoagulated. Amiodarone causes an increase in digoxin levels and inhibits warfarin metabolism, so appropriate adjustments to those medications should be made.
• Rate control is considered adequate between 60 and 80 bpm at rest and between 90 and 115 bpm during moderate exercise.

Three unique situations in managing rate control include the following:

• **AF in the setting of Wolff–Parkinson–White (WPW) syndrome** is a life-threatening arrhythmia due to the very rapid AV conduction across an accessory pathway. **AV nodal agents are contraindicated in WPW**, as they increase the ventricular rate via the accessory pathway, leading to hypotension or ventricular fibrillation. If the patient is hypotensive, DC cardioversion can be performed. In hemodynamically stable patients, procainamide or amiodarone can be given.
• **Patients with AF associated with sick sinus syndrome (SSS)** often have rapid AF alternating with significant sinus bradycardia and sinus pauses. The use of AV nodal

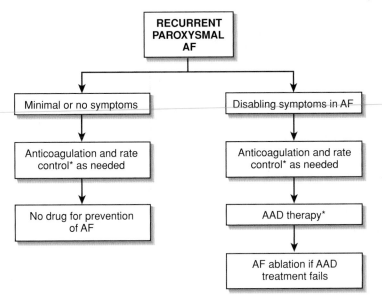

FIGURE 21-3. Management overview and algorithm with pharmacologic therapy for patients with recurrent paroxysmal AF. AAD, antiarrhythmic drug. (From Fuster V, Ryden LE, Cannom DS, et al. ACC/AHA/ESC 2006 Guidelines for the Management of Patients with Atrial Fibrillation. *J Am Coll Cardiol* 2006;48:e149, with permission.)

agents to control the rate of AF is difficult; in some cases, a permanent pacemaker may be needed.

• When pharmacologic therapy cannot control the heart rate and symptoms (**medically refractory AF**), alternative options include an ablation of the AV node with placement of a permanent pacemaker ("ablate and pace" strategy) or more aggressive rhythm control measures, such as pulmonary vein isolation (see below).

Rhythm Control

Some patients will require cardioversion and antiarrhythmic therapy to maintain sinus rhythm, control symptoms, improve exercise capacity, and improve cardiac function. Cardioversion can be performed with **synchronized DC electrical current and/or antiarrhythmic medications**. Because of the increased risk of thromboembolic events in the first several weeks after cardioversion, elective cardioversions should generally be performed with anticoagulation and continued for a minimum of 4 weeks thereafter. If the patient is hemodynamically unstable, urgent synchronized DC cardioversion is warranted without anticoagulation. Other situations where cardioversion can be performed without anticoagulation include short-duration AF (<48 hours) or after a TEE demonstrates absence of a left atrial thrombus. In the stable patient, if the AF has lasted longer than 48 hours, is of unknown duration, or there is coexisting mitral stenosis or a history of a thomboembolism, cardioversion should be delayed until anticoagulation can be maintained at appropriate levels (INR of 2.0–3.0) for 3 to 4 weeks or until TEE evaluation for thrombi of the left atrial appendage is performed.

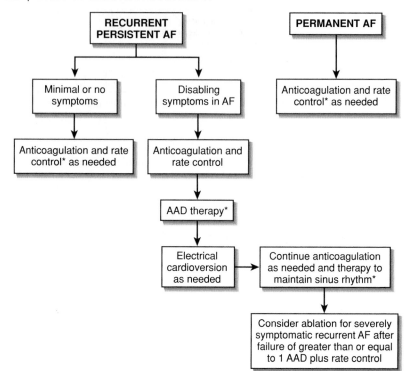

FIGURE 21-4. Management overview and algorithm with pharmacologic therapy for patients with recurrent persistent or permanent AF. AAD, antiarrhythmic drug. (From Fuster V, Ryden LE, Cannom DS, et al. ACC/AHA/ESC 2006 Guidelines for the Management of Patients with Atrial Fibrillation. *J Am Coll Cardiol* 2006;48:e149, with permission.)

There are multiple antiarrhythmic medications to achieve and maintain rhythm control; appropriate selection is based on safety, comorbidities, and the pattern of AF diagnosed (Fig. 21-5). Pharmacologic cardioversion is less effective than DC cardioversion, although there is evidence that pretreatment with certain antiarrhythmic medications can enhance the success of DC cardioversion. The choice of medication varies, but in general flecainide, sotalol, or propafenone is preferred in patients with no or minimal heart disease and amiodarone or dofetilide in patients with reduced LV function or heart failure. Proarrhythmic side effects require some of the medications to be initiated and titrated on an inpatient basis with continuous telemetry monitoring and routine ECGs. Potential organ toxicity requires frequent outpatient follow-up as well.

Despite rhythm control, many patients with AF experience a recurrence. Of those who are successfully cardioverted, only 20% to 30% continue in sinus rhythm for more than 1 year without antiarrhythmic therapy. Risk factors for recurrence include advanced age, heart failure, left atrial enlargement, hypertension, and rheumatic heart disease.

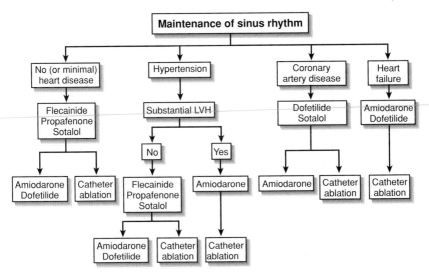

FIGURE 21-5. Management overview and algorithm for antiarrhythmic therapy to maintain normal sinus rhythm, based on various disease states, for patients with recurrent paroxysmal or persistent AF. (From Fuster V, Ryden LE, Cannom DS, et al. ACC/AHA/ESC 2006 Guidelines for the Management of Patients with Atrial Fibrillation. *J Am Coll Cardiol* 2006;48:e149, with permission.)

Three interesting findings of rhythm control strategies are as follows:

• When compared with a rate control-strategy in large trials with mostly older patients with asymptomatic persistent AF, there was no mortality benefit to a rhythm-control strategy (AFFIRM, RACE trials). In fact, there were trends toward improved survival and stroke risk with the rate-control strategy.

• Most patients with symptomatic AF prefer a rhythm-control strategy to achieve sinus rhythm. In asymptomatic patients, the differences in quality of life between the two strategies are not demonstrable in large studies.

• Embolic events take place with equal frequency in both methods of treatment, usually occurring when the patient is not taking warfarin or when the anticoagulation is subtherapeutic (see below).

Nonpharmacologic Treatments
The "gold-standard" surgical treatment for AF is the **Cox-Maze procedure**, which aims to eliminate all macroreentrant circuits that may develop in the atria. Initially this procedure involved many surgical incisions across both the right and left atrium ("cut and sew"); but more refined variations have used linear ablation lines with various energy systems, including radiofrequency energy, microwave, cryoablation, laser, and high-intensity focused ultrasound. Long-term success is reported to be >95%. It is generally performed for patients undergoing concomitant cardiac surgery but has been more recently used as a stand-alone procedure.

Because the triggers for atrial fibrillation are frequently found in or around the pulmonary veins (PV), **percutaneous PV isolation procedures** targeting this area have been developed. Advantages of a PV isolation procedure over the Cox-Maze procedure include quicker recovery and potentially lower procedural mortality. The main disadvantage is a considerably lower success rate (>60% with single procedures, >70% with multiple procedures for paroxysmal AF). Because of the modest risk profile associated with this complex procedure, **catheter ablation for the treatment of AF is recommended for symptomatic patients with AF that is refractory to at least one class I or class III antiarrhythmic medication.**

Anticoagulation
There is a significant risk of stroke in patients with AF due to the formation of a thrombus secondary to stasis of blood in the left atrial appendage. The annual risk of stroke from AF has been estimated at 1.5% in patients 50 to 59 years old and 23.5% in patients 80 to 89 years old. **Risk factors for thromboembolic events related to AF and yearly risk of stroke without anticoagulation can be estimated using the CHADS2 scoring system** (Table 21-2).

The overall goal of preventing thromboembolic events must be balanced with avoiding bleeding complications with warfarin anticoagulation. Because the risk/benefit ratio for warfarin is unique to each individual, variation exists in recommended anticoagulation strategies. The ACC/AHA/ESC recommendations are found in Table 21-3. Using the simplified CHADS2 scoring for patients at increased risk for stroke (CHADS2 score >1), anticoagulation therapy with warfarin is recommended. For patients with a lower risk for stroke (CHADS2 score 0), the risks of warfarin outweigh the benefit; thus aspirin is reasonable. Intermediate-risk patients (CHADS2 score 1) may use either aspirin or warfarin.

TABLE 21-2 STROKE RISK IN PATIENTS WITH NONVALVULAR AF NOT TREATED WITH ANTICOAGULATION ACCORDING TO THE CHADS2 INDEX

CHADS2 Risk Criteria	Score
Prior stroke or TIA	2
Age >75 years	1
Hypertension	1
Diabetes mellitus	1
Heart failure	1

Patients (N = 1733)	Adjusted Stroke Rate (%/y) (95% CI)	CHADS$_2$ Score
120	1.9 (1.2–3.0)	0
463	2.8 (2.0–3.8)	1
523	4.0 (3.1–5.1)	2
337	5.9 (4.6–7.3)	3
220	8.5 (6.3–11.1)	4
65	12.5 (8.2–17.5)	5
5	18.2 (10.5–27.4)	6

Source: From Fuster V, Ryden LE, Cannom DS, et al. ACC/AHA/ESC 2006 Guidelines for the Management of Patients with Atrial Fibrillation. *J Am Coll Cardiol* 2006;48:e149, with permission.

TABLE 21-3	ANTITHROMBOTIC THERAPY FOR PATIENTS WITH ATRIAL FIBRILLATION
Risk Category	**Recommended Therapy**
No risk factors	Aspirin, 81 to 325 mg daily
One moderate-risk factor	Aspirin, 81 to 325 mg daily, or warfarin (INR 2.0 to 3.0, target 2.5)
Any high-risk factor or more than 1 moderate-risk factor	Warfarin (INR 2.0 to 3.0 target 2.5)

Less Validated or Weaker Risk Factors	Moderate-Risk Factors	High-Risk Factors
Female gender	Age ≥75 years	Previous stroke, TIA or embolism
Age 65–74 years	Hypertension	Mitral stenosis
Coronary artery disease	Heart failure	Prosthetic heart valve
Thyrotoxicosis	LV ejection fraction 35% or less	
	Diabetes mellitus	

INR, International normalized ratio; LV, left ventricular; TIA, transient ischemic attack.
Source: From Fuster V, Ryden LE, Cannom DS, et al. ACC/AHA/ESC 2006 Guidelines for the Management of Patients with Atrial Fibrillation. *J Am Coll Cardiol* 2006;48:e149, with permission.

An additional option to minimize stroke risk is obliteration of the left atrial appendage, removing the most common site for thrombus formation. This procedure is performed surgically as adjunctive therapy during a Cox-Maze procedure, but percutaneous left atrial occluder devices are under investigation.

KEY POINTS TO REMEMBER

- AF is strongly associated with an increased risk of stroke.
- AF can be classified by frequency and duration of symptoms into paroxysmal, persistent, long-standing persistent, and permanent categories.
- The management for AF includes rate control, rhythm control, and anticoagulation to prevent thromboembolism.
- Rate control is achieved with beta blockers, calcium channel blockers, or digoxin. Amiodarone is a second-line agent.
- Rhythm control is achieved with antiarrhythmic drugs and synchronized DC cardioversion. Surgical and catheter-based therapies are available for select patients.
- Large studies of mostly asymptomatic patients with AF have shown that rate-control strategies are generally as safe as rhythm-control strategies provided that appropriate anticoagulation is achieved.
- The overall goal of preventing thromboembolic events with oral anticoagulation must be balanced against the bleeding risks. The CHADS2 risk score estimates yearly stroke risk based on underlying risk factors.

REFERENCES AND SUGGESTED READINGS

Almassi GH, Schowalter T, Nicolosi AC, et al. Atrial fibrillation after cardiac surgery: a major morbid event? *Ann Surg* 1997;226:501.

Calkins H, Brugada J, Packer DL, et al. HRS/EHRA/ECAS Expert Consensus Statement on Catheter and Surgical Ablation of Atrial Fibrillation: Recommendations for Personnel, Policy, Procedures and Follow-Up: A report of the Heart Rhythm Society (HRS) Task Force on Catheter and Surgical Ablation of Atrial Fibrillation. *Heart Rhythm* 2007;4:816.

Cameron A, Schwartz MJ, Kronmal RA, et al. prevalence and significance of atrial fibrillation in coronary artery disease (CASS Registry). *Am J Cardiol* 1988;61:714.

Chen SA, Hsieh MH, Tai CT, et al. Initiation of atrial fibrillation by ectopic beats originating from the pulmonary veins: electrophysiological characteristics, pharmacological responses, and effects of radiofrequency ablation. *Circulation* 1999;100:1879.

Echt DS, Liebson PR, Mitchell LB, et al. Mortality and morbidity in patients receiving encainide, flecainide, or placebo. The Cardiac Arrhythmia Suppression Trial. *N Engl J Med* 1991;324:781.

Fuster V, Ryden LE, Cannom DS, et al. ACC/AHA/ESC 2006 Guidelines for the Management of Patients with Atrial Fibrillation, A Report of the American College of Cardiology/American Heart Association Task Force on Practice Guidelines and the European Society of Cardiology Committee for Practice Guidelines (Writing Committee to Revise the 2001 Guidelines for the Management of Patients with Atrial Fibrillation). *J Am Coll Cardiol* 2006;48:e149.

Gage BF, Waterman AD, Shannon W, et al. Validation of clinical classification schemes for predicting stroke: results from the National Registry of Atrial Fibrillation. *JAMA* 2001;285:2864.

Gallagher MM, Guo XH, Poloniecki JD, et al. Initial energy setting, outcome, and efficacy in direct current cardioversion of atrial fibrillation and flutter. *J Am Coll Cardiol* 2001;38:1498.

Go AS, Hylec, EM, Philips KA, et al. Prevalence of diagnosed atrial fibrillation in adults: national implications for rhythm management and stroke prevention: The Anticoagulation and Risk Factors in Atrial Fibrillation (ATRIA) study. *JAMA* 2001;285:2370.

Haissaguerre M, Jais P, Shah DC, et al. Spontaneous initiation of atrial fibrillation by ectopic beats originating in the pulmonary veins. *N Engl J Med* 1998;339:659.

Krahn AD, Manfreda J, Tate RB, et al. The natural history of atrial fibrillation: incidence, risk factors, and prognosis in the Manitoba follow-up study. *Am J Med* 1995;98:476.

Nichol G, McAlister F, Pham B, et al. Meta-analysis of randomized controlled trials of the effectiveness of antiarrhythmic agents at promoting sinus rhythm in patients with atrial fibrillation. *Heart* 2002;87:535.

Page RL, Wilkinson WE, Clair WK, et al. Asymptomatic arrhythmias in patients with symptomatic paroxysmal atrial fibrillation and paroxysmal supraventricular tachycardia. *Circulation* 1994;89:224.

Pritchett EL. Management of atrial fibrillation. *N Engl J Med* 1992;326:1264.

Singer DE, Albers GW, Dalen JE, et al. antithrombotic therapy in atrial fibrillation: the seventh ACCP conference on antithrombotic and thrombolytic therapy. *Chest* 2004;126:429S.

Van Gelder IC, Hagens VE, Bosker HA, et al. A Comparison of Rate Control and rhythm control in patients with recurrent persistent atrial fibrillation. *N Engl J Med* 2002;347:1834.

Vaziri SM, Larson MG, Benjamin EJ, et al. Echocardiographic predictors of nonrheumatic atrial fibrillation: The Framingham Heart Study. *Circulation* 1994;89:724.

Wolf PA, Abbott RD, Kannel WB. Atrial Fibrillation as an independent risk factor for stroke: the Framingham Study. *Stroke* 1991;22:983.

Wyse DG, Waldo AL, DiMarco JP, et al. A comparison of rate control and rhythm control in patients with atrial fibrillation. The Atrial Fibrillation Follow-up Investigation of Rhythm Management (AFFIRM) investigators. *N Engl J Med* 2002;347:1825.

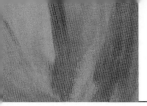

Peripheral Arterial Disease

Timothy W. Schloss and Jasvindar Singh

BACKGROUND

The term "peripheral arterial disease" (PAD) includes a group of disorders that lead to progressive stenosis, occlusion, or aneurysmal dilation of the aorta and its noncoronary branch arteries, including the carotid artery, upper extremity, visceral, and lower extremity arterial branches. "Peripheral vascular disease" is a much more inclusive term, including diseases that affect the arterial, venous, and lymphatic circulations. This chapter covers the vascular diseases caused primarily by atherosclerosis and thromboembolic processes that lead to ischemia of the lower extremity, kidney, and carotid artery territory. Diseases of the aorta are covered in Chapter 23.

Etiology

The most common cause of PAD is atherosclerosis. Identified risk factors include smoking, diabetes, hypertension (HTN), hyperlipidemia, and family history. Other etiologies are listed in Table 22-1.

Natural History

Although PAD can cause significant morbidity, the shared pathophysiology and risk factors between PAD and coronary artery disease (CAD) mean that the **majority of these patients will die from cardiovascular diseases such as myocardial infarction (MI) or ischemic stroke.** In fact, even minimally symptomatic patients with PAD are at relatively high risk for future cardiovascular events.

LOWER EXTREMITY PAD

Prevalence

Total prevalence of PAD has been estimated at 3% to 10% of the population, based on ankle–brachial testing. This increases to 15% to 20% in persons over 70 years of age. In a high-risk patient population greater than 50 years of age with a history of cigarette smoking or diabetes, the prevalence of PAD is estimated at 29%. Patients with lower extremity PAD have a two- to six-fold increased risk of death due to coronary heart disease events and are four to five times more likely to have a stroke or transient ischemic attack (TIA).

Risk Factors

The major cause of lower extremity PAD is atherosclerosis, with identified risk factors of smoking, diabetes, HTN, hyperlipidemia, hyperhomocysteinemia, and family history of CAD. Cigarette smoking is a significant dose-dependent contributor to the development of lower extremity PAD. **More than 80% of patients are current or former smokers,** and

TABLE 22-1 ETIOLOGY OF PAD

- Atherosclerosis
- Connective tissues diseases
  - Marfan Syndrome
  - Ehlers-Danlos syndrome
- Dysplastic disease
  - Fibromuscular dysplasia
- Vasculitic diseases
  - Large vessels: giant-cell (temporal) arteritis, Takayasu's arteritis
  - Medium-sized vessels: Kawasaki disease, polyarteritis nodosa
  - Small vessel disease (arterioles and microvessels), Wegener's granulomatosis, microscopic polyangiitis, Churg-Strauss syndrome, Henoch-Schönlein purpura, cryoglobulinaemic vasculitis
  - Thromboangiitis obliterans (Buerger's disease)
- Prothrombotic diseases
- Vasospastic diseases

a cigarette smoker is two to three times more likely to have lower extremity PAD than detectable CAD.

Clinical Presentation

Patients with lower extremity PAD range from those who are asymptomatic to those with acute limb-threatening emergencies. It is necessary for a clinician to differentiate between the severity of symptoms in deciding on further workup and the urgency of a treatment plan. Four general presentation categories are as follows:

- Asymptomatic
- Claudication
- Critical limb ischemia (CLI)
- Acute limb ischemia (ALI)

Asymptomatic lower extremity PAD does not necessarily mean that limb function is normal. Many of these patients do not have classic exertional limb discomfort but may have less typical symptoms. Patients with a low ankle–brachial index (ABI) but no symptoms of claudication may have decreased functional status—for example, affecting walking speed and balance. Because most of these patients have systemic atherosclerotic disease, they may be included in a high-risk category comparable to individuals with established CAD. Patients ≥50 years of age with cardiovascular risk factors and all patients ≥70 years should be asked about walking impairment, rest pain, and nonhealing wounds. These patients are at risk for PAD, and a resting ABI should be obtained so that therapeutic treatments known to reduce risk of MI, stroke, and death may be initiated.

"Claudication," derived from the Latin word meaning "to limp," is defined as fatigue, discomfort, or pain that occurs in a specific limb muscle group during effort; it is due to exercise-induced ischemia. Symptoms of chronic lower extremity atherosclerotic occlusion are variable but are frequently described as **reproducible cramping or fatigue with walking,** with resolution shortly after rest. Symptoms may occur anywhere in the lower extremity, including buttocks, thighs, or calves. An important distinction from intermittent claudication is pseudoclaudication from spinal stenosis. Classically, limb discomfort associated with spinal stenosis is not reliably reproduced with exertion; it is exacerbated by standing and relieved only by sitting. Occasionally, both disease states may coexist, and exercise testing along with noninvasive imaging of the spine will help guide therapy.

Critical limb ischemia (CLI) is defined as limb pain that occurs at rest or impending limb loss that is caused by severe compromise of blood flow to the affected extremity. This term should be used to describe all patients **with chronic pain at rest, ulcers, or gangrene** attributable to objectively proven arterial occlusive disease. Unlike claudication, the natural history of CLI leads to limb amputation, and the 1-year mortality for patients with CLI is >20%. CLI usually presents with rest pain, worse while lying in a supine position, and interfering with sleep. Patients will maintain limbs in a dependent position and are frequently unable to walk. The history should focus on identifying the chronicity of the disease and the region or level of underperfusion.

Acute limb ischemia (ALI) is caused by a sudden decrease in limb perfusion that threatens tissue viability. Symptoms occur as a result of thrombosis of an atherosclerotic plaque or a lower extremity embolism, frequently of cardiac or aortic origin. The typical symptoms and signs of acute limb ischemia include "the six P's:" **pain, paralysis, paresthesias, pulselessness, pallor, and polar (cold).**

Physical Exam

Every patient with risk factors for PAD should have a thorough examination of peripheral blood flow, including auscultation for bruits over major vascular beds as well as palpation of peripheral pulses over the femoral, popliteal, posterior tibial, and dorsalis pedis arteries. A quick screening maneuver is the **elevation-dependency test**, which can be performed by elevating the lower extremities to 60 degrees above horizontal while the patient is supine. The development of pallor in the skin of the sole of the foot indicates arterial disease in that extremity. Following elevation, the patient may sit up with extremities hanging off the examination table. Delayed return of color and venous engorgement in one extremity may help confirm inadequate circulation. With more advanced disease, a deep rubrous color develops along with dependent edema, so-called **dependent rubor**. Evidence of atheroembolization such as livido reticularis should be assessed, as well as note of ulcers, neuropathy, and infection. Additional findings include calf atrophy, alopecia over the dorsum of the foot, thickening of the toenails, and shiny, scaly skin due to loss of subcutaneous tissue.

Diagnostic Testing

Along with a vascular physical examination, all patients with symptomatic claudication should undergo measurement of the **ankle–brachial index (ABI)** to confirm the diagnosis and establish a baseline result (Fig. 22-1). Advanced age and long-standing diabetes mellitus contribute to vessel rigidity and make occlusion of the peripheral arteries with pressure cuffs difficult and the ABI test less reliable. When this occurs, a **toe–brachial index (TBI)** can be used instead. Toe pressures <30 mm Hg indicate ischemia, impaired wound healing, and increased risk of amputation. A toe–brachial index of <0.7 is considered diagnostic of lower extremity PAD.

If the resting ABI is normal and clinical suspicion is high, this examination should be repeated after exercise. If the patient cannot exercise, a **plantar flexion test** may be used instead. While standing, the patient raises his or her heels off the ground, standing "on tiptoe," and then returns to the normal position. When symptoms develop or after 50 repetitions, the ABI is repeated.

To further identify the location and extent of lower extremity PAD, a **segmental limb pressure exam** may be helpful. After an abnormal ABI, additional cuffs can be placed on

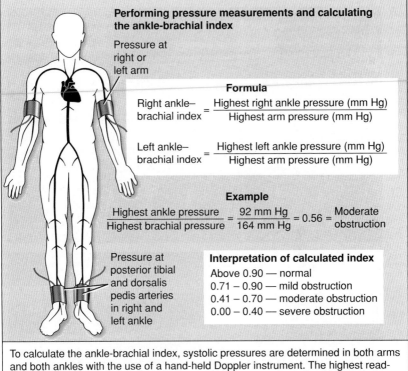

Performing pressure measurements and calculating the ankle-brachial index

Pressure at right or left arm

Formula

$$\text{Right ankle–brachial index} = \frac{\text{Highest right ankle pressure (mm Hg)}}{\text{Highest arm pressure (mm Hg)}}$$

$$\text{Left ankle–brachial index} = \frac{\text{Highest left ankle pressure (mm Hg)}}{\text{Highest arm pressure (mm Hg)}}$$

Example

$$\frac{\text{Highest ankle pressure}}{\text{Highest brachial pressure}} = \frac{92 \text{ mm Hg}}{164 \text{ mm Hg}} = 0.56 = \text{Moderate obstruction}$$

Pressure at posterior tibial and dorsalis pedis arteries in right and left ankle

Interpretation of calculated index

Above 0.90 — normal
0.71 – 0.90 — mild obstruction
0.41 – 0.70 — moderate obstruction
0.00 – 0.40 — severe obstruction

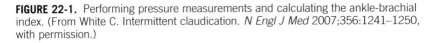

To calculate the ankle-brachial index, systolic pressures are determined in both arms and both ankles with the use of a hand-held Doppler instrument. The highest readings for the dorsalis pedis and posterior tibial arteries are used to calculate the index.

FIGURE 22-1. Performing pressure measurements and calculating the ankle-brachial index. (From White C. Intermittent claudication. *N Engl J Med* 2007;356:1241–1250, with permission.)

the upper thigh, lower thigh, and upper calf. A drop of 20 mm Hg in the systolic pressure between segments is consistent with arterial stenosis. **Pulse volume recordings** are frequently performed at the same time and are obtained with a cuff system that incorporates a pneumoplethysmograph, which identifies changes in pulse contour and amplitude. In the presence of arterial disease, the slope flattens, the pulse width widens, and the dicrotic notch is lost.

Duplex ultrasonography combines Doppler velocity and waveform analysis with gray-scale visualization of the arterial wall. A normal waveform is triphasic, with forward flow in cardiac systole followed by a brief flow reversal in early diastole followed by forward flow in late diastole. With arterial stenosis, distal blood flow velocities increase. In severe stenosis, the flow-reversal component is absent as well (Fig. 22-2). The degree of stenosis is determined by combining waveform analysis and measurement of the peak systolic velocity.

For specific anatomic delineation to guide revascularization, additional imaging with computed tomography (CT), magnetic resonance angiography (MRA), or digital subtraction angiography can be used. **Digital subtraction angiography** remains the "gold

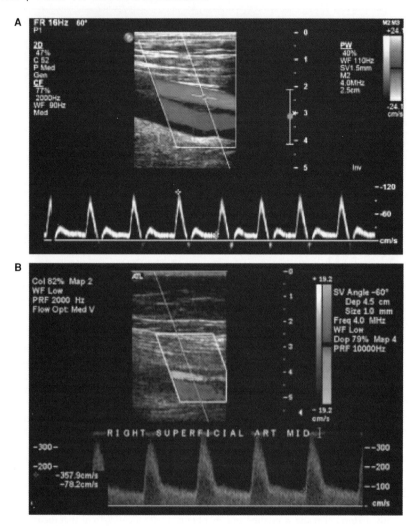

FIGURE 22-2. Doppler arterial waveforms from patients without (**A**) and with (**B**) PAD. In the setting of PAD, the peak systolic velocity increases and the diastolic flow reversal is lost. (From Begelman SM, Jaff MR. Noninvasive diagnostic strategies for peripheral arterial disease. *Cleve Clin J Med* 2006;73(Suppl 4):S22–S29, with permission.)

standard" test, but it is invasive and carries risks related to the use of contrast and radiation exposure. **CT angiography** is rapid and noninvasive but carries similar contrast and radiation risks. Calcium found in atherosclerotic lesions can create "blooming artifacts," rendering images less accurate. MRA carries fewer risks and gives detailed information, although prior stent placement can affect image quality.

Treatment

The goal should be prevention of the development of PAD through risk-factor modification, especially smoking cessation. When prevention fails, early detection and lifestyle modification, along with medical and, in some cases, mechanical reperfusion therapy should be combined to maintain and improve quality of life and to avoid limb- and life-threatening progression.

All patients with PAD, regardless of symptoms, should be treated with **aggressive risk-factor modification**, which includes:

- Lipid-lowering therapy (an HMG-CoA reductase inhibitor ["statin"] for a goal low-density-lipoprotein cholesterol level <100 mg/dL)
- Antihypertensive therapy (angiotensin converting enzyme [ACE] inhibitor and/or beta blocker for a goal blood pressure <140/90 or <130/80 with diabetes)
- Glucose control (hemoglobin A1c <7%)
- Daily foot inspection and proper foot care
- Smoking cessation
- Antiplatelet therapy (aspirin 75–325 mg daily or Plavix 75 mg daily)

In addition, patients suffering from claudication will benefit from a **supervised exercise program**. The improvements in functional capacity are gradual and occur over several months. When each exercise session lasts at least 30 minutes, takes place three times per week, and exercise is at near maximal pain, trials show a 150% improvement in maximal walking ability. **Cilostazol** (Pletal), a phosphodiesterase type 3 inhibitor, has both vasodilatory and platelet-inhibitory properties and has been shown to improve walking distance by ~50% compared with placebo. Because other phosphodiesterase inhibitors are associated with an increased mortality in patients with heart failure, care should be taken to avoid cilostazol in patients with left ventricular dysfunction.

For symptomatic patients with claudication that causes limitations in quality of life or vocational ability and who do not respond adequately to a supervised exercise program and medical management, a **revascularization procedure** may be considered. Because of the lower risk profile, initial revascularization strategies will usually rely on endovascular techniques, with surgical intervention reserved for unfavorable anatomy. Approximately 5% of patients with intermittent claudication will require a revascularization intervention for severe symptoms or progression to CLI, and only 2% will ultimately require amputation for distal ischemia. In contrast, nearly half of patients with CLI will require revascularization for limb salvage.

If the progression of disease has been fairly rapid, urgent referral to a vascular specialist is warranted to limit the extent of tissues necrosis and increase the chance of limb salvage. If signs of acute limb ischemia are present (the six P's), the vascular consult is emergent, and immediate concerns should address anticoagulation to prevent the propagation of thrombus material and initiate plans for urgent or emergent revascularization. It is important to keep in mind that patients frequently have concomitant severe CAD or cerebrovascular disease, which factors into the treatment plan. Endovascular treatments such as percutaneous transluminal angioplasty (PTA) with or without stenting, catheter-based thrombolysis, mechanical thrombectomy, and open surgical procedures are reasonable treatment options based on comorbidities and vascular anatomy.

RENAL ARTERIAL DISEASE

Background

The kidneys, through the renal arteries, receive ~20% of the total cardiac output. Renovascular HTN, secondary to inadequate renal perfusion, is the most common correctable

TABLE 22-2	CAUSES OF RENAL ARTERY STENOSIS

- Atherosclerosis
- Fibromuscular dysplasia
- Renal artery aneurysms
- Aortic or renal artery dissection
- Vasculitis
- Thrombotic or cholesterol embolization
- Collagen vascular disease
- Retroperitoneal fibrosis
- Trauma
- Posttransplantation stenosis
- Postradiation

cause of secondary HTN. In a study population of patients undergoing cardiac catheterization, renal artery stenosis (RAS) was detected in approximately 30% of the population, with lesions >50% found in 11% to 18% of the study population.

Renal hypoperfusion ultimately leads to activation of the renin-angiotensin system. Through the vasoactive properties of aldosterone and angiotensin II, RAS leads to volume expansion and elevated systemic blood pressures.

Etiology

More than 90% of all renovascular lesions are caused by atherosclerosis. Additional causes of RAS are listed in Table 22-2. Frequently, renal artery atherosclerosis involves the ostia of the renal artery and extends into the aorta. Fibromuscular dysplasia (FMD) is the second most common cause of RAS. Although occurring in both genders, the typical presentation of FMD is that of HTN in a young woman. In contrast to atherosclerotic renal artery stenosis, FMD involves the mid- and distal renal artery and may extend into the side branches. The characteristic "string of beads" appearance and location within the renal artery help to differentiate FMD from atherosclerotic RAS. FMD can also affect other arterial beds, especially the carotid and vertebral arteries. Because of the association with cerebral aneurysms, all patients with renal FMD should undergo screening MR or CT angiography of the head.

Clinical Presentation

Severe HTN and **fluid retention** are the hallmark findings of RAS. The clinical features that should prompt a search for RAS include:

- Onset of HTN before the age of 30 years
- Onset of severe HTN after the age of 55 years
- Accelerated HTN (sudden and persistent worsening of previously controlled HTN)
- Resistant HTN (HTN despite three drugs, one of which must be a diuretic)
- Malignant HTN (HTN with coexistent evidence of acute end-organ damage)
- Worsening renal function after the administration of an ACE inhibitor or angiotensin receptor blocker (ARB)
- An unexplained atrophic kidney or >1.5-cm size discrepancy between the two kidneys
- Sudden unexplained pulmonary edema

Diagnostic Testing

Duplex ultrasonography with Doppler is recommended as an initial test for the detection of RAS. This test is limited by body habitus, operator skill and experience. **CT or MRA** can define lesion characteristics and is helpful in imaging patients in whom ultrasonography proves difficult. CT uses nephrotoxic contrast, which can be particularly risky in a RAS population. MR uses gadolinium contrast, traditionally thought to be less nephrotoxic than CT contrast. However, a recently reported association with gadolinium and nephrogenic systemic fibrosis has raised concerns in patients with significant renal impairment. If initial tests are inconclusive or considered too risky, **catheter angiography** should be considered for definitive diagnosis. Owing to the high prevalence of atherosclerotic RAS in patients with lower extremity PAD and CAD, a nonselective renal angiogram should be considered in patients with CAD and clinical suspicion for RAS who are already undergoing invasive angiography.

Treatment

Medical treatment for atherosclerotic RAS focuses mainly on **controlling renovascular HTN**. Several classes of medication are effective and include ACE inhibitors, ARBs, calcium-channel blockers, and beta blockers. With the exception of beta blockers, all should be avoided in bilateral RAS, as they may contribute to worsening renal function and/or metabolic abnormalities. In particular, ACE inhibitors have been associated with worsening renal function, and careful monitoring of serum creatinine is warranted in initiating this class of medication.

Revascularization strategies for RAS are the subject of ongoing clinical trials. Initial percutaneous techniques with balloon angioplasty alone have, for the most part, been replaced by procedures involving balloon angioplasty followed by stent placement. This has resulted in a higher clinical success rate and lower restenosis rate, especially for ostial lesions. Patients with FMD are an exception; in such individuals, balloon angioplasty alone is the therapy of choice. In some situations, specifically macroaneurysmal disease and small, multiple renal arteries, the anatomy is unfavorable for percutaneous therapy and vascular surgical reconstruction may be the treatment of choice.

Determining which patients benefit from renal artery revascularization is the focus of active clinical investigation. Acknowledging the lack of convincing large randomized trial data, **revascularization may be considered** for the following groups of patients with hemodynamically significant RAS[1]:

- Accelerated HTN (sudden and persistent worsening of previously controlled HTN)
- Resistant HTN (HTN despite three drugs, one of which must be a diuretic)
- Malignant HTN (HTN with coexistent evidence of acute end-organ damage)
- HTN with an unexplained unilateral small kidney
- HTN with intolerance to medication
- Chronic kidney disease with bilateral RAS or a RAS to a solitary functioning kidney
- Recurrent, sudden unexplained pulmonary edema
- Recurrent angina in the setting of severe HTN

---

[1]Hemodynamically significant RAS is (1) ≥50% to 70% diameter stenosis by visual estimation with a peak translesional gradient of >20 mm Hg or a mean gradient ≥10 mm Hg with 5 Fr catheter or pressure wire or (2) any stenosis ≥70% diameter stenosis or (3) ≥70% diameter stenosis by intravascular ultrasound.

CAROTID ARTERY STENOSIS

Background

Like the detection of lower extremity PAD, the detection of carotid artery stenosis represents an opportunity to identify patients at high risk for adverse cardiovascular events. Nearly half of patients with atherosclerotic carotid artery disease have severe CAD. In addition to identifying high-risk patients for cardiovascular events, an ultimate goal of detecting carotid artery stenosis is to prevent cerebrovascular events. Stroke is the third leading cause of death in the United States and represents a major cause of long-term disability.

Prevalence

Localized carotid bruits are present in about 5% of patients over the age of 65. In the Cardiovascular Health Study, a carotid stenosis >50% was detected in 7% of the men and 5% of the women >65 years of age.

Clinical Presentation

Atherosclerotic carotid artery stenosis can present as an asymptomatic carotid bruit, TIA, or stroke. Although strokes and TIAs have multiple etiologies, ~80% are ischemic in origin. Of the ischemic strokes ~25% are due to a vascular stenosis or occlusion.

Risk Factors

Modifiable risk factors for stroke include HTN, tobacco use, dyslipidemia, and diabetes. The relative risk of stroke increases as the degree of stenosis progresses and with the development of symptoms. In several observational trials, patients with an asymptomatic carotid stenosis >60% have a 2%/year risk of stroke, while patients with symptomatic carotid stenosis >70% have a 13%/year risk of stroke.

Physical Examination

All patients presenting to a cardiovascular specialist should undergo auscultation of the carotid arteries. Most bruits detected will be during systole; if the bruit extends into diastole, this indicates a significant gradient in the carotid artery with stenosis of ~80%. During the physical examination, care should be taken to immediately notice a bradycardic event, which may be the result of carotid sinus sensitivity.

Treatment

Medical treatment should focus on control of the modifiable risk factors of cerebrovascular events. If not contraindicated, antiplatelet therapy with **aspirin** should be administered. For patients with a history of TIA or stroke, control of risk factors including HTN, diabetes, and cholesterol (with a **statin** medication) should be initiated.

Revascularization of the carotid artery is the subject of ongoing clinical investigation. Currently, the American Heart Association/American Stroke Association (AHA/ASA) recommends considering prophylactic carotid endarterectomy in highly selected patients with high-grade asymptomatic carotid stenosis performed by surgeons with <3% morbidity/mortality rates. For symptomatic patients, those with a recent TIA or ischemic stroke within the last 6 months with ipsilateral severe (70%–99%) carotid stenosis, endarterectomy by a surgeon with a perioperative morbidity and mortality of <6% is recommended. For symptomatic patients with a 50% to 69% stenosis, surgical recommendations depend on comorbidities and age. For patients who are poor surgical candidates, percutaneous carotid artery stenting is not considered to be inferior to surgical endarterectomy; it may therefore be considered as an alternative to surgery.

KEY POINTS TO REMEMBER

- Atherosclerosis is a systemic disease; patients with one affected vascular territory are at risk for complications of other territories, particularly CAD.
- Patients with lower extremity PAD should be stratified into one of four groups: asymptomatic, claudication, chronic limb ischemia, or acute limb ischemia.
- A reasonable vascular exam should include palpation of pulses, auscultation for bruits, and performance of the lower extremity elevation-dependency test.
- Aggressive atherosclerosis risk-factor modification is applicable to all forms of PAD.
- Revascularization strategies for all types of PAD depend on severity of symptoms, magnitude of vascular occlusion, risks of the procedure, patient comorbidities, and anatomic considerations.

REFERENCES AND SUGGESTED READINGS

Hirsch AT, Haskal ZJ, Hertzer NR, et al. ACC/AHA Guidelines for the Management of Patients with Peripheral Arterial Disease (lower extremity, renal, mesenteric, and abdominal aortic): A Collaborative Report from the American Association for Vascular Surgery/Society for Vascular Surgery, Society for Cardiovascular Angiography and Interventions, Society of Interventional Radiology, Society for Vascular Medicine and Biology, and the American College of Cardiology/American Heart Association Task Force on Practice Guidelines (Writing Committee to Develop Guidelines for the Management of Patients With Peripheral Arterial Disease). American College of Cardiology Website. Available at: http://www.acc.org/clinical/guidelines/pad/index.pdf.

Norgren L, Hiatt WR, Dormandy JA, Nehler MR, et al. TASC II Working Group. Inter-Society Consensus for the Management of Peripheral Arterial Disease (TASC II). TASC II: *J Vasc Surg* 2007:45:S1–S68.

Weber-Mzell D, Kotanko P, Schumacher M, et al. Coronary anatomy predicts presence or absence of renal artery stenosis. A prospective study in patients undergoing cardiac catheterization for suspended coronary artery disease. *Eur Heart J* 2002;21:1684–1691.

White C. Intermittent claudication. *N Engl J Med* 2007;356:1241–1250.

Diseases of the Aorta

23

Brian R. Lindman

INTRODUCTION

Aortopathies, or diseases of the aorta, can have acute and devastating consequences. Some patients are known to have an underlying disease process that puts them at risk for adverse aortic events. More often, patients have acute, life-threatening presentations that were not anticipated. There is growing awareness of the underlying aortic disease processes associated with aneurysm formation and dissection. This has led to enhanced surveillance of these patients and more aggressive medical and surgical interventions aimed at decreasing their risk. Ongoing investigation is clarifying the appropriate roles of medical, surgical, and endovascular management. Management of patients with aortic diseases largely depends on their presentation and the portion of the aorta involved (Fig. 23-1). The presentation is usually that of an **acute aortic syndrome** (including aortic dissection, rupture, or leak as well as intramural hematoma or penetrating atherosclerotic ulcer) or an asymptomatic **aortic aneurysm.**

Pathophysiology

The aorta is comprised of three layers: a thin intima, thick media, and thin adventitia. The media provides strength to the aorta and is composed of several sheets of elastic tissue. Most aortic pathology results from abnormalities in the intima and/or media. **Cystic medial degeneration** is the final common pathway for several underlying etiologies of thoracic aortic aneurysm (TAA) formation, as it causes weakness of the aortic wall, making it prone to dilate. **Atherosclerosis** plays the major pathologic role in descending TAAs and abdominal aortic aneurysms (AAAs). A tear in the intima due to shear forces and endothelial damage or an intimal ulceration caused by atherosclerotic changes can allow blood to enter into a weakened medial layer under systemic pressure and propagate a cleavage or dissection in the aortic wall.

CAUSES

Etiology

Several distinct diseases affect the aorta:

- **Bicuspid aortopathy:** Bicuspid aortic valve (BAV) occurs in ~1% of the population and is associated with increased risk of ascending aortic aneurysm, dissection, and coarctation of the aorta. Over half of patients with BAV have aortic dilatation, generally of the ascending aorta and root. This aortic enlargement is independent of valvular stenosis or regurgitation. Dissection is 10 times more common with BAV than in the normal population because of abnormalities of elastic tissue in the aorta and medial degeneration. Roughly 10% of first-degree relatives of patients with a BAV will have a BAV.
- **Marfan syndrome (MFS):** This is an autosomal dominant disease that affects 1 in 5000 to 10,000 individuals. It is caused by a mutation in the fibrillin-1 gene on

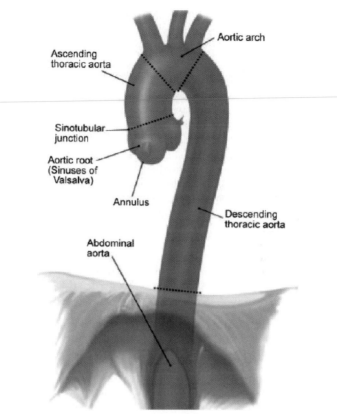

FIGURE 23-1. Anatomy of the thoracic and proximal abdominal aorta. (From Isselbacher EM. Thoracic and abdominal aortic aneurysms. *Circulation* 2005;111:816–828, with permission.)

chromosome 15. Fibrillin-1 is a structural protein that is the major component of microfibrils of elastin. Aortic root aneurysms are characteristically pear-shaped, being largest at the sinuses of Valsalva. MFS also affects the skeleton, lungs, dura, skin, and eye.

- **Loeys-Dietz syndrome (LDS):** This is an autosomal dominant aortic aneurysm syndrome characterized by hypertelorism (widely spaced eyes), a bifid uvula or cleft palate, and generalized arterial tortuosity with widespread vascular aneurysms. Patients have a high risk of aortic dissection or rupture at an earlier age and with smaller aortic sizes than in MFS.
- **Familial thoracic aortic aneurysm and dissection syndrome:** Accelerated cystic medial degeneration underlies these aneurysms in an autosomal dominant pattern, with variable age of onset and the absence of features of MFS or LDS.
- **Atherosclerosis:** The most common cause of descending thoracic and abdominal aortic aneurysms. Atherosclerosis predisposes patients to developing a penetrating atherosclerotic ulcer (PAU). Risk factors include type 2 diabetes, hyperlipidemia, smoking, hypertension, advanced age, and male gender.

- **Hypertension**: Accelerates the degeneration of elastic tissue in the media leading to cystic medial degeneration. Additionally, the high pressures increase the tension placed on the aortic wall, promoting dilatation and aneurysm formation.
- **Inflammatory aortitis**: Caused by diseases such as Takayasu arteritis, giant-cell arteritis, and the HLA-B27 spondyloarthropathies.
- **Infectious aneurysm**: Also called mycotic aneurysm, this can be caused by long-standing syphilis or by *Staphylococcus, Streptococcus,* or *Salmonella* species. The aneurysms tend to be saccular (asymmetric and outpouching).

Epidemiology

Over 75% of all aortic aneurysms are located in the abdominal aorta. In the United States each year, nearly 200,000 new AAAs are diagnosed and more than 15,000 people die of a ruptured aneurysm. The prevalence of 3- to 5-cm AAAs is 1.3% in 45- to 54-year-old men and 12.5% in 75- to 84-year-old men. The prevalence of the same size AAAs in women of the same age groups is nearly 0% and 5.2%, respectively.

Natural History

The main adverse outcome in patients with an **aortic aneurysm** is aortic rupture. Surface tension on the wall increases as a function of pressure and radius (Laplace's law), so the risk of rupture for both AAAs and TAAs is directly related to aortic dimension. Annual rates of rupture of AAAs are 0.3% (<4 cm aneurysm), 1% (4–5 cm), 6 to 10% (5–6 cm) and >15% (>6 cm). Most AAAs are related to atherosclerotic disease. Although AAA is more common in men, rupture occurs three times more often and at smaller aortic sizes in women. A ruptured AAA has a grave prognosis: 25% die suddenly; 50% die in the hospital before surgery can be performed; and the operative mortality of patients fortunate enough to live to surgery is 50%. Overall 30-day survival is ~10%.

Annual rates of rupture of thoracic aortic aneurysms are also size-dependent: 2% (<5-cm aneurysm); 3% (5–5.9 cm); and 7% (>6 cm). Adverse events typically occur at smaller aortic dimensions in patients with MFS, BAV, or other connective tissue disorders.

Aortic dissections tend to occur in the thoracic aorta and are not usually related to atherosclerotic disease. Dissections can be subdivided by location (Fig. 23-2):

- **Stanford type A dissection**
  - **Mortality ~1% per hour** during the first 24 to 48 hours
  - Medical management has ~50% to 60% in-hospital mortality
  - Surgical management has ~20% to 30% in-hospital mortality
- **Stanford type B dissection**
  - Medical management has ~10% in-hospital mortality
  - Surgical management has ~30% in-hospital mortality
  - Long-term survival with medical treatment is ~60% at 5 years and ~40% at 10 years

Two variants of aortic dissection that may present are **intramural hematomas (IMHs)** and **penetrating atherosclerotic ulcers (PAUs)** (Fig. 23-3). IMH is a hemorrhage in the medial layer of the aorta without an intimal tear, while PAU is a focal lesion, occurring at the site of an atherosclerotic plaque, characterized by erosion of the intima. While the natural history of PAU is largely debated, survival trends for IMH mimic those of aortic dissection:

- Type A: 18% to 36% (medically managed) versus 8% to 14% (surgically managed)
- Type B: 12% to 14% (medically managed) versus 17% to 20% (surgically managed)

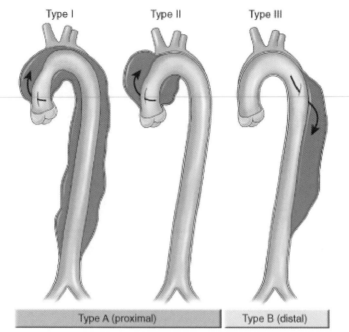

FIGURE 23-2. DeBakey type I: originates in the ascending aorta, propagates at least to the aortic arch and often beyond it distally; type II: originates in and is confined to the ascending aorta; type III: originates in the descending aorta and extends distally down the aorta or, rarely, retrograde into the aortic arch and ascending aorta. Stanford type A: ascending aortic involvement regardless of the site of origin; type B: no involvement of the ascending aorta. (From Isselbacher EM. Diseases of the aorta. In: Zipes DP, Libby P, Bonow RO, et al., eds. *Braunwald's Heart Disease: A Textbook of Cardiovascular Medicine,* 7th ed. Philadelphia: Elsevier Saunders; 2005:1403–1435, with permission.)

PRESENTATION

Clinical Presentation and History

Patients with sudden symptoms related to changes in aortic anatomy can be classified as having **acute aortic syndrome** (AAS) until more specifically defined. AAS includes symptomatic aneurysms, IMHs, PAUs, and aortic dissection, leak, or rupture. **Type A aortic pathology** affects the ascending aorta, potentially including the sinuses of Valsalva and/or aortic arch; it may or may not involve the descending aorta. **Type B aortic pathology** affects the descending aorta (distal to the origin of the left subclavian artery); it does not involve the ascending aorta or arch. A small number of patients may present with dissection isolated to the aortic arch. Patients with an acute aortic syndrome may describe:

- **Sudden onset severe chest and/or back pain** (acute aortic syndrome of the thoracic aorta). Classically, pain radiates to the neck with ascending aortic involvement and to the back between the scapulae with descending aortic involvement.
- **Steady, gnawing abdominal or back pain with pulsatile abdominal mass and hypotension** is a classic triad for AAA rupture (although this triad is more specific than sensitive). Patients with a ruptured AAA may have a rapid cardiovascular collapse.

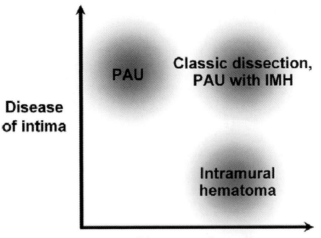

FIGURE 23-3. Acute aortic syndrome is caused by often overlapping aortic pathologies that are characterized by varying degrees of disease of the intima and/or media. (From Sundt TM. Intramural hematoma and penetrating atherosclerotic ulcer of the aorta. *Ann Thorac Surg* 2007;83:S835–S841, with permission.)

- Dyspnea
- Heart failure symptoms or hypotension from hemopericardium/tamponade and/or aortic regurgitation
- Stroke from compromise of cerebral vascular flow
- Syncope
- Paresis from compromise of spinal artery flow
- Abdominal, arm, or leg pain from compromise of arterial blood flow

Patients presenting with type A dissection may also present with ST-segment-elevation myocardial infarction (STEMI) due to proximal dissection involving the coronary ostia.

Patients presenting with a slowly enlarging aneurysm are often asymptomatic but may describe more chronic symptoms that will depend on the location of the aneurysm:

- Chronic chest and/or back pain related to compression of intrathoracic structures
- Dysphagia related to compression of the esophagus
- Dyspnea, cough, or wheezing related to compression of the trachea
- Heart failure symptoms from aortic regurgitation
- Abdominal pain or lower back pain with AAA

Family history is important to obtain, specifically to determine whether there is a family history of aortic aneurysm and/or dissection.

Physical Exam

A rapid exam should focus on the cardiovascular system, specifically looking for:

- Cardiac
  - Tachycardia
  - Hypertension or hypotension; widened pulse pressure with chronic aortic regurgitation (AR)

- Systolic ejection click (suggestive of a BAV)
- Diastolic decrescendo murmur (AR)
- Decreased heart sounds and elevated jugular venous pulse (suggestive of tamponade)
- **Vascular**
  - Unequal pulses and/or blood pressure (compromised vascular flow)
  - Cold, painful extremity
  - Pulsatile abdominal mass
- **Neurologic**
  - Focal neurologic deficit, usually due to an ischemic stroke (either from an embolic event or from compromised vascular flow due to a flap)
  - Paraplegia (from compromised blood flow to the spine)
- **Pulmonary**
  - Tachypnea ± hypoxia from heart failure
- **General**
  - Physical features suggestive of MFS or LDS

Diagnostic Evaluation

Rapid onset of severe symptoms or physical findings suggestive of acute aortic syndrome should prompt an emergent evaluation. For chronic symptoms, diagnostic workup may be less urgent. Tests are tailored to specific presentations and the resources available.

- **Chest x-ray (CXR)**: Findings include widened mediastinum, enlargement of aortic knob, tracheal deviation (**CXR may be normal in 10%–15% of acute dissections**; none of these signs is very sensitive nor specific).
- **Transthoracic echocardiography (TTE)**: Evaluates for the presence of aortic regurgitation (AR), pericardial effusion, proximal ascending aortic dimensions, and BAV. However, TTE is unable to reliably measure aortic dimensions beyond the proximal aortic root, and sensitivity is low for dissection.
- **Transesophageal echocardiography (TEE)**: Sensitivity of >95%, specificity 90% to 95% for most thoracic aortic pathology while giving similar functional information as TTE. Test of choice for diagnosing BAV. However, the distal ascending aorta and aortic arch vessels are often not seen well. Sedation is needed, which may be difficult or impossible in an unstable patient.
- **Computed tomography (CT)**: Rapid, readily available, and accurate. It is the test of choice for acute aortic syndromes in most hospitals. Sensitivity and specificity >95%. Dependent on adequate contrast bolus. Can detail the relationship to renal and visceral vessels for AAA. Does not detect aortic regurgitation. There are risks with IV contrast in patients with renal insufficiency.
- **Magnetic resonance imaging (MRI)**: Sensitivity and specificity >95%. The most complete test in terms of anatomic detail, aortic valve evaluation, and low-risk profile. However, it is often too time-consuming for an unstable patient.
- **Aortography**: Can diagnose a dissection (sensitivity 85%–90%, specificity 95%), but limited ability to detect IMH or PAU. Used primarily to evaluate for coronary disease prior to elective rather than emergent surgery.
- **Abdominal ultrasonography**: Used to diagnose and follow abdominal aortic aneurysm. Noninvasive but less accurate than CT.
- Although CT, MRI, and TEE provide excellent specificity and sensitivity for the diagnosis of acute aortic syndromes, none is perfect. If the initial test is inconclusive, then additional imaging may be warranted to definitively include or exclude the diagnosis.

TREATMENT

Acute Aortic Syndrome (AAS)

Medical

Patients with AAS are often tachycardic and hypertensive. The major goal of medical management is decreasing the heart rate (HR) and blood pressure (BP) to minimize the risk of further complications from the underlying aortic pathology. A HR of 60 and systolic BP of 100 to 120 or mean arterial pressure (MAP) of 60 to 75 are reasonable goals of therapy. Medications indicated in AAS include:

- **Beta blockers (BBs)**
  - First-line agents for AAS
  - Decrease HR, BP, and the force of left ventricular (LV) ejection (dP/dT)
  - Esmolol, a short-acting IV BB, is commonly used
  - Administer before agents that may decrease BP but induce reflex tachycardia (i.e., nitroprusside)
- **Calcium-channel blockers (CCBs)**
  - Verapamil or diltiazem
  - Second-line agents when BBs are not tolerated
- **Sodium nitroprusside**
  - IV medication used for additional lowering of BP when a BB or CCB provides inadequate control
- **Labetalol**
  - IV or PO medication with both beta- and alpha-blocking effects
  - Can be used as a single agent or in combination
- **Vasopressors**
  - If vasopressors are needed for hypotension, norepinephrine (Levophed) or phenylephrine (Neo-synephrine) are preferred, as they are less likely to increase dP/dT

Currently, medical treatment is the preferred management strategy for type B thoracic aortic pathology unless particular high-risk features are present, which may lead to surgical or (perhaps increasingly) endovascular management.

Surgical/Endovascular

Urgent surgical consultation is appropriate for most type A aortic pathology, complicated type B aortic pathology, and symptomatic AAA.

- **Type A aortic pathology**
  - Most hospitals will manage patients presenting with AAS and type A aortic pathology with emergent surgery; type A dissection certainly requires urgent surgical consultation.
  - Although controversial, a strategy endorsed in Asia is for early watchful waiting in patients with type A IMH and PAU: close monitoring and frequent imaging to evaluate for signs of progression that would trigger surgical repair.
  - The surgical procedure performed depends on the extent of aortic involvement and function of the aortic valve; generally the diseased portion of the aorta will be replaced with a graft and the aortic valve replaced as well if necessary.
- **Type B aortic pathology**
  - Type B aortic pathology is usually managed medically unless certain high-risk features are present
  - Indications for surgery (or endovascular or interventional treatment):
    - Vital organ or limb ischemia
    - Retrograde extension into the ascending aorta

- Rupture or impending rupture
- Uncontrolled pain or hypertension (HTN)
- Rapid expansion in aortic size or extension of a dissection
- Endovascular stent-graft placement may play a role for many patients with the high-risk features indicated above; it has less morbidity and mortality than open repair. Its role in the management of patients with acute and chronic type B dissection, IMH, and PAU is not yet clear.
- Percutaneous balloon fenestration ± stent implantation can be used for static or dynamic obstruction of branch vessels by a dissecting flap causing organ or limb ischemia.
- **Symptomatic AAA**
  - Symptomatic AAA requires urgent surgical consultation. Operative mortality for urgent AAA repair is ~20% and increases to 50% if the AAA has ruptured.

Asymptomatic Enlarging Aortic Aneurysm

Medical

Aggressive control of BP (goal systolic BP 105–120 mm Hg) is critical in minimizing the risk of rupture, dissection, and aneurysmal growth. BBs have been the most widely studied and have positive effects by lowering BP, reducing the force of each systole (dP/dt), and possibly improving connective tissue metabolism. Angiotensin receptor blockers (ARBs) may have a role in preventing aneurysm formation in patients with MFS. Additional risk-factor modification includes control of diabetes mellitus, tobacco cessation, and treatment of hyperlipidemia, particularly with HMG-CoA reductase inhibitors (statins).

Additionally, patients with a dilated aortic root or thoracic aneurysm should avoid activities that abruptly increase intrathoracic pressure and BP, such as weight lifting, climbing steep inclines, gymnastics, and pull-ups. Collision sports should also be avoided, as these may precipitate dissection or rupture. Aerobic exercise can be pursued, but at a decreased level of intensity. There is an increased risk of dissection during pregnancy in MFS and other genetically triggered thoracic aneurysm syndromes.

Surgical/Endovascular

Prophylactic aortic surgery is recommended when the expected benefit of preventing rupture outweighs the risk of the procedure. At experienced centers, the operative mortality for elective repair is 2% to 5% for ascending aortic surgery, 8% to 10% for descending and thoracoabdominal aneurysms, and 2% to 6% for AAAs. **Decisions regarding the timing of prophylactic surgery are mostly driven by aortic dimension with additional consideration to the underlying etiology and family history.** The exact criteria for surgery or endovascular repair will vary depending on institutional experience and patient comorbidities. Importantly, in patients with **symptomatic aneurysms**, surgery should not be delayed until the thresholds listed below are met.

Indications for Surgery for Asymptomatic Aortic Aneurysms

- **Ascending aorta** (see Fig. 23-4)
  - MFS and BAV
    - Dimension ≥5 cm (in some instances ≥4.5 cm)
    - Growth rate >0.5 cm/year
    - At the time of aortic valve replacement if aortic dimension is ≥4.5 cm (≥4 cm in some specialized centers)
  - Causes *other* than MFS or BAV
    - Dimension ≥5.5 cm
    - Growth rate ≥1 cm/year

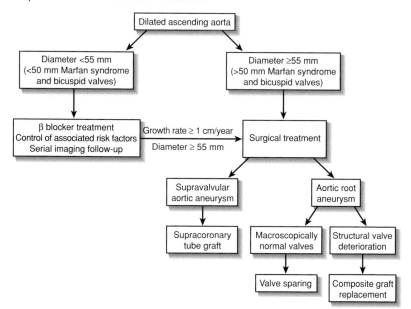

FIGURE 23-4. Medical and surgical management of an ascending aortic aneurysm. (From Nataf P, Lansac E. Dilation of the thoracic aorta: medical and surgical management. *Heart* 2006;92:1345–1352, with permission.)

- **Descending aorta**
  - ≥6 cm
  - Growth rate ≥1 cm/year
- **Abdominal aorta**
  - Males: 5.5 cm
  - Females: 4.5 to 5.0 cm can be considered
  - Growth rate ≥0.6 to 1 cm/year

Types of Surgical and Endovascular Procedures

In caring for patients who have undergone an aortic repair, it is essential to know the particular type of repair that was performed.

- **Ascending aorta**
  - Reduction aortoplasty with or without external synthetic wrapping
  - Replacement of the supracoronary ascending aorta with a synthetic tube graft (used for aneurysms that do not involve the sinuses of Valsalva)
  - Bentall procedure—replacement of the sinuses, ascending aorta, and aortic valve with a Dacron tube graft and prosthetic aortic valve sewn into the aortic annulus with the native coronary arteries (buttons) reimplanted into the Dacron graft (used for patients with significant valve disease and aortic aneurysms involving the root)
  - Valve-sparing root replacement—similar to the Bentall procedure except that the aortic valve leaflets are preserved and reimplanted within the graft (used for patients with normal aortic valve leaflets)
  - Ross procedure—excision of the aortic valve and root, replacing it with the patient's own pulmonary valve and root; the pulmonary root is replaced with a

cadaveric pulmonary or aortic homograft (often complicated by neoaortic root dilatation)
- Prosthetic arch graft—replacement of the aortic arch with reimplantation of the brachiocephalic vessels into a multilimbed prosthetic arch graft
- **Descending aorta**
  - Synthetic tube graft made of Dacron or Gore-Tex replaces the resected aneurysmal segment
  - Endovascular stent-grafts are investigational but may have a role in patients at high risk for aortic rupture but also at high risk for aortic surgery
- **Abdominal aorta**
  - Synthetic tube graft made of Dacron or Gore-Tex is constructed within aneurysmal aortic segment and can be extended down into iliac arteries if necessary
  - Endovascular stent graft
    - Roughly 50% of AAAs are anatomically suitable for endovascular repair
    - Considered particularly in older patients and those at high surgical risk
    - Frequent need for reintervention, often due to endoleaks, which continue to place the patient at risk for aortic rupture

PREVENTION

Surveillance Recommendations

The frequency of surveillance imaging of a patient's aorta depends on its current dimension, the rate of progression, and whether surgery has already been performed. After an initial diagnosis of an aortic aneurysm is made, the next evaluation of aortic dimension should be performed in 3 to 6 months to assess its growth rate. Depending on the growth rate and baseline size, subsequent imaging should be done every 6 to 12 months; as aneurysms get closer to surgical thresholds, the frequency of imaging may increase. It is important to image the aorta serially in those who have had surgical repair of a portion of the aorta, looking for the presence of pseudoaneurysm or aneurysms in unrepaired segments of the aorta. The imaging modality utilized to evaluate an aorta over time may vary depending on the anatomic location of the aorta being followed, the adequacy of a particular modality in a given patient, and the nature of the abnormality being followed. CT or MRI is most commonly used for TAA, but TTE can often be used to follow aneurysms of the aortic root. Ultrasound is the most commonly used screening tool for AAAs, with CT or MRI used mainly for larger AAAs to help guide decisions on specific surgical repair.

Screening Recommendations

- Patients with a known TAA should be screened at least once with an abdominal ultrasound for AAA, as up to 25% will have concomitant AAA.
- First-degree relatives of patients with a known familial aortopathy should undergo screening. TTE is usually sufficient to look at the aortic valve and aortic root dimension, but other imaging modalities may be indicated if one is interested in regions of the aorta beyond the root.
- Recommendations to screen for AAA vary considerably. In general, most experts agree that the physical exam has limited sensitivity for screening. The U.S. Preventive Services Task Force recommends one-time screening for abdominal aortic aneurysm (AAA) by ultrasonography in men 65 to 75 years of age who have ever smoked tobacco products, but it does not recommend screening women or lower-risk men. The Society for Vascular Surgery and the American Association for Vascular Surgery recommend ultrasound screening for all men 60 to 85 years of age, women 60 to 85 years of age with cardiovascular risk factors, and all patients over 50 years of age with a family history of AAA.

ACKNOWLEDGMENTS

Special thanks to Alan Braverman, MD, FACC; Professor of Medicine, Director of Marfan Syndrome Clinic, Cardiovascular Division, Washington University School of Medicine, for reviewing this chapter.

KEY POINTS TO REMEMBER

- Cystic medial degeneration is the most common underlying histologic abnormality leading to ascending aortic aneurysms, while atherosclerosis is the most common cause of aneurysms of the descending thoracic and abdominal aorta.
- Acute aortic syndrome should be considered in any patient with an acute onset of severe chest, back, or abdominal pain. Treatment requires aggressive control of heart rate and blood pressure with a beta blocker as the first-line agent and urgent surgical consultation.
- Type A acute aortic syndrome involves the ascending aorta and/or arch and is almost always managed surgically.
- Type B acute aortic syndrome is usually managed medically except when certain high-risk features are present.
- Decisions regarding prophylactic surgical repair of asymptomatic aortic aneurysms should be made based on specific aortic dimensions, location of the aneurysm, underlying etiology of the aortopathy, and patient-specific factors such as gender and comorbidities.

REFERENCES AND SUGGESTED READINGS

Boyer JK, Gutierrez F, and Braverman AC. Approach to the dilated aortic root. *Curr Opin Cardiol* 2004;19:563–569.

Braverman AC, Harris KM. Management of aortic intramural hematoma. *Curr Opin Cardiol* 1995;10:501–504.

Braverman AC. Aortic dissection. *Curr Opin Cardiol* 1997;12:389–390.

Braverman AC. Penetrating atherosclerotic ulcers of the aorta. *Curr Opin Cardiol* 1994;9:591–597.

Brewster DC, Cronenwett JL, Hallett JW, et al. Guidelines for the treatment of AAA: report of a subcommittee of the Joint Council of the American Association for Vascular Surgery and Society for Vascular Surgery. *J Vasc Surg* 2003;37:1106–1117.

Cecconi M, Nistri S, Quarti A, et al. Aortic dilatation in patients with bicuspid aortic valve. *J Cardiovasc Med* 2006;7:11–20.

Davies RR, Goldstein LJ, Coady MA, et al. Yearly rupture or dissection rates for thoracic aortic aneurysms: simple prediction based on size. *Ann Thorac Surg* 2002;73:17–28.

Habashi JP, Judge DP, Holm TM, et al. Losartan, an AT1 antagonist, prevents aortic aneurysm in a mouse model of Marfan syndrome. *Science* 2006;312(5770):117–121.

Hagan PG, Nienaber CA, Isselbacher EM, et al. The international registry of acute aortic dissection (IRAD): new insights into an old disease. *JAMA* 2000;283:897–903.

Ince H, Nienaber CA. Diagnosis and management of patients with aortic dissection. *Heart* 2007;93:266–270.

Isselbacher EM. Diseases of the aorta. In: Zipes DP, Libby P, Bonow RO, et al., eds. *Braunwald's Heart Disease: A Textbook of Cardiovascular Medicine,* 7th ed. Philadelphia: Elsevier Saunders; 2005:1403–1435.

Isselbacher EM. Thoracic and abdominal aortic aneurysms. *Circulation* 2005;111:816–828.

Kent KC, Zwolak RM, Jaff MR, et al. Screening for abdominal aortic aneurysm: a consensus statement. *J Vasc Surg* 2004;39:267–269.

Loeys BL, Schwarze U, Holm T, et al. Aneurysm syndromes caused by mutations in the TGF-β receptor. *N Engl J Med* 2006;355:788–798.

Maraj R, Rerkpattanapipat P, Jacobs LE, et al. Meta-analysis of 143 reported cases of aortic intramural hematoma. *Am J Cardiol* 2000;86:664–668.

Nataf P, Lansac E. Dilation of the thoracic aorta: medical and surgical management. *Heart* 2006;92:1345–1352.

Pretre R, Von Segesser LK. Aortic dissection. *Lancet* 1997;349:1461–1464.

Shiga T, Wajima Z, Apfel CC, et al. Diagnostic accuracy of transesophageal echocardiography, helical computed tomography, and magnetic resonance imaging for suspected thoracic aortic dissection: systematic review and meta-analysis. *Arch Intern Med* 2006;166:1350–1356.

Shores J, Berger KR, Murphy EA, et al. Progression of aortic dilatation and the benefit of long-term β-adrenergic blockade in Marfan's syndrome. *N Engl J Med* 1994;330:1335–1341.

Sundt TM. Intramural hematoma and penetrating atherosclerotic ulcer of the aorta. *Ann Thorac Surg* 2007;83:S835–S841.

von Kodolitsch Y, Csösz SK, Koschyk DH, et al. Intramural hematoma of the aorta: predictors of progression to dissection and rupture. *Circulation* 2003;107:1158–1163.

Deep Venous Thrombosis

Sitaramesh Emani and Phillip S. Cuculich

INTRODUCTION

Deep venous thrombosis (DVT) is a condition characterized by an appropriate activation of the clotting cascade leading to formation of venous thrombus, primarily in the extremities. DVT is part of a larger spectrum of clotting disorders collectively referred to as venous thromboembolism (VTE), which includes pulmonary embolism. It is estimated that 600,000 cases of VTE occur yearly in the United States, and two-thirds of these are from DVT alone.

Natural History

The classic environment for the development of DVT is Virchow's triad, which includes (1) disruption of normal blood flow (venostasis), (2) endothelial injury to a vessel wall, and (3) abnormal activation of the clotting cascade. Table 24-1 is a list of common risk factors for DVT and concomitant estimated relative risks for each condition. Patients with multiple risk factors have a much higher likelihood of forming a DVT than those with a single risk factor.

Clinical Presentation

Traditionally, the presentation of a DVT includes **tenderness, erythema, and swelling of an affected limb**. Other presentations of more advanced or long-standing disease are listed in Table 24-2. The most important reason to accurately diagnose and treat DVT is to prevent pulmonary embolism (PE). Distal venous thromboses (calf) often resolve spontaneously and infrequently cause PE. Unfortunately, **roughly 25% of untreated distal DVTs propagate to proximal veins**, and the **risk of PE from an untreated proximal venous thrombosis increases to near 50%**.

DIAGNOSTIC STUDIES

The most important feature in the diagnosis of DVT is the physician's degree of clinical suspicion (pretest probability). The Wells criteria (Table 24-3) constitute a validated method for identifying a patient's risk of having a DVT.

The choice of subsequent diagnostic testing to "rule in" or "rule out" DVT is greatly affected by the pretest probability.

- D-**dimer**—measurement of fibrinogen degradation. The normal D-dimer level (negative test) has a high negative predictive value in the evaluation of a DVT. Positive results are less useful, as many conditions can lead to an elevated D-dimer (sensitivity 96%–100%, specificity 50%).

TABLE 24-1	COMMON RISK FACTORS FOR DEVELOPMENT OF VENOUS THROMBOEMBOLISM IN VIRCHOW'S TRIAD	

Risk Factor	Estimated Relative Risk of VTE*
1. Venostasis	
• Recent surgery	5–200
• Recent hospitalization	5
• Extended travel (>8 hours)	3
2. Endothelial injury	
• Trauma	5–200
3. Propensity to clot	
• Prior history of VTE	50
• Inherited thrombophilias	
• Factor V Leiden mutation	50 (homozygous), 5 (heterozygous)
• Antithrombin deficiency	25
• Protein C deficiency	10
• Protein S deficiency	10
• Antiphospholipid antibodies	2–10
• Prothrombin G20210A mutation	2–3
• Hyperhomocysteinemia	1–3
• Estrogen use	
• Oral contraceptive	5
• Hormone-replacement therapy	2
• Selective estrogen-receptor modulator	3–5
• Age	
• Age >70	10
• Age >50	5
• Pregnancy	7
• Cancer	5
• Obesity	1–3

*Estimated risks vary greatly based on patient populations, severity of risk factors, methods of VTE diagnosis, and laboratory values to define risk factors.
Source: Adapted from Bates SM, Ginsberg JS. Treatment of deep-vein thrombosis. *N Engl J Med* 2004;351:269–277, with permission.

- **Venous ultrasound**—a combination of compression ultrasound (clot presence generally prevents compression) and Doppler flow evaluation (clot presence obstructs flow). For symptomatic patients with proximal vein thrombosis, the sensitivity (89%–96%) and specificity (94%–99%) are high. The sensitivity is considerably lower for patients without symptoms (42%–67%) or for patients with suspected calf DVT (50%).

TABLE 24-2	PRESENTATIONS OF DEEP VENOUS THROMBOSIS

- Local
  - Pain, erythema, edema
  - Postphlebitic syndrome/chronic venous insufficiency
  - Phlegmasia cerulea dolens (venous gangrene)
- Systemic
  - Pulmonary embolism
  - Chronic thromboembolic pulmonary hypertension

TABLE 24-3	WELLS CLINICAL MODEL FOR PREDICTING PRETEST PROBABILITY OF DEEP-VENOUS THROMBOSIS

Clinical Characteristic[†]	Score[*]
Active cancer (treatment ongoing, administered within previous 6 months or palliative)	1
Paralysis, paresis, or recent plaster immobilization of the lower extremities	1
Recently bedridden >3 days or major surgery within previous 12 weeks requiring general or regional anesthesia	1
Localized tenderness along the distribution of the deep venous system	1
Swelling of entire leg	1
Calf swelling >3 cm larger than asymptomatic side (measured 10 cm below tibial tuberosity)	1
Pitting edema confined to the symptomatic leg	1
Collateral superficial veins (nonvaricose)	1
Previously documented DVT	1
Alternative diagnosis at least as likely as DVT	−2

[*]A score of 2 or higher indicates that the probability of DVT is "likely"; a score of less than 2 indicates that the probability is "unlikely."

[†]In patients who have symptoms in both legs. the more symptomatic leg is used.

Source: From Wells PS, Anderson DR, Bormanis J, et al. Value assessment of pretest probability of deep-vein thrombosis in clinical management. *Lancet* 1997;350:1795–1798, and Scarvelis D, Wells PS. Diagnosis and treatment of deep-vein thrombosis. *CMAJ* 2006;175:1087–1092, with permission.

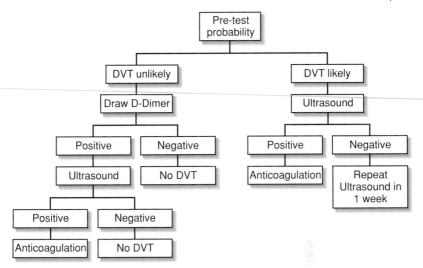

FIGURE 24-1. Diagnostic approach to deep venous thrombosis.

Therefore a patient with low pretest probability for DVT should receive a **D-dimer test to rule out** the diagnosis. A patient with a higher pre-test probability should have **venous ultrasound to rule in** the diagnosis. The decision tree shown in Figure 24-1 provides a recommended algorithm by which the appropriate test and diagnosis can be chosen.

TREATMENT

The treatment for a DVT is anticoagulation. Initiation of anticoagulation is outlined below:

- For suspected DVT, anticoagulation with low-molecular-weight heparin (LMWH) or unfractionated heparin (UFH) can be started before confirmatory results are available.
- In general, **subcutaneous LMWH is preferred over a continuous infusion of UFH for initiation of therapy**.
  - LMWH can be administered on an outpatient basis and requires less monitoring.
  - Intravenous UFH is preferred if contraindications to LMWH exist (e.g. renal impairment).
- Long-term oral anticoagulation with **warfarin should be started during initiation of therapy with LMWH/UFH,** and LMWH/UFH can be stopped when adequate oral anticoagulation has been established (target INR 2–3).
  - Initiating warfarin without UFH/LMWH increases the risk for a rare but serious complication of warfarin-induced skin necrosis.
  - Some evidence suggests that patients with antiphospholipid antibody (APA) would benefit from a higher target INR or longer duration of anticoagulation therapy.

- Patients with VTE and cancer are particularly thrombophilic, and data have suggested a greater benefit from long-term anticoagulation with LMWH rather than with warfarin.
- Patients on UFH or LMWH require monitoring of platelet values to **screen for heparin-induced thrombocytopenia (HIT)**, an immune response to platelet factor-4 (PF-4) that causes a markedly increased risk of thrombosis.
  - The diagnosis of HIT is strongly suspected if platelet counts decrease to <50% of the initial level or <100,000 in the setting of heparin exposure.
  - If HIT is suspected, UFH and LMWH should be stopped immediately.
  - Because of the increased risk of thrombosis, substitution of heparin with a direct thrombin inhibitor (lepirudin [Refludan] or argatroban) is essential.
  - A PF-4 antibody test should be ordered to confirm the diagnosis.

The **appropriate length of anticoagulation therapy is determined by underlying risk factors** (Table 24-4). Patients with identifiable and reversible risk factors are unlikely to have a spontaneous recurrence of DVT and should receive shorter courses of anticoagulation. Patients with idiopathic DVT or nonmodifiable risk factors are more likely to have recurrences and are treated longer.

In addition to anticoagulation, other treatments that help improve outcomes in patients with DVT include:

- Compressions stockings
  - Improve swelling and reduce the incidence of postphlebitic syndrome
  - Should be started early in the treatment course
  - Can be continued for up to 2 years postdiagnosis
- Ambulation
  - Patients with acute onset DVT should be encouraged to ambulate as tolerated.

Alternatives to anticoagulation therapy are available but are generally recommended only in certain situations:

- Inferior vena cava (IVC) filters
  - Removable IVC filters should be considered if anticoagulation is temporarily contraindicated (severe GI bleed, recent trauma, recent cranial surgery).

TABLE 24-4   DURATION OF ANTICOAGULATION THERAPY FOR DVT

Category	Recommended Length of Therapy
DVT in the setting of a reversible risk factor (limb immobilization, recent surgery)	3–6 months
DVT with 1 prothrombotic condition OR Idiopathic DVT (no identifiable risk factor)	6–12 months; consider indefinite therapy, but should weigh risk vs. benefit of anticoagulation
DVT with ≥2 prothrombotic conditions OR Recurrent DVT	12 months to indefinite
DVT in the setting of active cancer	Use of LMWH may be considered, 6 month minimum; if cancer is treated, continue 6 months after cure

DVT, deep venous thrombosis; LMWH, low-molecular-weight heparin.

- Permanent IVC filters can be considered in addition to anticoagulation for recurrent DVT despite anticoagulation therapy. Without anticoagulation, however, permanent IVC filters may increase the incidence of recurrent DVT.
- There is no evidence proving mortality benefits from IVC filters.
- Catheter-based thrombolytic therapy or venous thrombectomy is a recommended therapy for limb gangrene.

SECONDARY PREVENTION OF VTE

Prevention of a second VTE event involves three important steps: (1) **minimize modifiable risk factors**, (2) **implement age-appropriate cancer screening, and** (3) **identifying inherited thrombophilias.**

- Modifiable risk factors
  - Elimination of exogenous estrogen, if possible
  - Leg mobility exercises for extended trips
- Screening for malignancy
  - Up to 10% of patients with idiopathic DVT will be found to have an occult malignancy.
  - All patients should undergo age-appropriate cancer screening if not already performed.
  - Close clinical follow-up is recommended for at least 2 years.
  - Routine extensive screening for cancer without clinical signs may lead to more diagnoses of cancer but does not necessarily improve long-term outcomes.
- Screening for inherited thrombophilia
  - **Routine laboratory screening for thrombophilias in all patients with DVT is not recommended.**
  - Laboratory testing may be warranted if the following clinical features are present:
    - **Lack of identifiable risk factors**
    - **Multiple VTE events**
    - **Family history of VTE**
    - **Age <50**
    - **History of thrombosis in portal, hepatic, mesenteric, or cerebral veins**
    - **Personal history of premature fetal death in females**
  - Available laboratory studies can be divided into DNA tests, antibody titers, and factor activity levels.
  - **DNA tests** are not affected by treatment for VTE and may be ordered at any time during the workup; they include factor V Leiden and prothrombin 20210.
  - **Antibody titers** can be performed during treatment for VTE but should be repeated after several weeks to confirm their presence; they include anticardiolipin and lupus anticoagulant.
  - **Factor activity levels** are affected by the ongoing thrombosis. Low-activity test results can lead to a false diagnosis of thrombophilia and unnecessary anticoagulation. Generally these tests are ordered after anticoagulation has been completed: protein C activity, protein S activity, antithrombin-3 activity.

PRIMARY PREVENTION OF VTE

Roughly 25% of venous thromboembolism cases are associated with hospitalization. Because of the high risk of developing VTE in the hospital, **every hospitalized patient should undergo a risk assessment.** Pharmacologic prophylaxis is recommended for patients who are >40 years old, have had limited mobility for ≥3 days, and have at least one risk factor (Table 24-1).

Pharmacologic therapy can include (1) unfractionated heparin 5000 U SQ q8h; (2) enoxaparin 40 mg SQ daily; (3) dalteparin 5000 U SQ daily or; (4) fondaparinux 2.5 mg SQ daily. If patients cannot receive pharmacologic prophylaxis, the use of graduated compression stockings or pneumatic compression devices is recommended.

KEY POINTS TO REMEMBER

- DVT diagnosis is based on clinical suspicion (pretest probability).
- D-dimer is best used to rule out DVT in low-risk patients. Venous ultrasound is best used to rule in DVT in intermediate- and high-risk patients.
- Anticoagulation initially with LMWH or heparin, followed by long-term warfarin, is the preferred therapy.
- Duration of anticoagulation depends on the underlying risks of recurrence.
- Medical prophylaxis for VTE is strongly recommended for high-risk hospitalized medical patients.

REFERENCES AND SUGGESTED READINGS

Bates SM, Ginsberg JS. Treatment of deep-vein thrombosis. *N Engl J Med* 2004;351: 269–277.

Bauer KA. The thrombophilias: well-defined risk factors with uncertain therapeutic implications. *Ann Intern Med* 2001;135:367–373.

Büller HR, Agnelli GA, Hall RD, et al. Antithrombotic therapy for venous thromboembolic disease: the Seventh ACCP Conference on Antithrombotic and Thrombolytic Therapy. *Chest* 2004;126:401S–428S.

Du Breuil AL, Umland EM. Outpatient management of anticoagulation therapy. *Am Fam Physician* 2007;75:1031–1042.

Francis CW. Clinical practice: prophylaxis for thromboembolism in hospitalized medical patients. *N Engl J Med* 2007;356:1438–1444.

Kujovich J. Hormones and pregnancy: thromboembolic risks for women. *Br J Haematol* 2004;126:443–454.

Middeldorp S, Meinardi JR, Koopman MMW, et al. A prospective study of asymptomatic carriers of the factor V Leiden mutation to determine the incidence of venous thromboembolism. *Ann Intern Med* 2001;135:322–327.

Monreal M, Lensing AW, Prins MH, et al. Screening for occult cancer in patients with acute deep vein thrombosis or pulmonary embolism. *J Thromb Haemost* 2004;2: 876–881.

Piccioli A, Lensing AW, Prins MH, et al. Extensive screening for occult malignant disease in idiopathic venous thromboembolism: a prospective randomized clinical trial. *J Thromb Haemost* 2004;2:884–889.

Qaseem A, Snow V, Barry P, et al. Current diagnosis of venous thromboembolism in primary care: a clinical practice guideline from the American Academy of Family Physicians and the American College of Physicians. *Ann Intern Med* 2007;146:454–458.

Scarvelis D, Wells PS. Diagnosis and treatment of deep-vein thrombosis. *CMAJ* 2006;175:1087–1092.

Segal JB, Eng J, Tamariz LJ, et al. Review of the evidence in diagnosis of deep venous thrombosis and pulmonary embolism. *Ann Fam Med* 2007;5:63–73.

Segal JB, Streiff MB, Hofmann LV, et al. Management of venous thromboembolism: a systematic review for a practice guideline. *Ann Intern Med* 2007;146:211–222.

Snow V, Qaseem A, Barry P, et al. Management of venous thromboembolism: a clinical practice guideline from the American College of Physicians and the American Academy of Family Physicians. *Ann Intern Med* 2007;146:204–210.

Wells PS, Anderson DR, Bormanis J, et al. Value assessment of pretest probability of deep-vein thrombosis in clinical management. *Lancet* 1997;350:1795–1798.

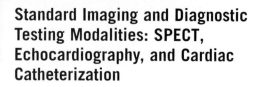
CARDIAC SPECT

Introduction

For assessment of myocardial perfusion and viability, the most commonly utilized modality in nuclear cardiology is single photon emission computed tomography (SPECT).

Physics

The basis for nuclear cardiac imaging is the administration of a radiotracer that is taken up by a viable cardiac myocyte and retained for a given period of time. The vast majority of SPECT studies use agents based on either **technetium-99m** (^{99m}Tc) (^{99m}Tc-sestamibi, ^{99m}Tc-tetrofosmin, ^{99m}Tc-teboroxime) or **thallium-201** (^{201}Tl). The uptake of radiotracer by the myocardium is directly proportional to myocardial perfusion. After uptake, gamma ray photons are emitted by the radiotracer. Thus, the amount of photon emission is directly proportional to myocardial perfusion.

A **gamma camera** (Fig. 25-1) captures the emitted photons and uses them to produce a digital image. The camera consists of the following:

- The **collimator,** which allows only those relatively few photons that are perpendicular to it to be captured. The majority of photons emitted by the radiotracer are not perpendicular to the collimator and thus ignored from an imaging standpoint.
- **Detector crystals,** which are struck by the perpendicular photons passing through the collimator. The collision of photons with detector crystals produces light (known as a **scintillation event**).
- **Photomultiplier tubes,** which sense scintillation events and convert the light into an electrical signal. The signal is then processed to record the energy and spatial location of the detected photon.

During a SPECT study, with the patient lying supine on the table, the radiotracer is administered intravenously. The gamma camera, placed near the patient, detects the photons emitted from the myocardium. The camera is then rotated to different positions to collect photons from different views. Multiple images, each comprising 20 to 25 seconds of emission data, are collected. Each one of the separate "projection" images constitutes a two-dimensional (2D) snapshot of myocardial perfusion from the angle at which the projection was acquired. Then, the imaging information from each of the angles is **back projected** onto an imaging matrix, creating a reconstruction of the heart (Fig. 25-2).

The gamma camera acquires SPECT data by rotating in an orbital path around the patient. Three modes are used for SPECT data acquisition:

Localization scintillation event signal from apex of heart

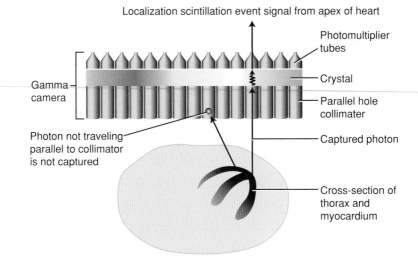

Photomultiplier tubes

Gamma camera

Crystal

Parallel hole collimater

Photon not traveling parallel to collimator is not captured

Captured photon

Cross-section of thorax and myocardium

FIGURE 25-1. Transmission of photons emitted from myocardium to gamma camera. (From Braunwald E, Zipes DP, Libby P, et al., eds. *Braunwald's Heart Disease: A Text-book of Cardiovascular Medicine,* 7th ed. Philadelphia: Elsevier; 2004, with permission.)

- **Step-and-shoot mode is the most common.** The camera rotates to predefined positions at discrete angles along the orbital path, acquires planar images for a fixed time, and then rotates to the next location. The camera does not detect counts while moving between positions.
- **Continuous step-and-shoot.** Counts are recorded as the camera moves to different positions. Spatial resolution is decreased slightly by movement of the camera, although only counts collected during the movement are affected.
- **In the continuous mode, the camera continually rotates around the radiation source, detecting photons while in motion.** There is a moderate decrease in spatial resolution as result of blurring from motion, but sensitivity is gained as more photons are detected.

SPECT orbits may be broadly classified as circular or noncircular. With **circular orbits,** the camera is at a fixed distance from the patient at all angles. With **noncircular orbits** (elliptical), the camera can be brought closer to the heart for some views. As the distance between the camera and the heart decreases, spatial resolution increases. Thus, noncircular orbits can be used as a method of attenuation correction to correct for decreased spatial resolution occurring at specific angles.

Circular orbits have been recommended by the 2006 guidelines of the American Society of Nuclear Cardiology, but the most important rule is to use a consistent approach to orbital selection.

The images are then acquired electronically. The long axis of the left ventricle is identified by special techniques, and then tomographic images in three standard planes (Fig. 25-3) are derived:

- **Short-axis images,** representing "donut-like" slices of the heart cut perpendicular to the long axis of the heart, are displayed beginning near the apex and moving toward the base. This view is similar to the short-axis view in two-dimensional echocardiography.

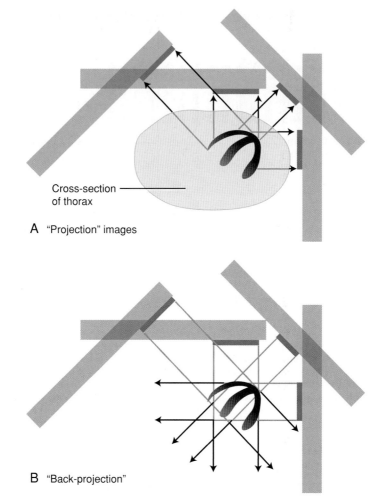

Cross-section of thorax

A "Projection" images

B "Back-projection"

FIGURE 25-2. Detection of photons by gamma camera. The camera is rotated to different angles to enable image acquisition from multiple views. (From Braunwald E, Zipes DP, Libby P, et al., eds. *Braunwald's Heart Disease: A Textbook of Cardiovascular Medicine,* 7th ed. Philadelphia: Elsevier; 2004, with permission.)

- **Vertical long-axis images** represent slices cut parallel to the long axis of the heart and also parallel to the long axis of the body; these are also termed vertical long-axis tomograms.
- **Horizontal long-axis images** represent slices also cut parallel to the long axis of the heart but perpendicular to the vertical long axis; these are also known as horizontal long-axis tomograms.

Applications

Uses for SPECT include **myocardial perfusion imaging (MPI), assessment of myocardial viability, and measurement of left ventricular (LV) volume and function**. MPI is by far the most common clinical application SPECT. It can be used in the setting of a stress test

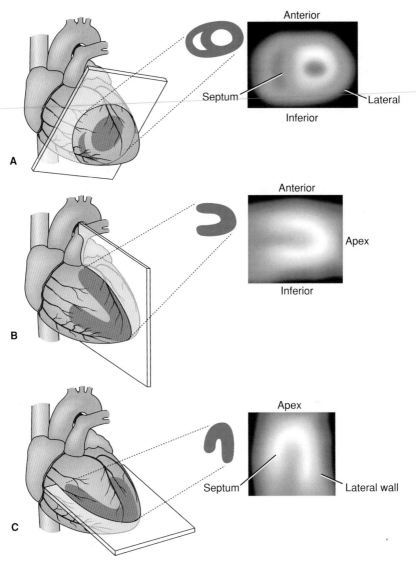

FIGURE 25-3. Tomographic views of the left ventricle. Short-axis view, vertical long-axis view, and horizontal long-axis view (top to bottom). (From Braunwald E, Zipes DP, Libby P, et al., eds. *Braunwald's Heart Disease: A Textbook of Cardiovascular Medicine,* 7th ed. Philadelphia: Elsevier; 2004, with permission.)

or as resting images only in a patient with active symptoms. Assessment of myocardial viability is less common, and the use of SPECT solely to determine LV volume and function is rare.

The goal of MPI is to identify normally perfused, ischemic, and infarcted myocardium. The most common way of performing SPECT MPI is as a stress test. The stress test examines coronary flow reserve by quantifying myocardial perfusion at rest and with stress. Stress can be accomplished by exercise or by administering a coronary vasodilator (adenosine or dipyridamole). A severe coronary stenosis at rest often has blood flow similar to a normal coronary vessel. When stress is applied, normal vessels show a physiologic increase in flow, whereas a significantly diseased vessel is unable to do so. Normally perfused myocardium shows normal perfusion during both rest and stress. Ischemic myocardium shows normal perfusion at rest but decreased perfusion with stress. Infarcted myocardium shows decreased perfusion at both rest and stress. There are considerable data showing poor outcomes in patients with large amounts of myocardial ischemia and infarction.

Understanding SPECT MPI requires understanding the properties of ^{201}Tl and ^{99}Tc. ^{201}Tl is biologically similar to potassium and taken up actively by myocytes. ^{201}Tl has greater myocardial extraction from the blood pool than ^{99}Tc agents and has a longer half-life. One of the most clinically important characteristics of ^{201}Tl is myocardial redistribution. A myocardial perfusion defect due to ischemic disease will initially have decreased ^{201}Tl uptake, but after 3 or 4 hours, ^{201}Tl will redistribute into the ischemic area by washout from normally perfused myocardium. However, ^{201}Tl will not wash out into infarcted myocardium. ^{99}Tc agents have slower myocardial uptake as well as shorter half-lives, and they do not significantly redistribute. Thus, imaging after the stress injection with ^{99}Tc is much more flexible than with ^{201}Tl, and image acquisition can be repeated if there is significant patient motion or instrument malfunction. **^{201}Tl is an optimal agent for detecting myocardial viability (rest imaging). ^{99}Tc agents are optimal for detecting myocardial ischemia (stress imaging).** Because the severity of coronary artery disease (CAD) needed to produce a detectable perfusion defect is less than that required to produce a wall motion abnormality, SPECT MPI tends to be more sensitive but less specific than stress echocardiography at detecting CAD.

Washington University/Barnes-Jewish Hospital uses a 1-day dual-radionuclide SPECT protocol. It consists of an injection of 3.0 to 3.5 mCi of ^{201}Tl at rest and an injection of 25 to 30 mCi of ^{99}Tc at peak stress. SPECT imaging starts immediately after the initial injection of ^{201}Tl at rest. Immediately following ^{201}Tl imaging, the patient undergoes the stress test. At peak exercise or vasodilator infusion, 25 to 30 mCi of ^{99}Tc is injected. SPECT imaging is repeated 15 to 30 minutes later. The entire exam takes ~90 minutes. In patients having active chest pain, a pain SPECT protocol can also be performed where only ^{99}Tc is injected, with imaging in 15 to 30 minutes. The presence of perfusion defects by ^{99}Tc pain imaging suggests either active ischemia or infarction, immediately placing a chest pain patient in a higher-risk category for CAD.

Myocardial viability can be assessed by using either ^{201}Tl or 18-fluorodeoxyglucose (FDG). ^{201}Tl is an excellent agent for viability, given its properties of redistribution and long half-life. If the goal of a SPECT examination is to assess myocardial viability, ^{201}Tl should ideally be performed 24 hours after injection, as this can detect an additional 8% to 15% of viable segments, which may be missed by 1-day rest–stress SPECT MPI alone. FDG is a PET radiotracer that can be used with SPECT. Two studies have demonstrated similar sensitivity to resting ^{201}Tl SPECT at detecting viable myocardium but increased specificity with FDG SPECT. Although the image quality and resolution of PET is clearly superior to those of SPECT, several studies have shown good correlations of viability between FDG PET and FDG SPECT.

The advent of ECG-gated SPECT enabled quantification of LV volume, ejection fraction, and wall motion abnormalities. These data are collected on almost all SPECT MPI studies. While they are clinically useful parameters, there is rarely a need to order a SPECT solely to acquire this information, as echocardiography can provide it in a faster, safer (no ionizing radiation), and more cost-efficient manner.

Limitations

While SPECT performs well in quantifying relative myocardial blood flow to the myocardium, it is unable to quantify absolute myocardial blood flow. SPECT does an excellent job at detecting single- and double-vessel CAD, but it can miss triple-vessel CAD, where myocardial perfusion will appear identical in all three coronary distributions. Again, this is because SPECT measures **relative blood flow**, not absolute rates of blood flow, and with triple-vessel CAD there may be balanced ischemia with global hypoperfusion. SPECT lacks the spatial and temporal resolution of PET. SPECT is also prone to attenuation. **Attenuation** occurs when emitted photons scatter in different directions as they travel through tissue in the body rather than moving directly in their initial trajectory. This decreases the spatial resolution of SPECT. Attenuation correction for PET is more reliable than for SPECT.

Conclusion

SPECT is a time-tested modality for assessing myocardial perfusion and viability. It can also provide some functional assessment (LV volume, ejection fraction, and wall motion). It is well validated for cardiovascular risk assessment and is also relatively cost-efficient. SPECT's main drawbacks are its ability to quantify only relative myocardial blood flow and miss triple-vessel CAD as well as its technical inferiority to PET.

Images

See Figures 25-4 through 25-7.

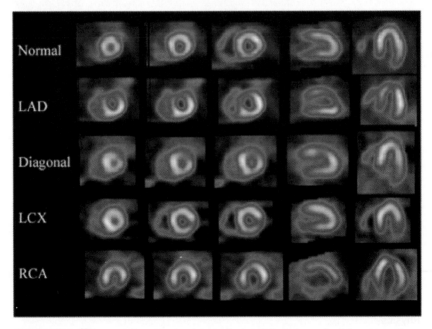

FIGURE 25-4. ^{99}Tc stress images showing perfusion defects in each of the respective coronary distributions. (From Fuster V et al., eds. *Hurst's The Heart,* 11th ed. New York: McGraw-Hill; 2005, with permission.)

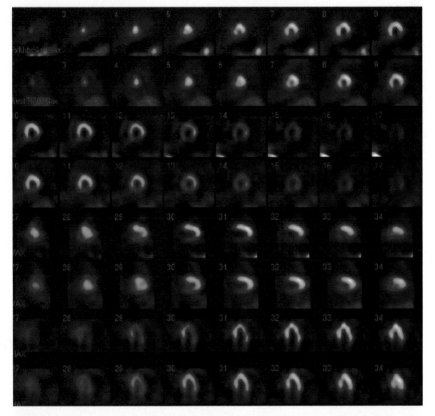

FIGURE 25-5. Rest and SPECT MPI images. Upper row represents stress images; lower row represents rest images. There is a large transmural infarction of the inferior wall and large, moderately severe ischemia of the inferolateral and lateral walls.

ECHOCARDIOGRAPHY

Introduction

Echocardiography, or ultrasound imaging of the heart, was the first medical application of ultrasound. Echocardiography initially began with single-dimensional (or M-mode) imaging but rapidly advanced to include 2D, continuous, and pulsed-wave Doppler, color Doppler, tissue Doppler, and three-dimensional (3D) imaging. Transthoracic echocardiography (TTE) involves placing an ultrasound transducer on the chest wall, while transesophageal echocardiography (TEE) uses an ultrasound transducer that is advanced through the mouth into the esophagus (see Fig. 25-8).

Physics

When sound waves are transmitted from one medium to another, they are either absorbed or reflected, based upon the difference in acoustic impedance between the two media. Echocardiography applies this phenomenon by using high-frequency (20,000 Hz) sound

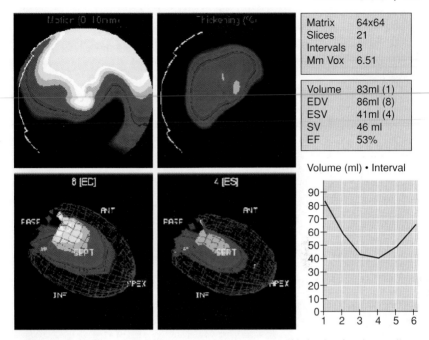

FIGURE 25-6. ECG-gated SPECT images used to measure LV ejection fraction, wall motion, and volume.

waves to image cardiovascular structures. The sound waves emitted by an echo machine originate from and return to a transducer, which converts electrical energy to mechanical energy and vice versa. This is done through the **piezoelectric effect**: the material of the transducer becomes mechanically deformed after application of an electrical current and vibrates, resulting in the production of sound waves.

These high-frequency waves (**ultrasound waves**) travel at a speed of 1540 m/s in the body; they pass easily through fluids but poorly through bone and air. This information is translated into a 2D image of reflected white echoes of varying intensity on a black background. **Hypoechoic structures** are seen on the screen as black regions, where the ultrasound is completely attenuated. Hypoechoic structures include blood, pericardial effusions, and pleural effusions. **Hyperechoic structures** are seen on the screen as gray regions of varying brightness. The brightness of these structures is directly associated with how well they reflect ultrasound waves. Hyperechoic structures include myocardium, valves, vessel walls, masses, thrombi, and vegetations. Although these images are typically displayed as 2D images, **M-mode** analysis can also be used. M-mode displays a thin slice of a 2D image graphically over time. Although M-mode is an older technique that is often difficult to interpret conceptually, it offers the advantage of improved temporal resolution (more frequent imaging of a structure in a given amount of time). 2D echocardiography and M-mode are commonly used for the measurement of ejection fraction, chamber quantification, and myocardial ischemia via stress echocardiography.

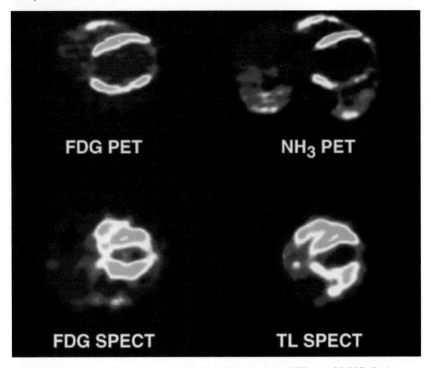

FDG PET

NH₃ PET

FDG SPECT

TL SPECT

FIGURE 25-7. Comparison of myocardial viability by both PET and SPECT. Both modalities demonstrate apical infarction with metabolically active myocardium in the other walls. Note the improved spatial resolution of PET over SPECT. (From Schiepers C, ed. *Diagnostic Nuclear Medicine,* 2nd ed. New York: Springer; 2006, with permission.)

In addition to assessing 2D structures, echocardiography can also be used to assess blood flow and tissue movement via **Doppler analysis**. **The Doppler effect** is the change in the frequency of a wave, resulting from either motion of the wave source or motion of the wave reflector. There are different types of Doppler analysis, including pulsed-wave Doppler, continuous-wave Doppler, color Doppler, and tissue Doppler. Pulsed-wave, continuous, and color Doppler all measure changes in blood flow by using red blood cells as the reflector.

Color Doppler quantifies blood flow direction by encoding blood flow on a color spectrum. Flow toward the transducer is displayed as red, while flow away from the transducer displayed as blue.

Pulsed-wave Doppler allows a sampling volume (or gate) to be positioned and then displays a graph of the full range of velocities and flow directions within the gate plotted as a function of time. Velocity measurement plays a crucial role in assessing the severity of valvular lesions and pressure estimation. However, pulsed-wave Doppler cannot measure velocities above the **Nyquist limit** (which results in an artifact called **aliasing**).

Continuous-wave Doppler, on the other hand, allows measurement of velocities above the Nyquist limit. But continuous-wave Doppler does not allow precise spatial localization

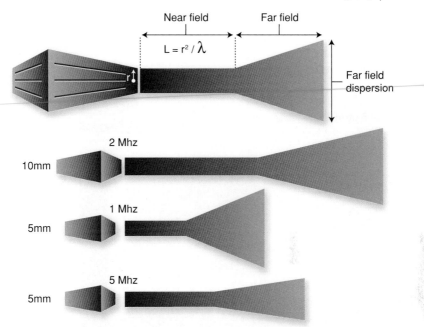

FIGURE 25-8. Schematic of a typical ultrasound transducer. The ultrasound transducer emits ultrasound from a series of piezoelectric crystals. The beam has several components, including a near field with relatively narrow beam width and a far field where there is divergence of the ultrasound beam. Ultrasound intensity decreases with distance from the transducer face. Higher frequencies preserve the length of the near field compared with lower frequencies, as do larger transducer diameters. (From Braunwald E, Zipes DP, Libby P, et al., eds. *Braunwald's Heart Disease: A Textbook of Cardiovascular Medicine,* 7th ed. Philadelphia: Elsevier; 2004, with permission.)

of blood flow. Thus pulsed- and continuous-wave Doppler have complementary roles in hemodynamic assessment.

Rather than quantifying blood flow, **tissue Doppler** quantifies the velocities of the myocardium during systole and diastole. Tissue Doppler is useful for the assessment of diastolic function as well as distinguishing pathologic entities, such as constriction versus restriction. Most recently, tissue Doppler has been used for detecting ventricular dyssynchrony and guiding cardiac resynchronization (i.e., biventricular pacing) therapy.

Three dimensional (3D) (Fig. 25-9) echocardiography is a technique that has existed for decades but is gaining increasing attention. Originally, sequential 2D images were obtained and reconstructed into a 3D data set offline. Unfortunately, this approach proved both time-consuming and cumbersome. Real-time 3D represented the next step in 3D echocardiography, and allowed the acquisition of real-time 3D volumetric data. The strengths of 3D echocardiography include measurement of LV volume and mass, RV volume and function, congenital malformations, and valvular pathology (particularly involving the mitral valve).

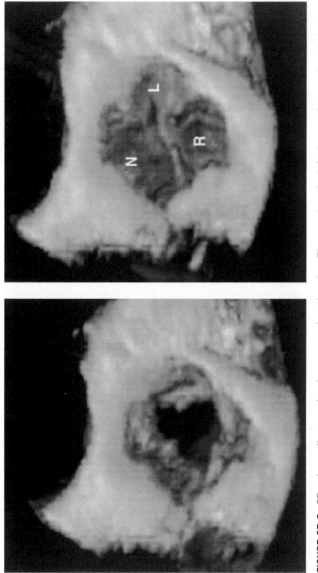

FIGURE 25-9. 3D echocardiogram showing a normal aortic valve. The panel on the left shows valve opening during systole. The right shows valve closure during diastole. The right (R), left (L), and noncoronary (N) cusps are clearly visualized. (From Braunwald E, Zipes DP, Libby P, et al., eds. *Braunwald's Heart Disease: A Textbook of Cardiovascular Medicine*, 7th ed. Philadelphia: Elsevier; 2004, with permission.)

Applications

In 2007, the American College of Cardiology, in collaboration with other groups, released appropriateness criteria for diagnostic echocardiography. The most common indications for TTE include investigation of dyspnea, shock, respiratory failure, murmur, fever, chest pain, congenital heart disease, stroke, and assessment of LV function for the placement of an implantable cardioverter-defibrillator (ICD). TEE is also useful for many of these indications but also allows better assessment of aortic pathology, left atrial thrombus formation, and mitral valve pathology.

Images

See Figures 25-10 through 25-12.

Transthoracic Echo

The images acquired by TTE (Figs. 25-13 through 25-18) are based on different views that depend on position of the ultrasound transducer. The standard views acquired in TTE include the **parasternal long axis, parasternal short axis (at the aortic, mitral, and papillary levels), apical four-chamber, apical two-chamber, subcostal, and suprasternal views.**

Transesophageal Echo

TEE is superior to TTE for visualizing left-sided and posterior structures, as the transducer is positioned posterior to the heart and uses a higher-frequency transducer to image through the thinner tissue of the esophagus. TEE is particularly effective in evaluating the aortic arch, left atrial appendage, mitral valve, aortic valve, and interatrial septum. It is also

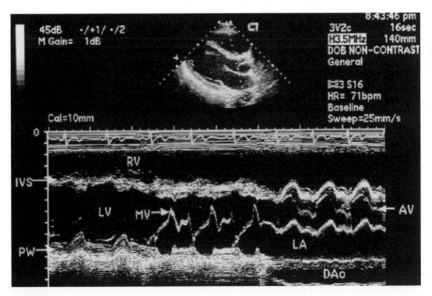

FIGURE 25-10. Normal M-mode echocardiogram in which the M-mode beam is swept from the aortic valve through the mitral valve and to the level of the papillary muscles. AV, aortic valve; DAo, descending aorta; LA, left atrium; LV, left ventricle; MV, mitral valve; RV, right ventricle. (From Braunwald E, Zipes DP, Libby P, et al., eds. *Braunwald's Heart Disease: A Textbook of Cardiovascular Medicine,* 7th ed. Philadelphia: Elsevier; 2004, with permission.)

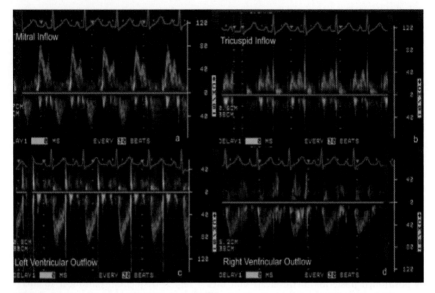

FIGURE 25-11. Composite pulsed wave Doppler tracings of normal flow in all four cardiac valves. (From Braunwald E, Zipes DP, Libby P, et al., eds. *Braunwald's Heart Disease: A Textbook of Cardiovascular Medicine,* 7th ed. Philadelphia: Elsevier; 2004, with permission.)

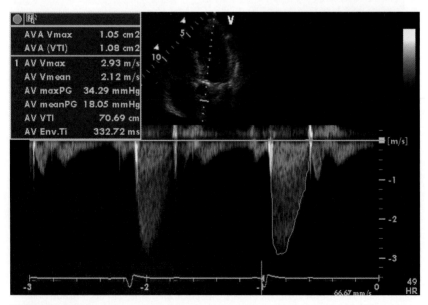

FIGURE 25-12. Continuous-wave Doppler interrogation of moderate aortic stenosis.

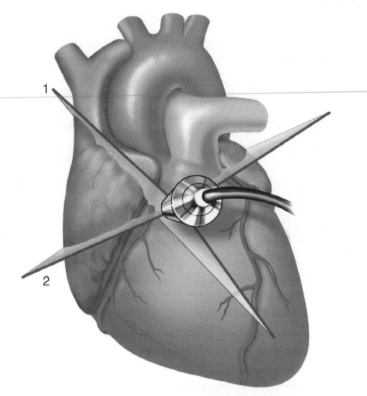

FIGURE 25-13. Transducer orientation used for acquiring parasternal views. Plane 1 represents a parasternal long-axis view. Scanning plane 2 is obtained by rotating the transducer 90 degrees and can be used to obtain a family of short-axis views of the heart. (From Feigenbaum H. *Echocardiography*, 4th ed. Malvern, PA: Lea & Febiger; 1986, with permission.)

useful for imaging nonbiologic structures such as mechanical valves and pacemaker leads. A variety of views are obtained by TEE. Unlike TTE, the TEE exam (Figs. 25-19 and 25-20) is generally goal-directed, with specific views obtained for a given clinical question.

Stress echocardiography involves a TTE that is performed before, during, and after cardiovascular stress. It is a cost-effective means for evaluating patients presenting with chest pain. Method of cardiovascular stress include exercise with treadmill or bicycle ergometry. The presence of exercise-induced wall motion abnormalities suggests inducible ischemia that can be assigned to specific coronary territory. For patients incapable of physical exercise, pharmacologic stress, most commonly employing a dobutamine infusion is used. These protocols rely on an incremental infusion protocol of 10, 20, 30, and 40 μg/kg/minute, which can be augmented by atropine to obtain an adequate heart rate response when necessary. A lower dose of 2.5 mcg/kg/minute can also be used to assess for myocardial viability and contractile reserve for ischemic and valvular cardiomyopathies. Images are obtained at each stage of dobutamine infusion. Patients with significant obstructive coronary disease develop regional wall motion abnormalities identical to those seen during physical stress. The safety record of dobutamine is excellent, and its accuracy appears equivalent to that of exercise

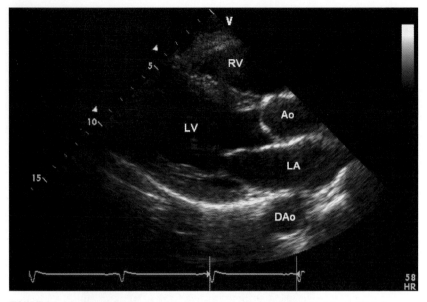

FIGURE 25-14. Parasternal long-axis view. Ao, aortic root; LA, left atrium; LV, left ventricle; DAo, descending aorta.

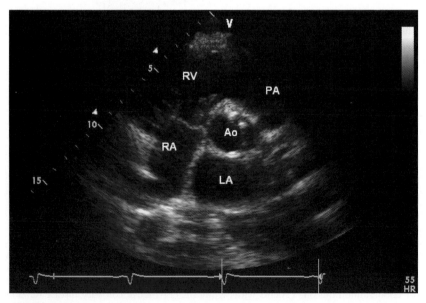

FIGURE 25-15. Short-axis 2D echocardiogram at the level of the aortic valve. Ao, aorta; LA, left atrium; PA, pulmonary artery; RA, right atrium; RV, right ventricle.

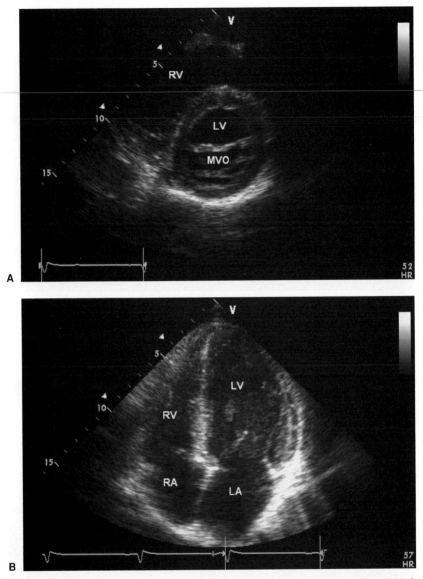

FIGURE 25-16. A: Short-axis 2D echocardiogram at the level of the mitral valve. LV, left ventricle; MVO, mitral valve orifice; RV, right ventricle. **B:** Apical four-chamber view of the left ventricle. LA, left atrium; LV, left ventricle; RA, right atrium; RV, right ventricle.

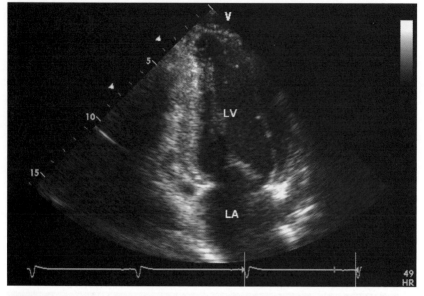

FIGURE 25-17. Apical two-chamber view of the left ventricle. LA, left atrium; LV, left ventricle.

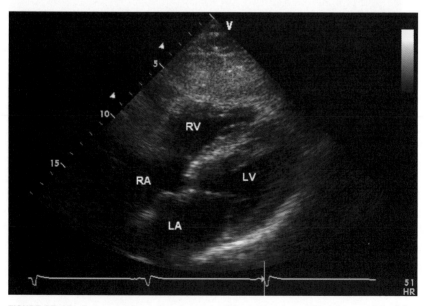

FIGURE 25-18. Subcostal four-chamber view. RA, right atrium; RV, right ventricle; LA, left atrium; LV, left ventricle.

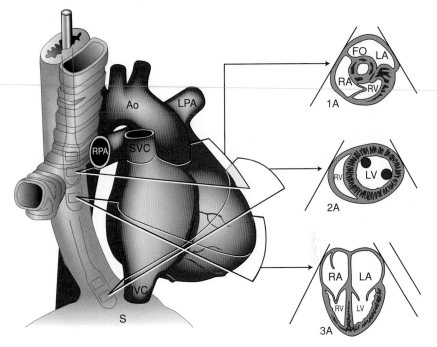

FIGURE 25-19. TEE views obtained in the horizontal transducer position. 3A is recorded in the gastric position, 2A from the midesophagus, and 1A from the upper esophagus. Ao, aorta; IVC, inferior vena cava; LA, left atrium; LAA, left atrial appendage; LUPV, left upper pulmonary vein; LV, left ventricle; RA, right atrium; RPA, right pulmonary artery; RV, right ventricle; S, stomach; SVC, superior vena cava. (From Feigenbaum H. *Echocardiography*, 4th ed. Malvern, PA: Lea & Febiger; 1986, with permission.)

echocardiography. In general, the sensitivity of SPECT tends to be slightly higher than that of exercise echocardiography, whereas the specificity of exercise echocardiography typically has been higher than that of SPECT: a greater degree of myocardial ischemia is needed to produce a wall motion abnormality than a perfusion defect alone.

Limitations

Although echocardiography offers a robust assessment of cardiac structure and function, it has limitations. Most notable is that image acquisition and interpretation are the most user-dependent of cardiac imaging modalities. Also, image quality is decreased by larger body habitus more than with other modalities. Hyperinflated lungs, as in patients with COPD, also diminish image quality. TEE usually requires intravenous sedation and is a semi-invasive procedure with associated risks.

Conclusion

Echocardiography is the workhorse noninvasive cardiac imaging modality. It offers a less expensive, portable method of imaging that provides anatomic, physiologic, and

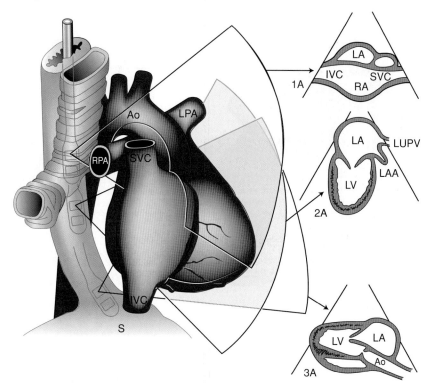

FIGURE 25-20. TEE views obtained in the longitudinal transducer position. 3A is recorded in the gastric position, 2A from the midesophagus, and 1A from the upper esophagus. Ao, aorta; IVC, inferior vena cava; LA, left atrium; LAA, left atrial appendage; LUPV, left upper pulmonary vein; LV, left ventricle; RA, right atrium; RPA, right pulmonary artery; RV, right ventricle; S, stomach; SVC, superior vena cava. (From Feigenbaum H. *Echocardiography*, 4th ed. Malvern, PA: Lea & Febiger; 1986, with permission.)

hemodynamic assessment. Its main drawbacks are the skill required for image acquisition and interpretation as well as its difficulties with increased patient body habitus and/or mechanical ventilation.

Images

See Figures 25-21 through 25-27.

CARDIAC CATHETERIZATION AND ANGIOGRAPHY

Introduction

Along with echocardiography, **cardiac catheterization** is one of the most widely used and comprehensive modalities of cardiac imaging. Cardiac catheterization yields information beyond the visual: pressure measurement and oximetry can be equally valuable in patient evaluation. Beyond image and data acquisition, cardiac catheterization also permits direct mechanical intervention of coronary and valvular lesions. With that understanding, this section focuses on the imaging aspects of cardiac catheterization.

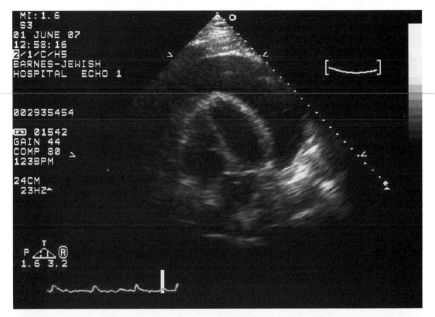

FIGURE 25-21. Apical four-chamber view demonstrating large pericardial effusion.

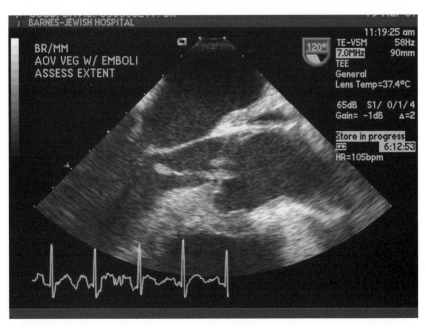

FIGURE 25-22. Transesophageal echocardiogram of the aortic root showing a large vegetation on the right coronary cusp of the aortic valve with aortic root abscess.

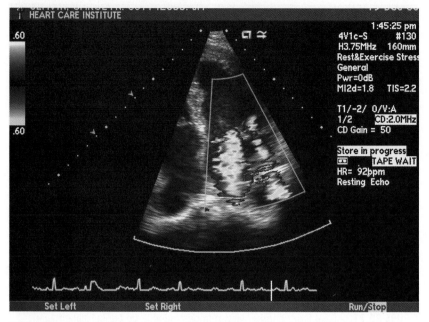

FIGURE 25-23. Apical four-chamber view showing multiple jets producing severe mitral regurgitation.

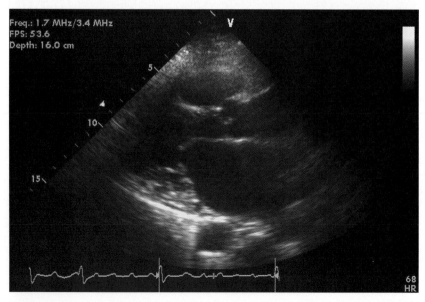

FIGURE 25-24. Parasternal long-axis view showing rheumatic mitral valve disease with the classic "hockey stick" appearance of the mitral valve leaflets and subsequent mitral stenosis.

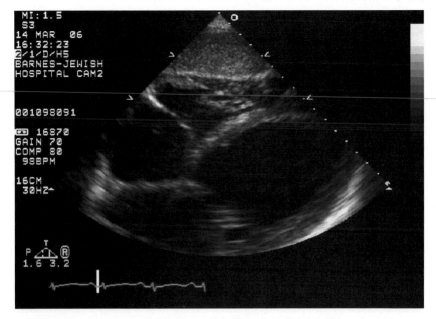

FIGURE 25-25. Subcostal view demonstrating dilated cardiomyopathy.

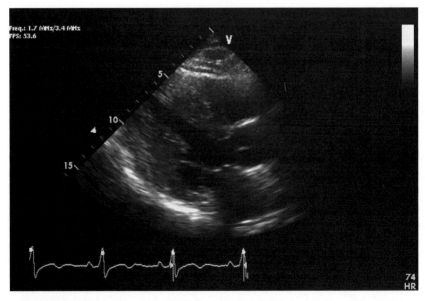

FIGURE 25-26. Parasternal long-axis view of patient with hypertrophic obstructive cardiomyopathy and subsequent left ventricular hypertrophy.

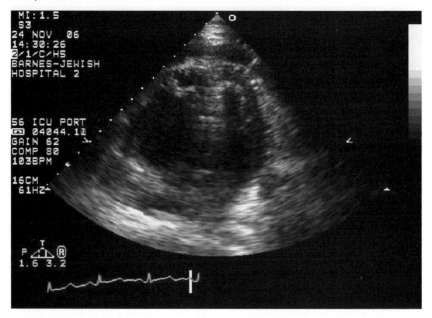

FIGURE 25-27. Apical four-chamber view demonstrating RV dilatation in a patient with pulmonary embolism.

Physics

Catheter-based angiography is performed using a **cinefluorographic system** (Fig. 25-28). Such a system produces an x-ray beam that projects through the patient at a desired angle. This projected x-ray beam is then detected after it passes through the patient and is transduced into a visible light image.

The basic components of a cinefluorographic system include a generator, x-ray tube, and image intensifier. The **generator** controls and delivers electrical power to the **x-ray tube**. The x-ray tube contains a filament that is heated by the generator to ultimately form the x-ray beam. The x-ray beam attenuates as it passes through tissue. The degree of attenuation varies with tissue density, projection angle and distance. After passing through the patient, the attenuated x-ray enters the **image intensifier (II)**. The image intensifier converts the attenuated x-ray beam into a visible light image. The image x-ray tube and II are positioned 180 degrees apart on a rotating gantry. Thus, the II always remains opposite the x-ray tube at various angles. It is convenient to think of the image intensifier as the camera that is taking pictures.

Cinefluorographic systems operate in two modes: **fluoroscopy and acquisition.** Fluoroscopy mode (often referred to as **"fluoro"**) provides a real-time x-ray image with adequate quality for guiding catheter manipulation. The acquisition mode (known as "cine") generates images of much greater visual quality which are then are recorded. However, most cinefluorographic systems are calibrated to give an x-ray dose that is 15 times greater during cine when compared with fluoro. Thus, fluoro is first used for catheter positioning and cine is then used to record dye injection after catheter placement.

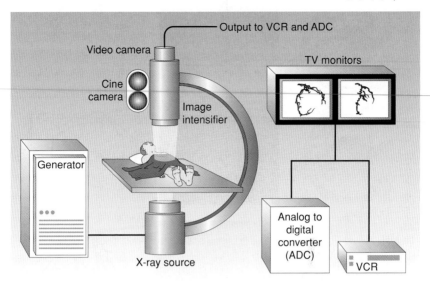

FIGURE 25-28. The cinefluorographic system. (From Braunwald E, Zipes DP, Libby P, et al., eds. *Braunwald's Heart Disease: A Textbook of Cardiovascular Medicine,* 7th ed. Philadelphia: Elsevier; 2004, with permission.)

Technique

Catheter placement requires **arterial or venous access**. Arterial access is typically obtained through the femoral, radial, or brachial arteries. Venous access is typically obtained through the femoral, internal jugular, or subclavian veins. Classically, an 18-gauge needle is inserted into the vessel at a 45-degree angle. After blood return is seen, a J-tipped wire is advanced into the vessel. The needle is then removed. A **sheath-dilator** combination is advanced over the wire into the vessel. The dilator is then removed leaving the sheath in place. The sheath secures the access site and acts as a door, allowing catheter insertion and removal.

Many different catheters are used for the various anatomic structures that are targets of contrast injection. The most common targets include the left main coronary artery (Judkins left and Amplatz left catheters), right coronary artery (Judkins right, Amplatz right, and WRP catheters), left ventricle (pigtail catheter), aortocoronary venous grafts (Judkins right, Amplatz right, right coronary bypass, left coronary bypass, and multipurpose catheters), left internal mammary artery (left internal mammary artery catheter and Judkins right catheter) and aorta (pigtail catheter). Less common targets include the right internal mammary artery, right ventricle, pulmonary artery, pulmonary veins, and surgical conduits for treatment of congenital heart disease.

After the target is successfully cannulated by catheter, contrast is injected. Contrast is a radiopaque substance that appears dark when viewed on a white fluoroscopic background. The purpose of contrast is to allow delineation of cardiac structures by temporarily opacifying them. All modern x-ray contrasts are exclusively iodine-based. Although the current generation of contrast is fairly safe, there are still risks. The two most common risks of using contrast are contrast-induced nephropathy and allergic reactions.

Angiograms are obtained at various angles to allow more complete visualization of 3D structures (Figs. 25-29 and 25-30). The nomenclature used describes the position of the image

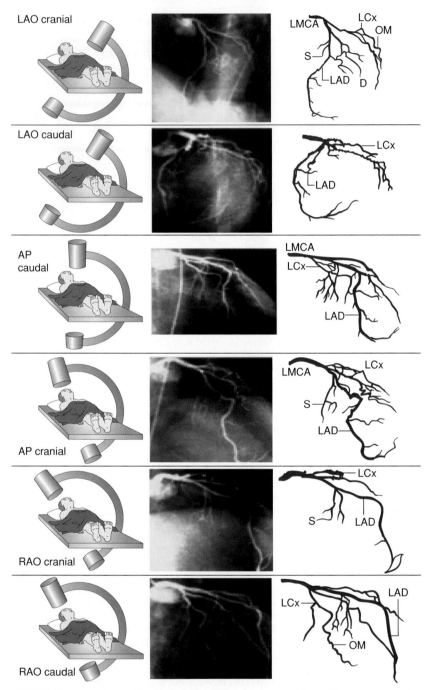

FIGURE 25-29. Angiographic views of the left coronary circulation. (From Braunwald E, Zipes DP, Libby P, et al., eds. *Braunwald's Heart Disease: A Textbook of Cardiovascular Medicine,* 7th ed. Philadelphia: Elsevier; 2004, with permission.)

intensifier (II) in relation to the patient. **AP** (anteroposterior) means that the II is directly over the patient. **Cranial** means that the II is angled superiorly. **Caudal** means that the II is angled inferiorly. **LAO** (left angle oblique) means that the II is angled to the patient's left. **RAO** (right angle oblique) means that the II is angled to the right of the patient. **Lateral** means that II is placed fully lateral to the patient.

Applications

The primary uses for cardiac catheterization are to assess the presence and/or severity of:

- Coronary artery disease
- Valvular heart disease
- Cardiomyopathy
- Congenital heart disease
- Pulmonary hypertension
- Aortic disease (aneurysm and dissection)

It is worth noting that for the first five indications, cardiac catheterization is considered the diagnostic "gold standard," as cardiac catheterization boasts both spatial and temporal resolution that surpasses those of cardiac computed tomography (CT) and magnetic resonance imaging (MRI).

Limitations

Cardiac catheterization does have several disadvantages. Most notably, it is invasive. Major complications are uncommon (<1%) after coronary angiography but include death (0.10%–0.14%), myocardial infarction (0.06%–0.07%), contrast agent reactions (0.23%), and local vascular complications (0.24%–0.1%).

Contrast-induced nephropathy (CIN) is another important complication of cardiac angiography. The mechanism of CIN is unclear. At least 5% of patients experience a transient rise in serum creatinine following coronary angiography, making CIN the third most common cause of hospital-acquired kidney failure. Most creatinine elevations are nonoliguric, peak within 1 to 2 days, and return to baseline in 7 days. It is very rare for patients to require chronic dialysis. CIN is associated with increased length of hospital stay and in-hospital mortality, which is even further increased if dialysis is required. The main measures to prevent CIN are to limit contrast volume and prehydration of the patient. There may be benefit to using sodium bicarbonate rather than saline for prehydration. The free-radical scavenger n-acetyl cysteine may have benefit as well.

Cardiac catheterization can also lead to allergic reactions to three materials: local anesthetic, iodinated contrast, or protamine sulfate. The most common allergic reactions (<1% of procedures) are caused by contrast. Symptoms vary on a spectrum including sneezing, urticaria, angioedema, bronchospasm, and even anaphylactic shock. If a severe reaction occurs, it should be treated with 10 μg boluses of epinephrine. If a patient has a known or suspected history of a contrast reaction, premedication with prednisone (20 mg PO tid × 24–48 hours), diphenhydramine (25 mg PO tid × 24–48 hours) and an H2 blocker (cimetidine or ranitidine) can reduce the risk of a second reaction to 5% to 10% and a severe reaction (bronchospasm or shock) to <1%.

The final limitation of coronary angiography is its inability to assess extraluminal manifestations of CAD. Luminal involvement is often the final stage of the progression of CAD. This drawback can be overcome by performing cardiac catheterization with intravascular ultrasound (IVUS) (see IVUS section in Chapter 26) to assess for extraluminal involvement. Nevertheless, cardiac CT and cardiac MRI both allow extraluminal assessment of the coronary arteries without additional cost.

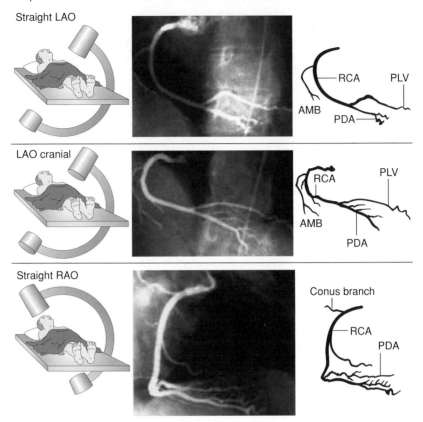

FIGURE 25-30. Angiographic views of the right coronary circulation. (From Braunwald E, Zipes DP, Libby P, et al., eds. *Braunwald's Heart Disease: A Textbook of Cardiovascular Medicine,* 7th ed. Philadelphia: Elsevier; 2004, with permission.)

Conclusion

Cardiac catheterization remains the gold standard for assessment of coronary lesions due to its superior spatial and temporal resolution. It also provides valuable hemodynamic information for assessing valvular, myopathic and congenital heart disease. Lastly, it allows direct mechanical intervention of coronary and peripheral artery disease. Its primary drawbacks are its low but non-negligible risks of vascular complications, renal failure and allergic reactions.

Images

See Figures 25-31 through 25-35.

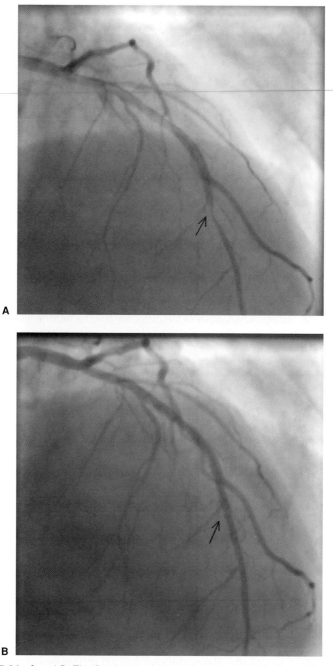

FIGURE 25-31. A and **B:** The first image shows a severe stenosis in the mid- left anterior descending artery (mid-LAD). The second image shows the results of successful stent placement in the diseased segment.

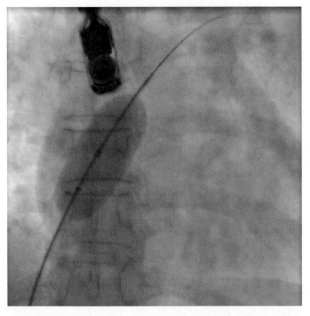

FIGURE 25-32. Balloon valvuloplasty of the pulmonic valve for treatment of pulmonic stenosis.

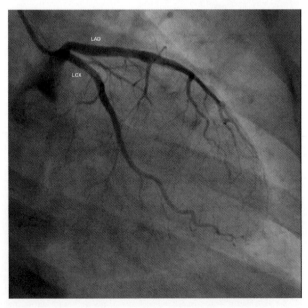

FIGURE 25-33. Coronary angiography demonstrating left anterior descending artery (LAD) and left circumflex (LCX) originating from separate coronary ostia ("double-barrel left main arteries").

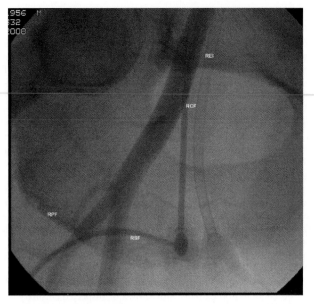

FIGURE 25-34. Peripheral angiogram of the right femoral vessels. REI, right external iliac artery; RCF, right common femoral artery; RSF, right superficial femoral artery; RPF, right profunda femoris artery.

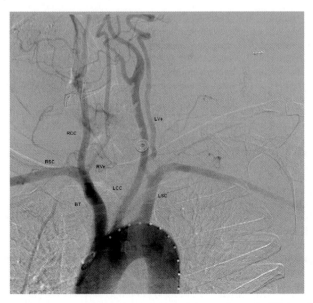

FIGURE 25-35. Digital subtraction angiography of the aortic arch. BT, brachio-cephalic trunk; RSC, right subclavian artery; RCC, right common carotid artery; RVe, right vertebral artery; LCC, left common carotid artery; LSC, left subclavian artery; LVe, left vertebral artery.

REFERENCES AND SUGGESTED READINGS

Baim DS. *Grossman's Cardiac Catheterization, Angiography and Intervention,* 7th ed. Baltimore: Lippincott Williams & Wilkins; 2006:53.

Bax JJ, Visser FC, Blanksma PK, et al. Comparison of myocardial uptake of fluorine-18-fluorodeoxyglucose imaged with PET and SPECT in dyssynergic myocardium. *J Nucl Med* 1996;37:1631–1636.

Berman D, Hachamovitch R, Lewin H, et al. Risk stratification in coronary artery disease: implications for stabilization and prevention. *Am J Cardiol* 1997;79(128):1–6.

Berman DS, Hachamovitch R, Kiat H, et al. Incremental value of prognostic testing in patients with known or suspected ischemic heart disease: a basis for optimal utilization of exercise technetium-99m sestamibi myocardial perfusion single-photon emission computed tomography. *J Am Coll Cardiol* 1995;26:639–647.

Berman DS, Kiat H, Friedman JD, et al. Separate acquisition rest thallium-201/stress technetium-99m sestamibi dual-isotope myocardial perfusion single-photon emission computed tomography: a clinical validation study. *J Am Coll Cardiol* 1993;22:1455–1464.

Birck R et al. Acetylcysteine for prevention of contrast induced nephropathy: meta-analysis. *Lancet* 2006;362;598–603.

Choosing a thallium-201 or technetium 99m sestamibi imaging protocol. *J Nucl Cardiol* 1994;1:S99–S108.

Chuah SC, Pellikka PA, Roger VL, et al. Role of dobutamine stress echocardiography in predicting outcome in 860 patients with known or suspected coronary artery disease. *Circulation* 1998;97:1474.

Crouse LJ, Harbrecht JJ, Vacek JL, et al. Exercise echocardiography as a screening test for coronary artery disease and correlation with coronary arteriography. *Am J Cardiol* 1991;67:1213.

Gibbons RJ, Hodge DO, Berman DS, et al. Long-term outcome of patients with intermediate-risk exercise electrocardiograms who do not have myocardial perfusion defects on radionuclide imaging. *Circulation* 1999;100:2140–2145.

Grundy SM, Pasternak R, Greenland P, et al. Assessment of cardiovascular risk by use of multiple-risk-factor assessment equations: A statement for healthcare professionals from the American Heart Association and the American College of Cardiology. *Circulation* 1999;100:1481–1492.

Hachamovitch R, Berman DS, Kiat H, et al. Exercise myocardial perfusion SPECT in patients without known coronary artery disease: incremental prognostic value and use in risk stratification. *Circulation* 1996;93:905–914.

Hachamovitch R, Berman DS, Shaw LJ, et al. Incremental prognostic value of myocardial perfusion single photon emission computed tomography for the prediction of cardiac death: Differential stratification for risk of cardiac death and myocardial infarction. *Circulation* 1998;97:535–543.

IMV Medical Information Division. 2003 Nuclear Medicine Market Summary Report. December 1, 2003. http://www.asnc.org/imageuploads/Imaging%20Guidelines.pdf.

Martin WH, Delbeke D, Patton JA, et al. FDG-SPECT: correlation with FDG-PET. *J Nucl Med* 1995;36:988–995.

McCullough PA et al. Acute renal failure after coronary intervention: incidence, risk factors and relationship to mortality. *Am J Med* 1997;103:368–375.

Merten GJ et al. The prevention of radiocontrast-agent-induced nephropathy with sodium bicarbonate: a randomized control trial. *JAMA* 2004;291:2328–2334.

Quinones MA, Verani MS, Haichin RM, et al. Exercise echocardiography versus 201Tl single-photon emission computed tomography in evaluation of coronary artery disease. Analysis of 292 patients. *Circulation* 1992;85:1026.

Scanlon P, Faxon D, Audet A, et al. ACC/AHA guidelines for coronary angiography. *J Am Coll Cardiol* 1999;33:1756.

Seward JB, Khandheria BK, Freeman WK, et al. Multiplane transesophageal echocardiography: image orientation, examination technique, anatomic correlations, and clinical applications. *Mayo Clin Proc* 1993;68:523.

Sharir T, Berman DS, Lewin HC, et al. Incremental prognostic value of rest-distribution Tl-201 single photon emission computed tomography. *Circulation* 1999;100:1964–1970.

Stevenson JG. Appearance and recognition of basic Doppler concepts in color flow imaging. *Echocardiography* 1989;6:451.

Takeuchi M, Araki M, Nakashima Y, et al. Comparison of dobutamine stress echocardiography and stress thallium-201 single-photon emission computed tomography for detecting coronary artery disease. *J Am Soc Echocardiogr* 1993;6:593.

Takuma S, Zwas DR, Fard A, et al. Real-time, 3-dimensional echocardiography acquires all standard 2-dimensional images from 2 volume sets: a clinical demonstration in 45 patients. *J Am Soc Echocardiogr* 1999;12:1.

Tommaso CL. Contrast-induced nephrotoxicity in patients undergoing cardiac catheterization. *Cathet Cardiovac Diagn* 1994;31:316.

Waggoner AD, Bierig SM. Tissue Doppler imaging: A useful echocardiographic method for the cardiac sonographer to assess systolic and diastolic ventricular function. *J Am Soc Echocardiogr* 2001;14:1143.

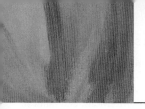

New Imaging and Diagnostic Testing Modalities (Cardiac CT, Cardiac MRI, PET, IVUS)

Sujith Kalathiveetil, Michael O. Barry,
Ibrahim M. Saeed, and Tillmann Cyrus

OVERVIEW

Over the last few decades, the cardiovascular disease community has witnessed an explosion in imaging modalities. These advances include the development of multiple different techniques including cardiac computed tomography (cardiac CT), cardiac magnetic resonance imaging (CMR), positron emission tomography (PET), and intravascular ultrasound (IVUS). Never has the clinician been offered more options and faced perhaps greater confusion in choosing a means to evaluate a patient's heart. In the sections that follow, we discuss these technologies in detail, with a focus on appropriate indications for their use. Indeed, the rapid expansion and availability of the first of these two imaging modalities, cardiac CT and CMR, have led to the publication of "appropriateness criteria" by multiple professional societies. Where possible, a brief discussion on technical aspects of each modality is included, but an in-depth discussion is beyond the scope of this book. For a more in-depth discussion about topics such as physics and image registration, the reader is referred to sources listed at the end of the chapter.

CARDIAC CT

Introduction

Cardiac CT is an imaging modality that has much to offer the cardiologist and internist alike. CT coronary angiography (CTCA), which involves imaging the coronary arteries, has been seen as a potential substitute for conventional diagnostic cardiac catheterization. It also allows the evaluation of cardiac chambers and surrounding structures. Additionally, coronary calcium screening has an important role in risk stratification for primary prevention of coronary artery disease.

When ordering a CT scan, it is important to have an understanding of differences between traditional scanners and multidetector CT (MDCT) as well as knowledge of basic imaging acquisition and, importantly, radiation exposure.

The thinnest image that can be reconstructed from the data collected is determined by the slice thickness of the scanner. It is the 64-slice scanner's ability to obtain thinner slice thickness that makes it superior to the traditional scanners (4- or 16-slice detector technology), as the imaging of submillimeter coronary vasculature requires very high spatial resolution.

Cardiac CT **image acquisition** must be timed with the cardiac cycle and is done via coupling image acquisition with electrocardiographic (ECG) triggering. The most commonly used method for CTCA is called retrospective gating, whereby the x-ray current is applied throughout the cardiac cycle. Although the coronary arteries fill during diastole, the additional radiation permits additional image acquisition during systole, thus enabling

TABLE 26-1	COMPARISON OF EFFECTIVE RADIATION DOSES IN CARDIAC IMAGING
Yearly background radiation	1 mSv
Standard chest x-ray	0.1 mSv
Diagnostic cardiac catheterization	5 mSv
Nuclear myocardial perfusion stress test	10–35 mSv
Nongated chest CT	8 mSv
Coronary calcium CT scan	1–1.5 mSv
Gated angiography (64-slice)	18–22 mSv
Dose-modulation gated coronary CT angiography (64-slice)	9–15 mSv

cine imaging (viewing cardiac motion throughout the entire cardiac cycle). This is useful for measuring ejection fraction, wall motion, and valvular orifice area.

CT radiation differs from that of a standard x-ray, in that the source of ionizing radiation rotates around the body. The potential radiation effects and magnitude of dose are dependent on many factors, but the effective dose or dose equivalent, defined in Sieverts (*Sv*), is the weighted sum of the radiation dose to a number of body tissues. It is important to remember that even noninvasive tests, which seem by nature benign, do expose the patient to substantial radiation. Table 26-1 lists the effective dose of multiple imaging techniques to allow comparison of radiation risk between medical imaging tests. It is important to remember that obese patients require increased current output from the x-ray tube for adequate tissue penetration and spatial resolution and thus receive greater radiation exposure.

Applications

Coronary CT Angiography

While coronary angiography during cardiac catheterization remains the reference standard for the diagnosis and quantification of coronary atherosclerosis, it has inherent limitations. It is by definition invasive. Another limitation of conventional coronary angiography is the inability to see beyond the vessel lumen. CTCA (Fig. 26-1) permits assessment of both the lumen and arterial wall. This enables assessment of positive remodeling, which occurs early in atherosclerosis. Positive remodeling has been defined as an expansion of the arterial cross-sectional area in an attempt to preserve the luminal area in response to increasing plaque burden. Positive remodeling is not well appreciated on conventional angiography.

The ability of CTCA to assess severity and extent of atherosclerosis in comparison to conventional angiography has been validated in multiple studies with both 16- and 64-slice scanners. Studies have shown that CTCA has a very strong negative predictive value to exclude significant coronary stenosis.

The role of cardiac CT in the assessment of acute chest pain in the emergency department (ED) is under investigation. CTCA should be considered in ED patients with chest pain and equivocal evidence of acute coronary syndrome (initial cardiac biomarkers nondiagnostic; absence of ST-segment elevation or new left bundle-branch block [LBBB] on ECG; the possibility of a noncoronary cause of chest pain, including pulmonary embolus, aortic dissection or pericarditis).

The uses of CTCA can be grouped as follows:

• Defining cardiac anatomy (congenital anomalies, pulmonary vein configuration, bypass graft location, tumors/thrombi)

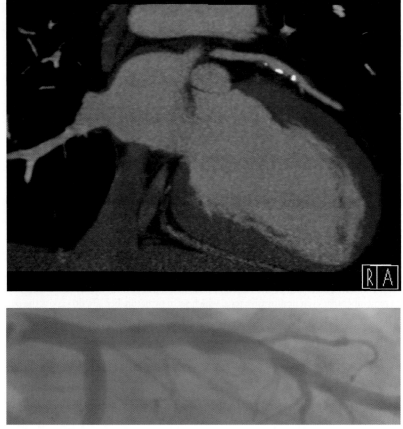

FIGURE 26-1. Atherosclerosis of the proximal LAD with positive remodeling. **A:** CTCA. **B:** conventional angiography.

- Atypical chest pain in a patient with coronary artery disease (CAD) risk factors and/or equivocal stress test results (elective CTCA)
- Acute chest pain assessment in the emergency department (the "triple rule-out")
- Screening asymptomatic high-risk Framingham individuals

Coronary Artery Calcification

An additional use of cardiac CT is quantification of coronary artery calcification (CAC). The theory of the vulnerable plaque, that nonobstructive plaques are at risk to rupture and promote subsequent thrombosis, is supported by the myriad of studies indicating that the majority of myocardial infarctions occur from nonobstructive plaques. It is overall atherosclerotic burden, rather than a specific stenosis, that may be more important in the prediction of long-term cardiovascular events (myocardial infarction and death). This is manifest by a strong correlation of atherosclerotic burden CAC.

Quantification of CAC (Fig. 26-2) is performed as a CAC score or Agatston score. This score is computer-generated by multiplying the calcium plaque area (in square

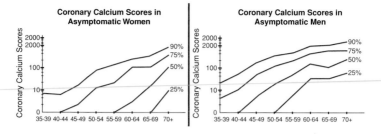

FIGURE 26-2. CAC Score. See text for description and details.

Calcium Score	Implication	Risk of Coronary Artery Disease
0	No identifiable plaque	Very low, generally less than 5 percent
1-10	Minimal identifiable plaque	Very unlikely, less than 10 percent
11-100	Definite, at least mild atherosclerotic plaque	Mild or minimal coronary stenosis likely
101-400	Definite, at least moderate atherosclerotic plaque	Mild coronary atery disease highly likely, significant stenosis possible
401 or Higher	Extensive atherosclerotic plaque	High likelihood of at least one significant coronary artery stenosis

millimeters) by the calcium plaque density (Hounsfield number). A high CAC score does not equate to a severely stenotic lesion but rather to a high atherosclerotic burden and therefore a higher risk of death and/or myocardial infarction. As a screening method, CAC scoring can risk-stratify patients using a limited amount of radiation, even in the setting of resting ECG abnormalities and without the use of medications, contrast, or exercise. Current data suggests that CAC has a role in the risk stratification of asymptomatic individuals, primarily those with intermediate Framingham risk scores (10%–20% risk of cardiovascular event at 10 years) and in symptomatic patients prior to an invasive diagnostic procedure. Importantly, patients can be risk-stratified based on both absolute CAC score ("cutpoints") as well as the expected CAC score for their age (quartiles). See Chapter 10 for further details.

Limitations of Cardiac CT

There are several **contraindications** to cardiac CT that need to be considered prior to scanning, including:

- Serum creatinine >1.5 mg/dL
- Pregnancy
- Breast-feeding
- History of severe allergy to IV contrast

Image quality will be reduced in patients with the following conditions:

- Irregular heart rhythms (atrial fibrillation/flutter and/or frequent premature atrial/ventricular contractions) with improper ECG triggering introducing slice misregistration and/or errors in radiation dose modulation

- High regular heart rates (>70 bpm) refractory to rate-lowering agents, causing motion artifact
- Extreme obesity (BMI >40 kg/m²), which leads to excessive radiation attenuation, with a subsequent reduction in the signal-to-noise ratio
- Metallic objects (surgical clips, mechanical heart valves, or the wires of a pacer/automatic implanted cardiac defibrillator), which are prone to radiation scatter, producing streaking artifacts). Coronary stent patency assessment is possible but not always reliable.

CARDIAC MRI

Introduction

Magnetic resonance imaging (MRI) uses a strong magnetic field and radiofrequency waves to provide detailed images of internal organs and tissues. A main advantage of this technology is the lack of x-rays, thus negating any DNA damage, which is important for patients requiring numerous imaging studies during the course of their disease. To improve image quality and reduce motion artifact during imaging of the heart and coronary arteries, simple breath-holding techniques and technologic advances including cardiac gating have been introduced. As limitations are still encountered, diagnostic utility can be improved by the use of adjunctive contrast agents. The physics behind MRI are truly fascinating but beyond the scope of this book. As a brief discussion will not do justice, the interested reader is referred to supplemental texts.

Applications

The high resolution of cardiovascular magnetic resonance (CMR) allows the examination of cardiac wall thickness and detailed structural analysis, which aids in the differentiation of cardiomyopathies, detection of iron in hemochromatosis, and visualization of other rare diseases such as ventricular noncompaction. The ability to provide images of motion facilitates the noninvasive assessment of the function of all cardiac valves, calculation of ejection fraction, and visualization of shunts. Importantly, MR technology yields high-resolution images regardless of body habitus. CMR can be used to determine myocardial viability at rest, and experienced centers routinely perform exercise (foot pedals) or dobutamine stress CMR. Another advantage of CMR is the ability to image flowing blood, which allows the examination of the arterial system without the contrast injection that is necessary in x-ray–based angiography. Yet another advantage of CMR is its ability to provide detailed images and reproducible quantitation of cardiac function independent of lung and scar tissues, which may obscure echocardiography images.

Indications

Congenital Heart Disease

CMR has traditionally played a significant role in the evaluation of congenital heart disease. The ability to generate 3D data sets to determine complex cardiac anomalies and lack of ionizing radiation has proven advantageous in young patients with complex cardiac anomalies who need sequential studies. CMR becomes especially valuable once children have undergone surgery, as the interposition of scar tissue and lungs as well as complex anatomy pose an increasing problem for echocardiography.

CMR plays an important role in the evaluation of many congenital anomalies, including:

- Anomalies of the visceroatrial sinus
  - Situs inversus or ambiguus
  - Malposition of the heart (dextro- or levocardia)

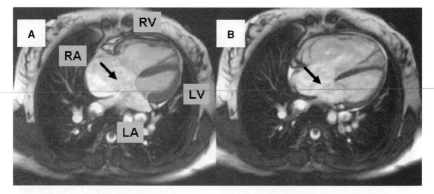

FIGURE 26-3. Ostium primum atrial septal defect: large ASD (arrow) depicted in systole **(A)** and diastole **(B)**.

- Identification of atrial septal defects and quantification of shunt size (Fig. 26-3)
- Isolated ventricular septal defects
- Complex anomalies such as:
  - Tetralogy of Fallot
  - Pulmonary atresia
  - Tricuspid atresia
  - Univentricular hearts and double-outlet ventricles
- Assessment of coarctation of the aorta before and after surgery
- Sinus of Valsalva aneurysms
- Aortic dilatations associated with Marfan and Ehler–Danlos syndromes
- Patency of systemic-to-pulmonary shunts and extracardiac conduits
- Anomalies in the origin and course of coronary arteries

Cardiomyopathies

CMR is well established to evaluate left and right ventricular mass and function. The CMR-derived quantitative parameters for both the left ventricle (LV) and right ventricle (RV) have been shown to be superior to those of 2D and M-mode echocardiography. CMR may be used to evaluate for many different types of cardiomyopathies, including:

- **Arrhythmogenic RV dysplasia/cardiomyopathy**
- **Infiltrative cardiomyopathies** such as
  - Amyloid heart disease
  - Hemochromatosis
  - Sarcoidosis
- Focal inflammatory changes in **myocarditis**
- Serial assessment of rejection episodes following **heart transplantation**
- **Pericardial thickening** in the evaluation of constrictive pericarditis (Fig. 26-4)
- **Identification of fibrotic areas** linked to the risk of sudden cardiac death and development of heart failure
- **LV noncompaction**, the failure of loosely arranged muscle fibers to form mature compacted myocardium during the embryonic development, which is increasingly recognized during high-resolution MR studies
- **Tumor infiltration** into the pericardium with differentiation of cystic tumors, fatty tumors, melanoma metastasis, hemorrhage, and vascular tumors (Fig. 26-5)

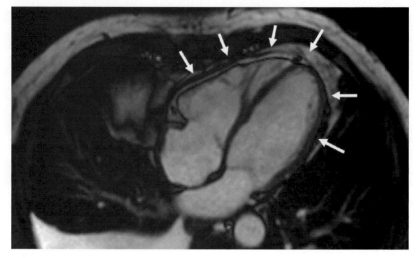

FIGURE 26-4. Pericardial constriction: concentric pericardial thickening and constriction around the LV and RV (*arrows*).

Valvular Heart Disease

For routine evaluation of valvular heart disease, transthoracic (TTE) and transesophageal echocardiography (TEE) are cost-effective and widely available. CMR allows the morphologic and functional assessment of any valve regardless of the poor acoustic windows that may be encountered in TTE and is a valuable alternative when a TEE procedure is not

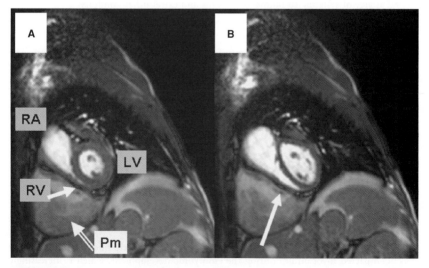

FIGURE 26-5. RV compression. **A:** Pericardial mass (Pm; *double arrow*) compressing the RV (*white arrow*) during systole. Right atrium is enlarged. **B:** Ability of the RV to fill during diastole is significantly impaired.

desired by the patient. Because of its accuracy, high-resolution CMR is also a favorable modality in serial imaging. CMR can be used to measure peak velocity within the core of a jet and, as with echo, the modified Bernoulli equation is used to estimate the pressure gradient to evaluate the severity of AS and PR. Most prosthetic valves are safe for imaging with most magnets, but focal artifacts may obscure the images.

Vascular Disease

CMR further distinguishes itself from traditional x-ray angiography by its ability to image many aspects of the vessel wall, including the assessment of dissection, thrombus, inflammation, and atherosclerotic plaque. Magnetic resonance angiography (MRA) may be done without contrast injection using "time-of-flight" techniques or with intravenous gadolinium. This makes MRA is especially useful in patients with contraindications to x-ray contrast agents or renal insufficiency. **However, a rare but significant side effect of gadolinium contrast agents, nephrogenic systemic fibrosis (NSF), has recently been described in patients with severe renal insufficiency; therefore caution is warranted in these patients** (see below). CMR angiography combined with vascular wall imaging is valuable in the detection of thoracic and abdominal aortic aneurysms and dissection. CMR is an ideal modality for monitoring aortic changes in Marfan syndrome and for postsurgical follow-up.

Coronary Artery Disease

The direct visualization of coronary arteries with coronary MRA has significantly improved in recent years but still faces technical challenges, mainly due to motion artifacts. CMR is also useful in the assessment of myocardial perfusion both in the detection of acute and chronic myocardial infarction as well as for ischemia. Myocardial infarction can be detected using late gadolinium-enhanced CMR. Images are acquired before and 20 minutes after IV injection of gadolinium. Because gadolinium is an extracellular contrast agent, it is not retained in normal myocardium; but since infarcted myocardium has a larger extracellular compartment, there is slower washout of the contrast agent from the infarcted region. The retained gadolinium shows up as a bright signal during the late enhancement scan. Furthermore, CMR is valuable in the detection of regional wall motion abnormalities at rest and during exercise or in dobutamine stress testing. Detection of atherosclerotic plaque and imaging of the vascular wall is possible (see "Vascular Disease," above) but is largely done in research studies.

Contrast Enhancement

Like other imaging technologies, MRI benefits from the use of contrast agents. Conventional MR contrast agents generate contrast effects by altering the local magnetic field and relaxation parameters within the tissue that is imaged. The most commonly used contrast agents are gadolinium chelates.

Anaphylactoid reactions with these agents have been observed in less than 0.1% of cases. In distinction to the iodine-based agents used in x-ray angiography, gadolinium chelates have a much lower incidence of nephrotoxicity and thus have been an alternative for patients that could not undergo contrast-enhanced x-ray exams. However, a rare but serious complication termed **nephrogenic systemic fibrosis (NSF)** has recently been described after certain gadolinium chelates were given. This resulted in a FDA request, in May 2007, for a boxed warning for all gadolinium-based contrast agents. NSF has occurred in patients with severe renal insufficiency, and the current recommendation is to consider the risks and benefits of gadolinium-based contrast agents in patients with acute or chronic severe renal insufficiency, renal dysfunction of any severity due to the hepatorenal syndrome, or in the perioperative liver transplantation period. In these patients, gadolinium-based contrast agents should be avoided unless the diagnostic information is essential and not available with non-contrast-enhanced MRI. Dialysis patients should receive gadolinium agents only when this is essential, and dialysis should be performed as soon as possible after completion of the MRI scan.

Pregnancy

Not enough data exist on the effects of MR on the developing fetus. Current guidelines recommend that a pregnant woman should undergo MR imaging only when essential and ideally after the first trimester, when organogenesis is completed. Although no harmful effects on the fetus have been demonstrated, the fetus may be more sensitive to the effects of heating and noise. Importantly, gadolinium compounds cross the placenta and are not recommended for use in pregnancy.

Contraindications

Absolute (with exceptions as noted):

- **Pacemakers/implanted cardiac defibrillators** (ICDs) and other electronic implants are usually considered an absolute contraindication mainly owing to inappropriate electronic function rather than the magnetic field's effect on the implant.
- **Metallic fragments** in the eye are not held in place by scar tissue and can dislocate even many years after deposition into the eye. If a metal fragment is suspected to be in the eye, an orbital x-ray should be performed prior to MRI.
- **Aneurysm clips** in the brain are not protected by scar tissue and may dislocate in the magnetic field.

Relative

- Orthopedic implants are usually stable if embedded for several weeks, but cause artifacts when adjacent to the area of interest.
- Staples are considered safe when embedded for several weeks.
- Acoustic noise is due to the currents in the wires of the gradient magnets, which are rapidly switched on and off, causing expansions and contractions of the coil itself. The stronger the main field, the louder the noise will get. In 3T scanners, depending on the imaging techniques, the noise can reach more than 130 dB. Thus, appropriate ear protection is mandatory.

POSITRON EMISSION TOMOGRAPHY

Introduction

While single photon emission computed tomography (SPECT) has been the dominant nuclear modality in clinical practice, positron emission tomography (PET) has transitioned from a valuable research technique to an important clinical modality—one that may be superior to SPECT.

A basic review of the principles of PET is needed to understand its clinical utility. Positrons are positively charged particles that are identical in mass to electrons. PET tracers (that is, the metabolic compounds used in PET imaging) decay by emission of positrons. When a positron and an electron are in close proximity to each other, **annihilation** occurs, resulting in the conversion of their masses into two gamma-ray photons traveling in opposite directions. PET scanners detect pairs of gamma rays formed by annihilation. By determining where these gamma rays originated, the PET scanner can create an image showing where in the body the annihilation occurred.

There are many tracers that emit positrons. The two that are most often used in nuclear cardiology are **fluorine-18** (^{18}F) and **rubidium-82** (^{82}Rb). ^{18}F is used to produce FDG (18-fluorodeoxyglucose). FDG is taken up by cells for glucose metabolism at a rate proportional to the cells' metabolic demands. ^{82}Rb is a potassium analog that follows blood flow. Both are very specific to the myocardium.

Applications

PET is used for the assessment of myocardial perfusion, viability, metabolism, innervation, and receptor density.

The goal of PET **myocardial perfusion imaging** (Fig. 26-6) is to detect myocardial infarction and ischemia. The most common radiotracers used for evaluating myocardial perfusion are nitrogen-13 (^{13}N), rubidium-82 (^{82}Rb), and oxygen-15 (^{15}O). As in the case of SPECT, resting images are obtained initially. Next, a pharmacologic stress agent (adenosine or dipyridamole) is administered to test coronary flow reserve. Because these three radiotracers have very short half-lives, an exercise stress test cannot be performed.

^{18}FDG is the tracer most commonly used for assessing **myocardial viability.** Ischemic myocardium that is viable remains metabolically active (utilizes glucose). Thus, myocardial viability is assessed by administering ^{18}FDG with either ^{13}N, ^{82}Rb, carbon-11 (^{11}C), or ^{15}O or by utilizing a SPECT study. The PET perfusion/SPECT radiotracers will assess myocardial perfusion while ^{18}FDG and ^{11}C will assess myocardial metabolism. Classically,

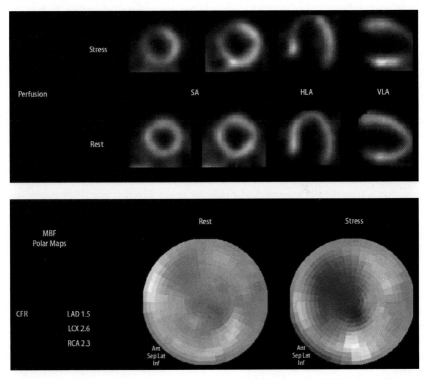

FIGURE 26-6. Myocardial perfusion study showing 13N-ammonia PET at rest with adenosine-stress images. The upper images demonstrate a reversible perfusion defect involving the septum, anterior wall, and apex. The lower images show quantification of absolute myocardial blood flow with reduced flow reserve in the territory of the LAD (From Valk PE. *Positron Emission Tomography: Clinical Practice.* New York: Springer; 2006, with permission.)

ischemic but viable tissue will show a mismatch pattern, with decreased perfusion but preserved glucose or fatty acid metabolism.

As a result of the nearly unlimited availability of biomolecules for labeling with radiotracers, PET has played a prominent role in the study of **substrate utilization in myocardial metabolism**. Agents used for the assessment of substrate utilization have included ^{18}FDG (glucose transport), ^{11}C glucose (glucose metabolism), ^{11}C acetate (citric acid cycle metabolism), ^{11}C palmitate (fatty acid metabolism), ^{18}F-thioheptadecanoic acid (fatty acid uptake), and ^{11}C lactate (lactate utilization).

^{11}C-hydroxyephedrine (HED), ^{11}C-epinephrine (EPI), and ^{123}I-meta-iodobenzylguanidine (MIBG) are radiotracers used in the assessment of **myocardial innervation**. These radiotracers are taken up by sympathetic neurons and have been used in the study of sympathetic reinnervation of cardiac allografts posttransplant as well as the effects of sympathetic innervation in patient populations at risk for cardiac arrhythmias.

Limitations

The major disadvantages of PET are cost and convenience. PET studies cost significantly more than SPECT studies. SPECT radiotracers are also more convenient to use than PET radiotracers. ^{18}F must be produced by a cyclotron that, owing to its 2-hour half-life, must be located in the vicinity of the PET scanner. Other shorter-lived radiotracers, such as ^{11}C compounds, actually require an on-site cyclotron. ^{82}Rb has a very short half-life (76 seconds) but can be produced from a longer-lived strontium-82 (^{82}Sr). Lastly, pharmacologic means must be used to assess coronary flow reserve with PET. The time needed for exercise testing is incompatible with the short half-lives of PET radiotracers. This eliminates the valuable physiologic information that can be gained from assessing exercise capacity.

INTRAVASCULAR ULTRASOUND (IVUS)

Introduction

Intravascular ultrasound (IVUS) is a catheter-based ultrasound modality that provides real-time high-resolution images, allowing precise tomographic assessment of lumen area, plaque size, and composition of a segment of a coronary artery. The first true IVUS system was designed by Bom and coworkers in Rotterdam in 1971 as an improved technique for visualizing cardiac chambers and valves. The first transluminal images of human arteries were recorded by Yock and colleagues in 1988. IVUS is now routinely used in cardiac catheterization laboratories for guidance of interventional and electrophysiologic procedures.

An IVUS catheter integrates a miniaturized ultrasound probe to obtain high-resolution ultrasound images of the coronary walls and intracardiac structures. Ultrasound waves are emitted from the catheter tip, usually in the 10- to 20-MHz range, which then return to the transducer and are sent out to external computerized ultrasound equipment. A real-time ultrasound image of the structures surrounding the catheter tip is reconstructed from the returning ultrasound waves.

Applications

IVUS is frequently used to determine the degree of stenosis in situations where angiographic imaging is considered unreliable, as for ostial coronary lesions, left main stenosis, or overlapped segments (Figs. 26-7 and 26-8). IVUS is also used to evaluate complex lesions before percutaneous revascularization and before stent deployment within a coronary artery in the setting of intervention. If a stent is not adequately expanded flush against the wall of the vessel, turbulent flow may occur between the stent and the wall of the vessel, thus creating a nidus for acute stent thrombosis. Another interventional application is

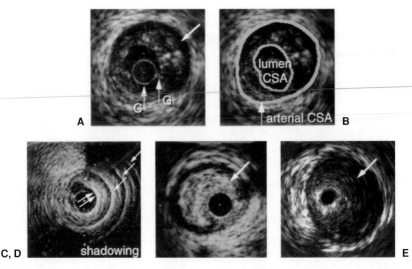

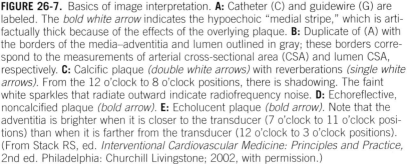

FIGURE 26-7. Basics of image interpretation. **A:** Catheter (C) and guidewire (G) are labeled. The *bold white arrow* indicates the hypoechoic "medial stripe," which is artifactually thick because of the effects of the overlying plaque. **B:** Duplicate of (A) with the borders of the media–adventitia and lumen outlined in gray; these borders correspond to the measurements of arterial cross-sectional area (CSA) and lumen CSA, respectively. **C:** Calcific plaque *(double white arrows)* with reverberations *(single white arrows)*. From the 12 o'clock to 8 o'clock positions, there is shadowing. The faint white sparkles that radiate outward indicate radiofrequency noise. **D:** Echoreflective, noncalcified plaque *(bold arrow)*. **E:** Echolucent plaque *(bold arrow)*. Note that the adventitia is brighter when it is closer to the transducer (7 o'clock to 11 o'clock positions) than when it is farther from the transducer (12 o'clock to 3 o'clock positions). (From Stack RS, ed. *Interventional Cardiovascular Medicine: Principles and Practice,* 2nd ed. Philadelphia: Churchill Livingstone; 2002, with permission.)

for guidance of percutaneous closure of an atrial septal defect or patent foramen ovale. IVUS is also used by cardiac electrophysiologists to guide cannulation of the coronary sinus from the right atrium.

IVUS has been used as a research tool for examining characteristics of lesions that predispose patients to myocardial infarctions and to assess the benefit of pharmacologic interventions on atheroma size and volume. Motorized transducer pullback through a stationary imaging sheath permits accurate length and volume measurements by generating a 2D image. This technique is available only with mechanical IVUS catheters. Cross-sectional IVUS measurements using pullback have been validated with multiple in vitro studies.

The lumen is typically a dark (echolucent) area adjacent to the imaging catheter. The coronary artery vessel wall is bright (echogenic) and appears as three layers: intima, media, and adventitia. Segmentation of IVUS images to isolate the intima–media and lumen provides important information about the degree of vessel obstruction as well as the shape and size of plaques. Although IVUS cannot provide accurate biochemical information regarding plaque composition, IVUS imaging can separate lesions into subtypes according to echodensity.

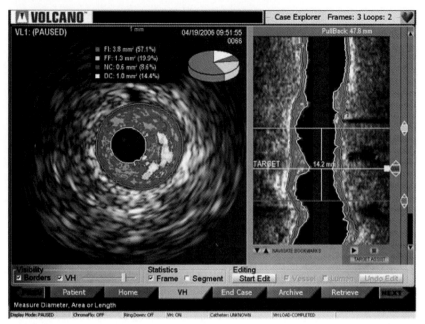

FIGURE 26-8. An IVUS image of a coronary artery (A) and a 2D map of the vessel by pullback (B). The length of a given target segment can then be measured for choosing appropriate stent length. (Images obtained from Volcano Corporation IVUS website: http://www.volcanocorp.com/products/ivus-imaging/s5-imaging.asp. Volcano and the Volcano Logo are registered trademarks of Volcano Corporation.)

Limitations

The primary disadvantages of routine use of IVUS in the cardiac catheterization laboratory are expense, increase in the time of the procedure, and near exclusive use by interventional cardiologists and electrophysiologists.

KEY POINTS TO REMEMBER

Cardiac CT

- Cardiovascular CT is a powerful evolving tool that can provide excellent anatomic assessment of cardiac structures and coronary arteries including intralaminal detail.
- Coronary artery calcium scores can also be used for risk stratification.
- The primary disadvantages of this modality are radiation dose, contrast load poor visualization with rapid irregular heart rates, and lack of physiologic assessment.

Cardiac MRI

- Cardiovascular MRI provides a vast array of clinical applications from noninvasive assessment and serial evaluation of congenital heart disease to sophisticated imaging of cardiac function, differentiation of cardiomyopathies and myocarditis, support of electrophysiology studies, and advanced ischemia detection.

KEY POINTS TO REMEMBER (Continued)

- Cardiovascular MRI has the unique ability to define cardiac and vascular anatomy in great detail and to utilize angiography without the use of nephrotoxic contrast agents and ionizing radiation, as necessary in x-ray–based imaging.
- Cardiovascular MRI is useful to determine cardiac dimensions, structural abnormalities, wall motion, ejection fraction, shunts, and valvular function.
- Late-enhancement imaging allows determination of myocardial viability, similar to nuclear imaging studies.
- Cardiovascular MRI is a safe procedure with a low rate of side effects, mainly claustrophobia and rarely systemic fibrosis after gadolinium contrast in patients with severely impaired kidney function.

PET

- PET is a powerful research tool with both clinical and research applications.
- It is technically superior to SPECT.
- The main drawbacks preventing its widespread use are its significantly higher cost and the difficulties involved in using PET radiotracers (cyclotron availability and very short half-lives).

IVUS

- IVUS is a useful but highly specialized tool for imaging coronary vasculature and intra-cardiac structures.
- The diagnostic benefits of using IVUS must be weighed against its drawbacks of additional cost, time, and potential risk.

REFERENCES AND SUGGESTED READINGS

Achenbach S, Giesler T, Ropers D, et al. Detection of coronary artery stenoses by contrast-enhanced, retrospectively electrocardiographically gated, multislice spiral computed tomography. *Circulation* 2001;103:2535–2538.

Assomull RG, Pennell DJ, Prasad SK. Cardiovascular magnetic resonance in the evaluation of heart failure. *Heart* 2007;93:985–992.

Bacharach SL, Bax JJ, Case J, et al. PET myocardial glucose metabolism and perfusion imaging. Part 1: Guidelines for data acquisition and patient preparation. *J Nucl Cardiol* 2003;10:543–556.

Barkhausen J, Ruehm SG, Goyen, M, et al. MR evaluation of ventricular function: true fast imaging with steady-state precession versus fast low-angle shot cine MR imaging: feasibility study. *Radiology* 2001;219:264–269.

Bax JJ, Valkema R, Visser FC, et al. FDG SPECT in the assessment of myocardial viability. Comparison with dobutamine echo. *Eur Heart J* 1997;18(suppl D): D124–D129.

Bengel FM, Ueberfuhr P, Schiepel N, et al. Effect of sympathetic reinnervation on cardiac performance after heart transplantation. *N Engl J Med* 2001;345:731–738.

Bom N, Lancee CT, van Egmond FC. An ultrasonic intracardiac scanner. *Ultrasonics* 1972;10:71–76.

Bruce CJ, Packer DL, Seward JB. Transvascular imaging: feasibility study using a vector phased array ultrasound catheter. *Echocardiography* 1999;16:425.

Cademartiri F, Runza G, Mollet NR, et al. Impact of intravascular enhancement, heart rate, and calcium score on diagnostic accuracy in multislice computed tomography coronary angiography. *Radiol Med* (Torino) 2005;110:42–51.

Cyrus T, Lanza GM, Wickline SA. Molecular imaging by cardiovascular MR. *J Cardiovasc Magnet Res* 2007;9:827–843.

Dayanikli F, Grambow D, Muzik O, et al. Early detection of abnormal coronary flow reserve in asymptomatic men at high risk for coronary artery disease using positron emission tomography. *Circulation* 1994;90:808–817.

Depre C, Vanoverschelde JL, Gerber B, et al. Correlation of functional recovery with myocardial blood flow, glucose uptake, and morphologic features in patients with chronic left ventricular ischemic dysfunction undergoing coronary artery bypass grafting. *J Thorac Cardiovasc Surg* 1997;113:371–378.

Di Carli MF, Tobes MC, Mangner T, et al. Effects of cardiac sympathetic innervation on coronary blood flow. *N Engl J Med* 1997;336:1208–1215.

DiCarli MF, Asgarzadie F, Schelbert HR, et al. Quantitative relation between myocardial viability and improvement in heart failure symptoms after revascularization in patients with ischemic cardiomyopathy. *Circulation* 1995;92:3436–3444.

DiMario C, The SH, Madretsma S, et al: Detection and characterization of vascular lesions by intravascular ultrasound: an in vitro study correlated with histology. *J Am Soc Echocardiogr* 1992;5:135–146.

Dirksen MS, Jukema JW, Bax JJ, et al. Cardiac multidetector-row computed tomography in patients with unstable angina. *Am J Cardiol* 2005;95:457–461.

Djavidani B, Debl K, Lenhart M, et al. Planimetry of mitral valve stenosis by magnetic resonance imaging. *J Am Coll Cardiol* 2005;45:2048–2053.

Feigenbaum H. *Echocardiography*, 5th ed. Malvern, PA: Lea & Febiger; 1994.

Fuessl RT, Mintz GS, Pichard AD, et al: In vivo validation of intravascular ultrasound length measurements using a motorized transducer pullback device. *Am J Cardiol* 1996;77:1115–1118.

Gambhir SS, Schwaiger M, Huang SC, et al. Simple noninvasive quantification method for measuring myocardial glucose utilization in humans employing positron emission tomography and fluorine-18 deoxyglucose. *J Nucl Med* 1989;30:359–366.

Garcia MJ, Lessick J, Hoffmann MH et al. Accuracy of 16-row multidetector computed tomography for the assessment of coronary artery stenosis. *JAMA* 2006;296 (4):403–411.

Giesler T, Baum U, Ropers D, et al. Noninvasive visualization of coronary arteries using contrast-enhanced multidetector CT: influence of heart rate on image quality and stenosis detection. *AJR Am J Roentgenol* 2002;179:911–916.

Gould K, Goldstein R, Mullani N, et al. Clinical feasibility, sensitivity and specifically of positron cardiac imaging without a cyclotron using generator produced Rb-82 for the diagnosis of coronary artery disease. *J Nucl Med* 1986;27:976.

Gropler RJ, Geltman EM, Sampathkumaran K, et al. Comparison of carbon-11-acetate with fluorine-18-fluorodeoxyglucose for delineating viable myocardium by positron emission tomography. *J Am Coll Cardiol* 1993;22:1587–1597.

Gussenhoven EJ, Essed CE, Lancee CT, et al. Arterial wall characteristics determined by intravascular ultrasound imaging: an in vitro study. *J Am Coll Cardiol* 1989;14: 947–952.

Hendel RC, Patel MR, Kramer CM, Poon M. ACCF/ACR/SCCT/SCMR/ASNC/ NASCI/SCAI/SIR 2006 appropriateness criteria for cardiac computed tomography and cardiac magnetic resonance imaging: a report of the American College of Cardiology Foundation/American College of Radiology, Society of Cardiovascular Computed Tomography, Society for Cardiovascular Magnetic Resonance, American Society of Nuclear Cardiology, North American Society for Cardiac Imaging, Society for

Cardiovascular Angiography and Interventions, and Society of Interventional Radiology. *J Am Coll Cardiol* 2006;48:1475–1497.

Herrero P, Weinheimer CJ, Dence C, et al. Quantification of myocardial glucose utilization by PET and 1-carbon-11-glucose. *J Nucl Cardiol* 2002;9:5–14.

Herzog C, Britten M, Balzer JO, et al. Multidetector-row cardiac CT: diagnostic value of calcium scoring and CT coronary angiography in patients with symptomatic, but atypical, chest pain. *Eur Radiol* 2004;14:169–177.

Hodgson JMcB, Eberle M, Savakus A. Validation of a new real time percutaneous intravascular ultrasound imaging catheter [Abstract]. *Circulation* 1988;78:II-21.

Kaul T, Agnohotri A, Fields B, et al. Coronary artery bypass grafting in patients with an ejection fraction of twenty percent or less. *J Thorac Cardiovasc Surg* 1996;111:1001–1012.

Knez A, Becker CR, Leber A, et al. Usefulness of multislice spiral computed tomography angiography for determination of coronary artery stenoses. *Am J Cardiol* 2001;88:1191–1194.

Kopp AF, Schroeder S, Kuettner A, et al. Non-invasive coronary angiography with high resolution multidetector-row computed tomography: results in 102 patients. *Eur Heart J* 2002;23:1714–1725.

Kramer CM, Budoff MJ, Fayad ZA, et al. ACCF/AHA Clinical Competence Statement on Vascular Imaging with Computed Tomography and Magnetic Resonance. A report of the American College of Cardiology Foundation/American Heart Association/American College of Physicians Task Force on Clinical Competence and Training. *J Am Coll Cardiol* 2007;50:1097–1114.

Kuettner A, Kopp AF, Schroeder S, et al. Diagnostic accuracy of multidetector computed tomography coronary angiography in patients with angiographically proven coronary artery disease. *J Am Coll Cardiol* 2004;43:831–839.

Leber AW, Knez A, von Ziegler F, et al. Quantification of obstructive and nonobstructive coronary lesions by 64-slice computed tomography: a comparative study with quantitative coronary angiography and intravascular ultrasound. *J Am Coll Cardiol* 2005;46:147–154.

Leschka S, Alkadhi H, Plass A, et al. Accuracy of MSCT coronary angiography with 64-slice technology: first experience. *Eur Heart J* 2005;26:1482–1487.

Levine GN, Gomes AS, Arai AE, et al. Safety of Magnetic Resonance Imaging in Patients with Cardiovascular Devices. An American Heart Association Scientific Statement From the Committee on Diagnostic and Interventional Cardiac Catheterization, Council on Clinical Cardiology, and the Council on Cardiovascular Radiology and Intervention. Endorsed by the American College of Cardiology Foundation, the North American Society for Cardiac Imaging, and the Society for Cardiovascular Magnetic Resonance. *Circulation* 2007;116:2878–2891, published online Nov. 19, 2007.

Mallery JA, Tobis JM, Griffith J, et al. Assessment of normal and atherosclerotic arterial wall thickness with an intravascular ultrasound imaging catheter. *Am Heart J* 1990;119:1392–1400.

Marwick T, Shan K, Patel S, et al. Incremental value of rubidium-82 positron emission tomography for prognostic assessment of known or suspected coronary artery disease. *Am J Cardiol* 1997;80:865–870.

Matar FA, Mintz GS, Farb A, et al. The contribution of tissue removal to lumen improvement after directional coronary atherectomy. *Am J Cardiol* 1994;74:647–650.

McVeigh ER, Guttman MA, Lederman RJ. Real-time interactive MRI-guided cardiac surgery: aortic valve replacement using a direct apical approach. *Magn Reson Med* 2006;56:958–964.

Merlet P, Delforge J, Syrota A, et al. Positron emission tomography with ^{11}C CGP-12177 to assess beta-adrenergic receptor concentration in idiopathic dilated cardiomyopathy. *Circulation* 1993;87:1169–1178.

Mollet NR, Cademartiri F, Nieman K, et al. Noninvasive assessment of coronary plaque burden using multislice computed tomography. *Am J Cardiol* 2005;95: 1165–1169.

Nandalur KR, Dwamena BA, Choudhri AF, et al. Diagnostic performance of stress cardiac magnetic resonance imaging in the detection of coronary artery disease. *J Am Coll Cardiol* 2007;50:1343–1353.

Nicholls SJ, Sipahi I, Schoenhagen P, et al. Application of intravascular ultrasound in anti-atherosclerotic drug development. *Nat Rev Drug Disc* 2006;5(6):485–492.

Nicholls SJ, Tuzcu EM, Sipahi I, et al. Intravascular ultrasound in cardiovascular medicine. *Circulation* 2006;114(4):e55–e59.

Nieman K, Resning B, van Geuns RJ, et al. Usefulness of multislice computed tomography for detecting obstructive coronary artery disease. *Am J Cardiol* 2002;89: 913–918.

Nishimura RA, Edwards WD, Warnes CA, et al. Intravascular ultrasound imaging: in vitro validation and pathologic correlation. *J Am Coll Cardiol* 1990;16:145–154.

Oemrawsingh PV, Mintz GS, Schalij MJ, et al. Intravascular ultrasound guidance improves angiographic and clinical outcome of stent implantation for long coronary artery stenoses: final results of a randomized comparison with angiographic guidance (TULIP Study). *Circulation* 2003;107:62.

Packer DL, Stevens CL, Curley MG, et al. Intracardiac phased-array imaging: methods and initial clinical experience with high resolution, under blood visualization: initial experience with intracardiac phased-array ultrasound. *J Am Coll Cardiol* 2002; 39:509.

Patterson RE, Eisner RL, Horowitz SF. Comparison of cost-effectiveness and utility of exercise ECG, single photon emission computed tomography, positron emission tomography, and coronary angiography for diagnosis of coronary artery disease. *Circulation* 1995;91:54–65.

Peterson LR, Herrero P, Schechtman KB, et al. Effect of obesity and insulin resistance on myocardial substrate metabolism and efficiency in young women. *Circulation* 2004; 109:2191–2196.

Potkin BN, Bartorelli AL, Gessert JM, et al. Coronary artery imaging with intravascular high-frequency ultrasound. *Circulation* 1990;81:1575–1585.

Raff GL, Gallagher MJ, O'Neill WW, et al. Diagnostic accuracy of noninvasive coronary angiography using 64-slice spiral computed tomography. *J Am Coll Cardiol* 2005;46:552–557.

Rahimtoola SH. The hibernating myocardium. *Am Heart J* 1989;117:211–221.

Reant P, Lederlin M, Lafitte S, et al. Absolute assessment of aortic valve stenosis by planimetry using cardiovascular magnetic resonance imaging: comparison with trans-esophageal echocardiography, transthoracic echocardiography, and cardiac catheterization. *Eur J Radiol* 2006;59:276–283.

Sato Y, Matsumoto N, Kato M, et al. Noninvasive assessment of coronary artery disease by multislice spiral computed tomography using a new retrospectively ECG-gated image reconstruction technique. *Circ J* 2003;67:401–405.

Schelbert HR, Beanlands R, Bengel F, et al. PET myocardial perfusion and glucose metabolism imaging. Part 2: Guidelines for interpretation and reporting. *J Nucl Cardiol* 2003;10:557–571.

Schlosser T, Malyar N, Jochims M, et al. Quantification of aortic valve stenosis in MRI. *Eur Radiol* 2007;17:1284–1290.

Schoenhagen P, Nissen SE. Intravascular ultrasonography: using imaging end points in coronary atherosclerosis trials. *Cleve Clin J Med* 2005;72(6):487–496.

Selvanayagam JB, Hawkins PN, Paul B, et al. Evaluation and management of the cardiac amyloidosis. *J Am Coll Cardiol* 2007;50:2101–2110.

Sipahi I, Tuzcu EM, Schoenhagen P, et al. Static and serial assessments of coronary arterial remodeling are discordant: an intravascular ultrasound analysis from the Reversal of Atherosclerosis with Aggressive Lipid Lowering (REVERSAL) trial. *Am Heart J* 2006;152(3):544–550.

Stack RS, ed. *Interventional Cardiovascular Medicine: Principles and Practice,* 2nd ed. Philadelphia: Churchill Livingstone; 2002.

Suzuki J, Caputo GR, Kondo C, et al. Cine MR imaging of valvular heart disease: display and imaging parameters affect the size of the signal void caused by valvular regurgitation. *Am J Roentgenol* 1990;155:723–727.

Tobis JM, Mallery JA, Gessert J, et al. Intravascular ultrasound cross-sectional arterial imaging before and after balloon angioplasty in vitro. *Circulation* 1989;80:873–882.

Topol EJ. *Textbook of Interventional Cardiology,* 4th ed. Philadelphia: Saunders; 2003.

Vogl TJ, Abolmaali ND, Diebold T, et al. Techniques for the detection of coronary atherosclerosis: multi-detector row CT coronary angiography. *Radiology* 2002;223:212–220.

Von Birgelen C, van der Lugt A, Nicosia A, et al. Computerized assessment of coronary lumen and atherosclerotic plaque dimensions in three-dimensional intravascular ultrasound correlated with histomorphometry. *Am J Cardiol* 1996;78:1202–1209.

Warnes CA. Transposition of the Great Arteries. *Circulation* 2006;114:2699–2709.

Weber OM, Higgins CB. MR evaluation of cardiovascular physiology in congenital heart disease: flow and function. *J Cardiovasc Magnet Res* 2006;8:607–617.

Wenguang L, Gussenhoven WJ, Zhong Y, et al. Validation of quantitative analysis of intravascular ultrasound images. *J Card Imaging* 1991;6:247–253.

Wood JC. Anatomical assessment of congenital heart disease. *J Cardiovasc Magnet Res* 2006;8:595–606.

Yi-qun Y, Fang-ling L, Jun T, et al. Assessment of autopsic samples of carotid atherosclerosis in the aged by intravascular ultrasound. *Chin Med J* 1994;107:750–754.

Yock PG, Johnson EL, Linker DT. Intravascular ultrasound: development and clinical potential. *Am J Card Imaging* 1988;2:185–193.

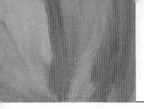

Procedures in Cardiovascular Critical Care

Michael O. Barry and Andrew M. Kates

INTRODUCTION

The care of the critically ill patient can be very challenging. Altered ventricular filling, poor myocardial perfusion, abnormal cardiac rhythms, and severe valvular lesions all contribute in a complex interaction. There are several procedures that, when used appropriately, can both stabilize and help treat the cardiac patient. This chapter discusses the rationale and technique of three of these: utilization of the intra-aortic balloon pump, pulmonary artery catheter, and temporary transvenous pacemaker.

INTRA-AORTIC BALLOON PUMP

Introduction

The intra-aortic balloon pump (IABP), the first hemodynamic support device, was developed in the 1960s. It provides improvements in the myocardial O_2 supply/demand ratio and circulatory support. It remains the most widely used mechanical cardiac-support device because of its simplicity, ease of insertion, and long clinical track record.

Hemodynamic Effects of Counterpulsation

The intra-aortic balloon exerts its hemodynamic effects through counterpulsation (Fig. 27-1, Table 27-1). The balloon rapidly inflates during diastole and deflates during systole. The inflation and deflation provide two specific hemodynamic effects:

- Rapid expansion in early diastole (i.e., just after aortic valve closure), produces an increase in diastolic pressure, which translates into a marked increase in coronary perfusion pressure.
- Abrupt deflation during isovolumetric contraction (just before the opening of the aortic valve), which removes effective aortic volume. This decreases the aortic systolic pressure and subsequently resistance, allowing for greater left ventricular (LV) systolic ejection and effectively decreasing myocardial O_2 requirements through afterload reduction.

Technique

An understanding of balloon insertion technique aids in understanding its clinical utility as well as possible complications. The patient must first be assessed for evidence of contraindications to balloon insertion (see below). Then an appropriate-sized balloon is determined by patient size. Needle access to the common femoral artery is obtained. A guidewire is passed through the needle into the abdominal aorta, making sure no resistance is encountered. Placement of the wire is confirmed by fluoroscopy. A 7- to 9-Fr introducer sheath is placed over the wire by the modified Seldinger technique. A small amount of contrast dye

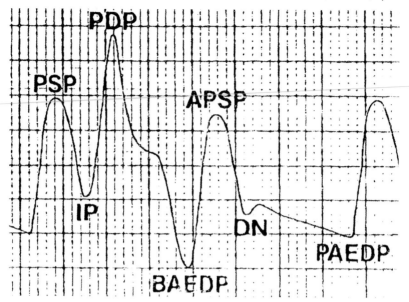

FIGURE 27-1. Normal arterial waveform with intra-aortic balloon pump (IABP) set at 1:2 pulsation (with every other beat, the balloon inflates and deflates). APSP, assisted peak systolic pressure; BAEDP, balloon aortic end-diastolic pressure; DN, dichrotic notch; IP, inflation point; PAEDP, patient aortic end-diastolic pressure; PDP, peak diastolic pressure; PSP, peak systolic pressure. (From Sorrentino M, Feldman T. Techniques for IABP timing, use, and discontinuance. *J Crit Illn* 1992;7[4]:597–604, with permission.)

TABLE 27-1 INTRAAORTIC BALLOON PUMP TERMINOLOGY

Terminology (at a 1:2 pumping rate)	Effects
Peak systolic pressure	Systolic pressure without activity related to the balloon pump
Inflation point	Point on the arterial pressure tracing where balloon inflation originates, just after the dicrotic notch
Peak diastolic pressure	Augmented increase in diastolic pressure that occurs when the balloon inflation displaces aortic blood volume due to counterpulsation
Balloon aortic end-diastolic pressure	Lowest pressure in the aorta, reflecting balloon deflation
Assisted peak systolic pressure	Systolic peak that reflects the afterload reduction produced by the balloon pump
Dicrotic notch	Landmark on the downslope of the arterial pressure waveform that signals aortic valve closure and the beginning of diastole

is injected through the sheath and, using cineangiography, the suitability of the ileofemoral arterial system is assessed, as severe vascular disease precludes placement of the IABP. Of note, some IABP systems allow placement over a long wire without a sheath. In emergent situations, when fluoroscopy is not available, the procedure can be done at the bedside. Confirmation by chest x-ray of IABP tip position just below the aortic arch (distal to the left subclavian artery) is essential. The balloon line is connected to the pump, which injects helium, and the blood port is connected to the pressure transducer.

Indications

- Cardiogenic shock: acute myocardial infarction, acute mitral regurgitation, ventricular septal defect (VSD), myocarditis, stress-induced cardiomopathy ("takotsubo cardiomyopathy"), or drug toxicity
- Unstable angina
- Prophylaxis in the setting of high-risk intervention
- Severe symptomatic aortic stenosis, especially when associated with heart failure
- Severe multivessel or left main coronary artery disease (CAD) requiring urgent cardiac or noncardiac surgery

Contraindications

- Significant aortic regurgitation
- Abdominal aortic aneurysm
- Aortic dissection
- Septicemia
- Uncontrolled bleeding
- Severe bilateral peripheral vascular disease
- Bilateral femoropopliteal bypass grafts for severe peripheral vascular disease

Complications

- **Limb ischemia** is related to simple mechanical obstruction by the balloon catheter at the insertion site. Balloon removal generally alleviates the problem.
- **Iatrogenic retrograde arterial dissection** may occur as a result of wire advancement and usually presents with severe back pain.
- **Cholesterol embolization** usually manifests as bilateral, painful, cold, mottled limbs (livedo reticularis) with associated eosinophilia, eosinophiluria, and thrombocytopenia as well as renal failure secondary to cholesterol emboli.
- **Embolic cerebrovascular accident** may occur if the IABP's central lumen has been flushed vigorously due to thrombus formation. Therefore the central lumen of the IABP should not be used as a source of arterial blood.
- **Sepsis** is a rare complication.
- **Balloon rupture** occurs due to calcification in the aorta. The ruptured balloon may produce thrombus within the balloon, making percutaneous removal impossible and requiring consultation from a vascular surgeon. Rarely, balloon rupture may be associated with helium embolization.

Troubleshooting

Late Balloon Inflation

- If the balloon inflates **late** after the aortic valve closes, the diastolic augmentation period is shortened, which translates into reduced coronary perfusion time.

Early Balloon Inflation

- If the balloon inflates before the aortic valve closes, myocardial stress is increased because of increased afterload.

- Therefore balloon inflation should coincide with the dicrotic notch on the arterial waveform.

Early Balloon Deflation

- If the balloon deflates before isovolumetric contraction, the aorta refills with blood before ventricular ejection.

Late Balloon Deflation

- If the balloon deflates late after the aortic valve opens, ejection fraction is reduced and myocardial work increased.
- Therefore balloon deflation should coincide with the onset of isovolumetric contraction on the arterial waveform.

PULMONARY ARTERY CATHETERIZATION

The decision to place a pulmonary artery (PA) catheter (also called a "right heart" catheter or Swan-Ganz catheter) should be preceded by a specific question regarding the patient's hemodynamic status. As placement of a PA catheter is not without risk, the answer to this question must have significant bearing on the management of the patient. During routine right-heart catheterization, measurements of pressures and O_2 saturations in the vena cava, right atrium, right ventricle (RV), and pulmonary artery (PA) can be obtained; in addition, pulmonary capillary wedge pressure (PCWP) and cardiac output (CO) quantified. O_2 saturations may be used to assess the location and magnitude of an intracardiac shunt occurring in the presence of an atrial septal defect or ventricular septal defect or possibly a patent ductus arteriosus. The PCWP usually provides an accurate estimation of left atrial pressure which, in the absence of mitral stenosis, reflects LV end-diastolic pressure and is a measurement of preload. Right-heart catheterization allows for evaluation of the severity of tricuspid or pulmonic stenosis, pulmonary hypertension, calculation of pulmonary vascular resistance (PVR), and determination of the etiology of shock (Table 27-2).

Risks and complications associated with right-heart catheterization include:

- Air embolism
- Endocarditis/sepsis
- PA rupture
- Bleeding
- Cardiac tamponade/perforation
- Pulmonary infarction

TABLE 27-2	SHOCK: ETIOLOGY-DEPENDENT HEMODYNAMICS			
Etiology of Shock	**PCWP**	**RAP**	**CO**	**SVR**
Cardiogenic	High	High	Low	High
Septic	Low	Low	High/normal	Low
Pulmonary embolism/ pulmonary HTN	Normal	High	Low	High/ normal
Hypovolemic	Low	Low	Low	High

CO, cardiac output; HTN, hypertension; PCWP, pulmonary capillary wedge pressure; RAP, right arterial pressure; SVR, systemic vascular resistance.

- Right bundle-branch block (complete heart block if there is underlying left bundle-branch block)
- Pneumothorax (if the superior approach is used)
- Sustained ventricular arrhythmias
- Thromboembolism

Access and Catheterization Technique

Choice of access site should be determined individually according to the risks and benefits of each location. Nevertheless, the left subclavian and the right internal jugular approaches permit easiest passage of the catheter into the PA. Femoral veins are often used but require more skill in placement and are associated with a higher risk of infection or deep venous thrombosis if the catheter is left in place. Placement via a femoral vein is most often done under fluoroscopic guidance. Use of fluoroscopy for patients with intracardiac devices such as permanent pacemakers (PPMs) or implantable cardioverter-defibrillators (ICDs) is also strongly encouraged.

The technique of insertion of the 7- to 8-Fr introducer (also called a **sheath**) is the same as that for any central venous access—the Seldinger technique. The PA catheter is passed through the introducer into the vein and the balloon is inflated when the tip of the catheter exits the sheath. Continuous pressure tracing and fluoroscopy aid with establishment of catheter tip position. When the catheter is being advanced, the balloon should be fully inflated. As the catheter is advanced through the tricuspid valve, the pressure tracing records a dramatic change to the higher pressures seen in the RV. This location is associated with the greatest risk for arrhythmias; thus, proceed without delay. Arrival at the PA is heralded by the appearance of the dicrotic notch on the pressure tracing. Also, the diastolic pressure is greater than that of the RV. From the PA, **slowly** advance the inflated balloon catheter until a fall in the systolic pressure is noted compared with the pressure in the PA; this is the PCWP. The balloon may now be deflated and the PA tracing should reappear. The balloon should then be **slowly** reinflated. If too little balloon volume is required to reach the wedge position, the catheter tip is positioned too distally, and further inflation risks PA rupture. Perform a chest x-ray to confirm the position of the PA catheter. The tip should be no more than 3 to 5 cm from the midline. Ideally, the catheter tip should be in zone III of the lung, where arterial pressure exceeds venous and alveolar pressure, thereby creating a column of blood to the left atrium. **The balloon should always be maintained in the deflated position except when a PCWP measurement is being made.**

Hemodynamic Measurements

Pressure Measurement and Waveforms

Once the catheter has been positioned in the desired cardiac chamber, it is connected directly through fluid-filled tubing to a pressure transducer. This transducer transforms a pressure signal into an electrical signal. See **Table 27-3** for normal hemodynamic values.

Errors in pressure measurements can result from several sources, such as inaccurate zero referencing of the manometer.

Right Atrial Tracing

- Right atrial systole follows the P wave on the electrocardiogram (ECG) and produces the *a* wave of the right atrial pressure tracing. With relaxation, there is a decline in the pressure, known as the *x* descent.
- Filling of the right atrium from the venous circulation and retrograde movement of the tricuspid valve annulus during RV systole produces the *v* wave. When the tricuspid valve opens, blood from the right atrium empties into the RV, thus causing a decline in the right atrial pressure and producing the *y* descent.
- Typically, the pressure of the peak *a* wave is higher than that of the peak *v* wave.

TABLE 27-3	NORMAL HEMODYNAMIC VALUES
Cardiac index (L/min per m^2)	2.6–4.2
PCWP (mm Hg)	6–12
PA (mm Hg)	16–30/3–12
Mean	10–16
RV (mm Hg)	16–30/0–8
RA (mm Hg)	0–8
SVR (dynes/sec/cm^{-5})	700–1600
PVR (dynes/sec/cm^{-5})	20–130

PA, pulmonary artery; PCWP, pulmonary capillary wedge pressure; PVR, pulmonary vascular resistance; RA, right atrium; RV, right ventricle; SVR, systemic vascular resistance.

Right Ventricular Tracing

Right ventricular systole follows the QRS complex, which gives rise to a rapidly increasing systolic pressure waveform. With ventricular relaxation, the pressure waveform declines and reaches a nadir.

Pulmonary Artery Tracing

The normal PA pressure consists of a systolic wave that coincides with RV systole. The decline in the pressure wave is usually interrupted by the **dicrotic notch**, which corresponds to the pulmonic valve closure. The nadir of the decline represents the end-diastolic pressure (Fig. 27-2).

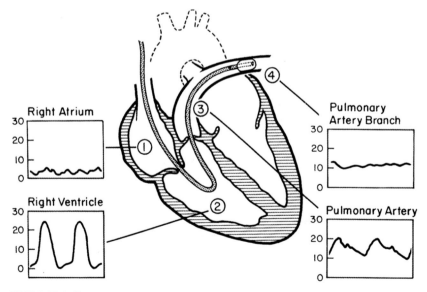

FIGURE 27-2. Pressure tracing exhibited in the various chambers and positions during right-heart catheterization. (From Marino PL. *The ICU Book,* 2nd ed. Philadelphia: Lippincott Williams & Wilkins; 1997:157, with permission.)

Pulmonary Capillary Wedge Tracing

- The pressure waveform obtained is a transmitted left atrial pressure. The tracing is similar to the right atrial waveform. There is an *a* wave, an *x* descent, a *v* wave, and a *y* descent; these correspond with left atrial systole, relaxation, filling, and emptying, respectively.
- Typically, the *v* wave is greater than the *a* wave.

Cardiac Output

Cardiac output (CO) is defined as liters of output per minute, whereas the cardiac index (CI) is the magnitude of CO proportional to the body surface area. The two commonly used methods of measuring CO are the **Fick method and the thermodilution technique.**

The Fick method is based on the hypothesis that the consumption of oxygen ($\dot{V}O_2$) by an organ is the product of the blood flow to that organ and the regional arteriovenous concentration difference of the substance.

$$\text{CO (L/minute)} = O_2 \text{ consumption (mL/minute)/arteriovenous } O_2 \text{ difference}$$
$$(\text{A}\dot{V}O_2) \text{ across the lungs (mL/L)}$$

To measure CO in humans, this principle is applied to the lungs. By measuring the amounts of O_2 extracted from inspired air and the $\text{A}\dot{V}O_2$ across the lungs, one can calculate the pulmonary blood flow. Pulmonary blood flow is equal to systemic blood flow; therefore, in the absence of a significant shunt, it can be extrapolated as CO. In many labs, the O_2 consumption is estimated from a nomogram. Determining $\text{A}\dot{V}O_2$ differences across the lungs requires blood from the PA and pulmonary vein to be analyzed for O_2 content. Because the O_2 content of the pulmonary venous blood is similar to that of the systemic arterial blood (in the absence of a right-to-left interatrial shunt), these values may be interchanged. The Fick method is **most accurate for patients with a low CO** and least accurate in patients with a high CO or significant shunts.

With the **thermodilution technique** to determine CO, a known amount of indicator is injected into the circulation and allowed to mix completely in the blood; then its concentration is measured over time (Fig. 27-3). A time–concentration curve is generated, and the area under the curve, as calculated by minicomputers, corresponds to the CO. The indicator most often used is cold saline. A balloon-tipped, flow-direct catheter with a thermistor at the tip is used. The distal tip with the thermistor is advanced to the PA, and the proximal port is within the right atrium. Next, 5 to 10 mL of iced fluid is injected through the proximal port, and the temperature change at the distal thermistor is recorded as time. This allows for a thermodilution curve to be formulated and converted into CO. This technique is inexpensive, easy to perform, and does not require arterial sampling; **however, certain conditions may render the results unreliable, such as tricuspid regurgitation, pulmonic regurgitation, or intracardiac shunts and low CO.**

Vascular Resistance

The resistance of a vascular bed is calculated by dividing the pressure gradient across the bed by the flow through it.

$$\text{Systemic vascular resistance (SVR)} = (\text{mean systemic arterial pressure}$$
$$- \text{ mean right atrial pressure})/\text{CO}$$

- Increased SVR is usually present in patients with systemic hypertension. It also may be seen in patients with low a CO who have compensatory vasoconstriction.
- Reduced SVR is seen with inappropriately increased CO (e.g., sepsis, arteriovenous [AV] fistulas, anemia, fever, thyrotoxicosis).

$$\text{Pulmonary vascular resistance (PVR)} = (\text{mean pulmonary arterial pressure}$$
$$- \text{ mean PCWP})/\text{CO}$$

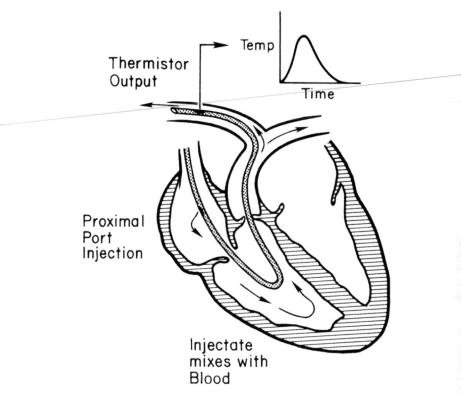

FIGURE 27-3. The thermodilution technique for determining cardiac output. (From Marino PL. *The ICU Book,* 2nd ed. Philadelphia: Lippincott Williams & Wilkins; 1997:179, with permission.)

- Elevated PVR is seen in pulmonary diseases and Eisenmenger syndrome, or a significant left-sided valvular lesion or wall motion defect.

Shunt Calculation

The magnitude and direction of any shunt can be calculated by oximetry, using the following equation:

$$\dot{Q}p/\dot{Q}s = (SAO_2 - MVO_2)/(PVO_2 - PAO_2)$$

Where $\dot{Q}p$ is pulmonary blood flow, $\dot{Q}s$ is systemic blood flow, **SAO_2 is systemic arterial oxygen saturation, MVO_2 is myocardial oxygen consumption, PVO_2 is mixed venous oxygen pressure, and PAO_2 is partial pressure of oxygen in arterial blood.**

MVO_2 is usually equal to the PAO_2 unless there is a shunt and/or congenital anomaly. In this case, MVO_2 is calculated as follows:

$$MVO_2 = [(3 \times SVCO_2) + (IVCO_2)]/4$$

where $SVCO_2$ is the oxygen saturation of the superior vena cava and $IVCO_2$ is that of the inferior vena cava. The PVO_2 can be drawn from the catheter tip in the wedge position (carefully!), although a true PVO_2 is drawn from the left atrium. A $\dot{Q}p/\dot{Q}s > 1$ suggests a net left-to-right shunt; <1 is right-to-left shunt.

Temporary Transvenous Pacing

Initially, temporary cardiac pacing was solely used to increase heart rate, although improvements in our understanding of electrophysiology and pacing electrodes have meant that temporary cardiac pacing can be used as a technique to control both bradyarrhythmias and tachyarrhythmias. The anatomy of the conduction system is described in detail in Chapter 19. Briefly, the normal heartbeat arises from the sinoatrial (SA) node, located in the right atrium near its junction with the superior vena cava. The predominant blood supply to the SA node is from the SA nodal artery, which arises either from the the right coronary artery (60%) or the left circumflex coronary artery (40%). The atrioventricular (AV) node is located posteriorly in the right atrium, adjacent to the tricuspid annulus. The AV node's blood supply arises from the distal right coronary artery (RCA) in 90% of people and the left circumflex coronary artery in 10% of people. There is a delay within the AV node allowing for atrial contraction, then the blood travels through the His bundle to the Purkinje system and the ventricular myocardium. Both the SA and AV nodes are richly innervated by the autonomic nervous system.

The relative balance between the parasympathetic and sympathetic nervous system accounts for the resting autonomic tone. Increased parasympathetic output (i.e., increased vagal tone) can result in clinically significant bradycardia. Common vagal stimuli include:

- Intubation
- Suctioning
- Increased intracranial pressure
- Markedly increased blood pressure
- Urination or defecation
- Vomiting
- Sleeping

Causes

Bradyarrhythmias can be caused by intrinsic disease of the conduction system or by extrinsic factors acting on the conduction system (Table 27-4).

It is important to note that myocardial infarction can cause block at any level of the conduction system. The location of the infarct has a large influence on the prognosis and treatment of conduction disease. In general, proximal (AV-nodal) conduction disease is associated with an infarct of the RCA. This causes a transient AV block and often does not warrant immediate placement of a temporary pacemaker. One exception is AV block in the setting of RV infarction, where restoration of AV synchrony can improve RV filling and thus cardiac output. Distal (infranodal) conduction disease is frequently associated with an left anterior descending (LAD)/septal infarct and is more lasting and life-threatening. Immediate pacing efforts should be pursued.

Temporary Treatment for Bradycardia

Medical treatment with atropine, epinephrine, or dopamine is useful in emergency situations requiring immediate intervention until pacing can be initiated. **Transcutaneous pacing**, first introduced by Zoll in 1952, is the oldest form of pacing. Pacing is achieved by stimulation through electrodes placed on the chest wall. Limitations of this procedure include pain with impulse delivery. There is also limited ability of the electrical impulse to capture the ventricle owing to heavy interference caused by the skeletal muscles and chest wall. Epicardial pacing is frequently used in patients after cardiac surgery. The leads are placed on the epicardium during surgery and can be readily removed at any time. **Epicardial pacing wires** serve both diagnostic and therapeutic functions. Since these wires record atrial and/or ventricular electrical activity, they allow differentiation between ventricular and supraventricular arrhythmias. Epicardial pacing can also be used to terminate certain atrial and ventricular tachyarrhythmias by overdrive pacing. This is done by pulse generators capable of pacing above the tachycardia rate to **"overdrive" the heart.**

TABLE 27-4	EXTRINSIC AND INTRINSIC CAUSES OF CONDUCTION DISEASE

Extrinsic causes
Medications
Beta blockers; calcium-channel blockers; digoxin; class IA, IC, and III antiarrhythmics
Acute MI
Hyperkalemia
Hypothyroidism
Infectious causes
Endocarditis, Lyme disease, AV block, sepsis
Autonomic excess
Increased vagal output or carotid hypersensitivity
Surgical trauma
Aortic or mitral valve rings

Intrinsic causes
Degenerative idiopathic disease
CAD
Cardiomyopathy
Hypertensive heart disease
Myocarditis
Collagen vascular disease
Infiltrative diseases
Amyloid, sarcoid, neoplasm, hemochromatosis, radiation treatment

AV, atrioventricular; CAD, coronary artery disease; MI, myocardial infarction.

TRANSVENOUS PACING

Technique

Transvenous pacing involves the insertion of a pacing catheter, typically into the right atrium or ventricle to directly stimulate the myocardium. Briefly, a percutaneous entry site is chosen, usually the right internal jugular vein or the femoral vein. The left-sided central veins should be left uncontaminated if possible, since, if a permanent pacer is required, they are the preferred sites of access and should be free of hardware. The modified Seldinger technique allows placement of a 6-Fr introducer sheath. A bipolar pacing lead is introduced into the RV under the aid of a balloon-tipped catheter, which allows easy flotation of the pacing wire to the apex of the RV. Special J-shaped wires are also available to allow atrial stimulation in dual-chamber temporary pacing. Guidance systems to assure proper placement of the bipolar pacing lead include fluoroscopy (most common), catheter-tip electrogram, or ECG-rhythm strip during pacemaker stimulation. A prosthetic tricuspid valve is a relative contraindication to placement of a transvenous pacer. The femoral vein should not be used if the patient has an inferior vena cava filter in place.

Indications

Indications for the insertion of a temporary pacemaker and the clinical situations for its use are shown in Table 27-5. Remember that certain medications—such as beta blockers, nondihydropyridine calcium-channel blockers, and digoxin (causing toxicity)—commonly lead to high-degree heart block in the hospitalized patient.

TABLE 27-5	COMMON INDICATIONS FOR TRANSVENOUS TEMPORARY PACING
Condition	**Setting**
Third-degree AV block	Symptomatic congenital complete heart block
	Symptomatic acquired complete heart block
	Postoperative symptomatic complete heart block
Second-degree AV block	Symptomatic Mobitz I or II AV block
Acute MI	Symptomatic bradycardia
	High-grade AV block (trifascicular block)
	Complete AV block
Sinus node dysfunction	Symptomatic bradyarrhythmias
Tachycardia prevention/treatment	Bradycardia-dependent arrhythmias
	Long-QT syndrome with ventricular arrhythmias

AV, atrioventricular; MI, myocardial infarction.

Complications

- Pneumothorax
- Myocardial perforation
- Bleeding
- Ventricular ectopy/nonsustained ventricular tachycardia (VT)
- Thromboembolism
- Infection

Using the Pacemaker

Once the introducer sheath has been established and the lead is in a good position, it is sutured in place at the skin surface. The lead is attached to a pacing generator after confirmation of placement by fluoroscopy. The pacing generator's sensitivity may be set on demand (synchronous) mode or fixed (asynchronous) mode. In **demand mode**, the lead "senses" the heart's intrinsic electrical activity; in the absence of conduction, the pulse generator delivers an impulse at a preset adjustable voltage. This impulse initiates depolarization and contraction of the ventricles. **Fixed (asynchronous) mode** delivers a set amount of impulses per time, regardless of the underlying native conduction. This fixed pacing mode is rarely used, as it may precipitate ventricular arrhythmias via an R-on-T phenomenon. A **pacing threshold** must be established; this is defined as the least amount of current (in milliamperes) necessary to depolarize or capture the ventricle. The threshold gives the operator an idea of the proximity of the pacing lead to the ventricular wall. Therefore the lower the threshold, the closer the pacing wire is to the ventricular wall. The optimal pacing threshold is <1 mA. The voltage delivered by the pulse generator is usually set at least 2 mA above the pacing threshold. The **set rate** depends on the clinical scenario. Usually, it is set at 40 to 50 bpm as a backup to the intrinsic heart rate unless the CO is very low. In this setting, AV pacing may be required. For tachyarrhythmia prevention, pacing is usually set at ~100 bpm until the underlying predisposition is corrected. The **pacer threshold** should be checked twice daily; if the threshold is >2 mA, the patient should be restricted to bed rest and repositioning of the lead should be considered.

    Pacing failure may be as simple as the disconnection of a loose wire, but the most common cause is failure of the lead to initiate sufficient voltage to pace the ventricle (i.e., failure of the ventricle to capture). Failure to capture is illustrated on the rhythm strip as pacer spikes that do not initiate capture (i.e., there is no ventricular depolarization). This is most likely due to displacement of the lead, which means that the pacing threshold will have increased beyond the voltage delivered by the pulse generator. The generator voltage should be increased immediately until appropriate pacing is seen, and the lead should be repositioned. **Other reasons for failure to pace** include fracture of the lead or an overly sensitive pacing generator that detects impulses traveling from the chest muscles that inhibit the pulse generator. This can be corrected by reducing the sensitivity of the pulse generator. **Diaphragmatic pacing** is a complication associated with a high preset voltage; as a result, the phrenic nerve is stimulated through the wall of the RV. It also may indicate a perforation of the RV wall, with the lead stimulating the diaphragm directly. Beware of a patient hiccupping at a rate identical to the pacer rate.

KEY POINTS TO REMEMBER

- Right-heart catheterization, temporary transvenous pacemaker implantation, and IABP placement are three of the most common procedures in the cardiac intensive care unit.
- A careful decision with regard to necessity and site of insertion must be made.
- These procedures require the assistance of those trained in the procedure in order to avoid complications and initiate rapid, appropriate action in the setting of complications.

REFERENCES AND SUGGESTED READINGS

Gore JM. *Handbook of Hemodynamic Monitoring.* Boston: Little, Brown; 1985.

Gregoratos G, Cheitlin MD, Gonill A, et al. ACC/AHA guidelines for implantation of cardiac pacemakers and antiarrhythmia devices: executives summary. A report of the American College of Cardiology/American Heart Association Task Force on Practice Guidelines (Committee on Pacemaker Implantation). *Circulation* 1998;97:1325–1335.

Grossman W. *Cardiac Catheterization and Angiography,* 4th ed. Philadelphia: Lea & Febiger; 1996:113–125.

Kaushik V, Leon A, Forrester J, et al. Bradyarrhythmias, temporary and permanent pacing. *Crit Care Med* 2000;28(10):N121–N128.

Keenan J. Cardiology update. Temporary cardiac pacing. *Nurs Stand* 1995;9(20):50–51.

Lumia FJ, Rios JC. Temporary transvenous pacemaker therapy: an analysis of complications. *Chest* 1973;64:604–608.

Marino P. *The ICU Book,* 2nd ed. Philadelphia: Lippincott Williams & Wilkins; 1997.

Mueller HS. Role of intra-aortic counterpulsation in cardiogenic shock and acute myocardial infarction. *Cardiology* 1994;84:168.

O'Rourke MF, Sammel N, Chang VP. Arterial counterpulsation in severe heart failure complication acute myocardial infarction. *Br Heart J* 1979;41:308.

Putterman C. The Swan-Ganz catheter: a decade of hemodynamic monitoring. *J Crit Care* 1989;4:127.

Sasayama S, Osakada G, Takahash M, et al. Effects of intraaortic balloon counterpulsation on regional myocardial function during acute coronary occlusion in the dog. *Am J Cardiol* 1979;43:59.

Topol E. *Textbook of Cardiovascular Medicine.* Philadelphia: Lippincott–Raven; 1998:1957–1969.

Zoll PM. Resuscitation of the heart in ventricular standstill by external electric stimulation. *N Engl J Med* 1952;247:768–781.

Cardiovascular Diseases in Special Populations

28

Stacy Mandras

INTRODUCTION

Cardiologists care for a broad spectrum of patients. This chapter focuses on the cardiovascular issues specific to women, the elderly, minorities, cancer patients, and patients with HIV.

CARDIOVASCULAR DISEASE IN WOMEN

Prevalence and Presentation

Cardiovascular disease (CVD) is the leading cause of death in women worldwide, accounting for one-third of all deaths. In the United States, 38.2 million women (34%) are living with CVD. The incidence of CVD rises sharply after menopause to nearly equal that of men. Therefore women present approximately 10 years later in life than men, and the clinical picture is different enough that the diagnosis is often delayed or even missed. Women (and their physicians) frequently attribute their chest pain to anxiety, stress, and other psychological problems, which further delays time to diagnosis.

While chest pain is the most common presenting symptom in both men and women with acute myocardial infarction (MI), chest pain in men is more predictive of coronary artery disease (CAD) than it is in women. A 60-year-old man with typical angina has a 90% chance of having obstructive CAD, whereas a woman presenting with the same chest pain has a 60% chance. Women are more likely than men to present with **atypical** symptoms, including back, jaw, and neck pain, nausea and/or vomiting, dyspnea, palpitations, indigestion, dizziness, fatigue, loss of appetite, and syncope.

CAD in women presents most often as stable angina rather than an acute ST-segment-elevation MI (STEMI). However, when women do present with STEMI, they have higher postrevascularization complication rates and higher in-hospital mortality.

Overall, the **prognosis of CAD is worse in women**, with 42% mortality in the year following MI versus 24% mortality in men. In addition, women who survive an MI have a greater likelihood of developing chronic heart failure, partially because of a higher prevalence of diabetes and hypertension in this population as well as later age of disease onset.

Diagnosis

As with any medical condition, the diagnosis of CAD and CVD in women begins with taking a careful **history**. Focus should be on characterizing the patient's chest pain and assessing the presence of risk factors. While the same risk factors are present in both men and women, certain risk factors—including diabetes, decreased high-density-lipoprotein cholesterol (HDL-C), elevated triglycerides, and depression—are more ominous in women. **Physical exam** should include measurement of blood pressure, body mass index, and waist circumference.

Treadmill electrocardiography (ECG) testing is the oldest and most studied test in women. For women, treadmill ECG exercise testing has a higher false-positive rate (38%–67% compared with 7%–44% in men) but a lower false-negative rate. While routine ECG exercise testing has its limitations, it has been shown to reduce procedures without a loss of diagnostic accuracy and can reliably exclude CAD when the test is negative.

Combining exercise or pharmacologic stress with **echocardiography or radionuclide imaging** increases accuracy over stress and ECG alone. However, breast tissue can cause anterior attenuation artifacts, which may be mistaken for perfusion defects suggestive of ischemia.

The definitive diagnosis of CAD is made by **coronary angiography**. Studies have shown that women are 40% to 50% less likely to undergo angiography than men and are less likely to be revascularized and/or to receive secondary preventative pharmacologic therapy. Proposed reasons for this disparity include lower perceived risk of CAD in women, differences in physician–patient interaction, and description or perception of symptoms.

Treatment

Women have been underrepresented in randomized trials of new therapies for CAD. Overall, the therapies used to treat CAD in men are equally efficacious in women, including antiplatelet agents, beta blockers, nitroglycerin, thrombolytics, angiotensin-converting enzyme (ACE) inhibitors, and statins. Women do have a higher risk of bleeding complications from antiplatelet agents, anticoagulants, and thrombolytics, most likely due to failure to adjust dosage for smaller body size and advanced age.

Success rates of coronary stenting and atherectomy appear similar in men and in women. Women are less likely than men to undergo coronary artery bypass grafting (CABG) and more likely to undergo percutaneous revascularization (PCI). This may be because of the higher prevalence of comorbidities and advanced age in the women presenting with CAD, and with this the perception of higher perioperative risk.

Prevention of CVD in Women

In February 2007, the American Heart Association (AHA) published new guidelines for the prevention of CVD in women. Their recommendations are evidence-based and focus on reducing lifetime risk using the Framingham risk-assessment tool. These new guidelines are summarized below.

Lifestyle Interventions

- **Smoking cessation.**
- **Physical activity:** A minimum of 30 minutes of moderate-intensity activity on most, preferably all, days of the week. For those who need to lose weight, 60 to 90 minutes daily.
- **Rehabilitation:** Women with recent acute coronary syndrome (ACS) or coronary intervention should participate in a comprehensive risk-reduction regimen or physician-guided home- or community-based exercise training program.
- **Dietary intake:** Recommend a diet rich in fruits and vegetables, whole grains, high-fiber foods, and fish (especially oily fish) at least twice a week; limit saturated fat and cholesterol, consume <1 drink of alcohol/day, and limit sodium to <2.3 g/day.
- **Weight maintenance/reduction:** Goal BMI 18.5–24.9, waist circumference ≤35 inches.
- **Omega-3 fatty acids:** in addition to diet, 850 to 1000 mg EPA and DHA in women with CAD and 2 to 4 g for those with hypertriglyceridemia.
- **Depression:** Screen and treat when indicated.

Major Risk-Factor Interventions

- **Blood pressure:** Optimally <120/80 mm Hg achieved through lifestyle modifications. Pharmacotherapy when blood pressure is ≥140/90 mm Hg or even lower in setting of chronic kidney disease or diabetes (goal with diabetes is ≤130/80 mm Hg). Thiazides are a reasonable first-line agent for most patients; high-risk women should receive beta blockers and/or an angiotensin-converting enzyme (ACE) inhibitor or angiotensin-receptor blocker (ARB).
- **Lipid and lipoprotein levels:** Goal low-density-lipoprotein cholesterol (LDL-C) <100 mg/dL, HDL-C >50 mg/dL, triglycerides <150 mg/dL, non–HDL-C <130 mg/dL. Lifestyle modification and lipid-lowering drug therapy should be used simultaneously to reach these goals. Reduction of LDL-C to <70 mg/dL is reasonable in women with CAD at very high risk and may require combination drug therapy.
- **Diabetes mellitus (DM):** Lifestyle changes and pharmacotherapy should be used to achieve a HbA1c <7%.

Preventative Drug Interventions

- **Aspirin: High-risk patients** with established CAD, cerebrovascular disease, peripheral arterial disease, abdominal aortic aneurysm, end-stage or chronic renal disease, diabetes mellitus, or a 10-year Framingham risk >20% should receive 75 to 325 mg of aspirin daily unless contraindicated.
- **Aspirin for other at-risk or healthy women:** For women ≥65 years of age, consider 81 to 100 mg aspirin daily or every other day if blood pressure is controlled and benefit for ischemic stroke/MI prevention is likely to outweigh risk of gastrointestinal bleeding and hemorrhagic stroke.
- **Beta blockers:** Use indefinitely in all women after MI, acute coronary syndrome, or left ventricular dysfunction with or without symptoms of heart failure (HF) unless contraindicated.
- **ACE inhibitors/ARBs:** Use in women after MI, in those with HF or left ventricular ejection fraction (LVEF) ≤40%, and those with diabetes mellitus unless contraindicated.
- **Aldosterone blockade:** Use after MI in women with LVEF ≤40% with symptoms of HF, who are already receiving therapeutic doses of an ACE inhibitor and beta blocker, and who do not have significant renal dysfunction or hyperkalemia.

Class III Interventions (Not Useful/Effective and May Be Harmful) for CAD or MI Prevention in Women

- **Menopause therapy:** See "Hormone Replacement Therapy," below.
- **Antioxidant supplements:** Supplements such as vitamins E and C and beta carotene should not be recommended for primary or secondary prevention of CAD owing to lack of supporting evidence for these indications.
- **Folic acid:** With or without B6 and B12 supplementation, should not be recommended for primary or secondary prevention of CAD owing to lack of supporting evidence for these indications.
- **Aspirin is not recommended for MI prevention in women <65 years old at low risk for CAD.**

Hormone Replacement Therapy

Early observational studies and early data from the Heart and Estrogen/Progestin Replacement study (HERS) suggested a protective effect of hormone replacement therapy (HRT) on CHD risk in postmenopausal women. However, post hoc analysis showed a statistically significant time-dependent trend with more CHD events in the first year of treatment in those patients taking HRT and fewer events in the third to fifth years.

HERS II, conducted to determine if this protective effect persisted over an additional 2.7 years of follow-up, showed that the protective effects seen in the later years of HERS did not persist. The **Women's Health Initiative,** a randomized trial that included 27,347 women, demonstrated an increased risk of CHD events in women treated with estrogen alone or estrogen plus progestin.

The bottom line: HRT should not be prescribed for the purpose of reducing risk of CHD in women. The pros and cons of HRT must be weighed prior to initiating HRT, particularly in women more distant from menopause.

Heart Disease and Pregnancy

Multiple cardiovascular issues arise during pregnancy. This section focuses on the most common and most life-threatening, including arrhythmia, peripartum cardiomyopathy, and pregnancy occurring in women with congenital heart disease.

Normal Hemodynamics of Pregnancy

An understanding of the normal physiologic changes that occur with pregnancy is necessary before attempting to evaluate a pregnant woman with a cardiovascular condition.

In the fifth to sixth weeks of pregnancy, cardiac output begins to rise because of a 40% to 50% increase in blood volume. This increase is associated with an increase in left ventricular end-diastolic volume and atrial stretch. During the third trimester, cardiac output is approximately 7 L/minute and increases further to 10 to 11 L/minute during delivery. Despite a marked fall in vascular resistance, arterial blood pressure remains unchanged, as does ventricular contractility.

In addition, there is a decrease in serum protein concentration and altered protein-binding affinity as well as increased renal perfusion and liver metabolism, all of which affect the pharmacokinetics of drugs administered during pregnancy. There is also an increase in plasma catecholamines and adrenergic receptor sensitivity, which further increases cardiac demands.

Most healthy women are able to meet these demands without difficulty; however, many with an underlying cardiovascular condition may not.

Maternal Arrhythmias During Pregnancy

Any arrhythmia can occur during pregnancy in women with and without known heart disease. The **pathogenesis** of arrhythmia is likely multifactorial, and includes hemodynamic and neurohormonal changes mentioned above. **Anemia, hyperthyroidism, and electrolyte imbalances** as well as exogenous factors such as **tobacco, caffeine, and illicit drug use** may exacerbate previously identified arrhythmias or initiate new arrhythmias.

Women can present with palpitations, fatigue, dyspnea, chest pressure, dizziness, presyncope, or syncope. These symptoms can be frightening to the pregnant patient, and making the correct diagnosis is critical before initiating therapy. Certain elements in the history—including onset, severity, frequency, and duration—as well as a comprehensive physical examination and baseline ECG are essential to making the correct diagnosis. An algorithm for the management of arrhythmias is shown in Figure 28-1.

Potential arrhythmias include the following:

- **Sinus tachycardia** is common, related to altered vascular resistance.
- **Atrial premature beats** occur frequently and are benign.
- **Paroxysmal supraventricular tachycardia** (SVT).
- **Atrial fibrillation/flutter** (AF/AFl) is unusual.
- **Ventricular tachycardia** (VT) and **ventricular fibrillation** (VF) also occur but are rare and predominantly seen in women with structurally abnormal hearts.
- **Symptomatic bradycardia** is rare. It is usually related to supine hypotensive syndrome of pregnancy, in which the uterus compresses the inferior vena cava and causes a paradoxical slowing of the sinus node.
- **Complete heart block** is uncommon. Temporary pacing may be required during delivery.

Treatment of maternal arrhythmias includes both pharmacologic and nonpharmacologic methods. Most antiarrhythmic agents are safe to use during pregnancy, but there are

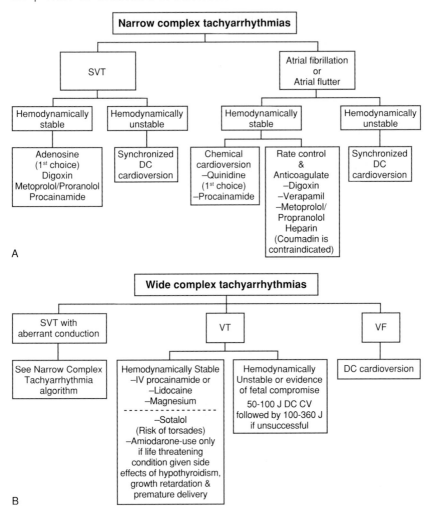

FIGURE 28.1. Tachycardia management in pregnancy. SVT, supraventricular tachycardia; DC, direct current; J, joules; VT, ventricular tachycardia; VF, ventricular fibrillation.

exceptions, and all cross the placenta. Algorithms for the management of narrow- and wide-complex tachyarrhythmias are shown.

Permanent pacemakers and internal defibrillators can be implanted during pregnancy if necessary; this is done either with echocardiographic guidance or with fluoroscopy, using a shield to protect the fetus.

Fetal arrhythmias also occur and can carry a significant risk of morbidity and mortality, but this subject is beyond the scope of this chapter.

Peripartum Cardiomyopathy

Peripartum cardiomyopathy (PPCM) is defined as left ventricular systolic dysfunction presenting in the last month of pregnancy or the first 5 months postpartum. To meet the diagnostic criteria for PPCM, there must be no preexisting LV dysfunction and no alternative diagnosis for the patient's heart failure (HF).

In the United States, PPCM occurs in 1 in 3000 to 4000 pregnancies. **Risk factors** include advanced maternal age, multiparity, multiple pregnancy, preeclampsia, and gestational hypertension. There is a higher risk in African American women, but this may be confounded by the higher prevalence of hypertension in this population.

The **etiology** of PPCM remains unclear. There is evidence to support a **viral etiology,** including coxsackievirus, parvovirus B19, adenovirus, and herpesvirus. **Fetal microchimerism**—in which fetal cells escape into the maternal circulation and induce an autoimmune myocarditis—has also been a suggested cause. Last, a role for abnormalities in oxidative stress has been suggested.

Clinically, women with PPCM present with signs and symptoms of HF. Of course dyspnea on exertion and lower extremity edema are common in late pregnancy; therefore PPCM may be difficult to recognize. Cough, orthopnea, and paroxysmal nocturnal dyspnea are warning signs that PPCM may be present, as is the presence of a displaced apical impulse and a new mitral regurgitation (MR) murmur on exam. Most commonly, patients present with New York Heart Association (NYHA) class III and IV HF, although both mild cases and sudden cardiac arrest may occur.

Diagnosis requires echocardiographic evidence of LV systolic dysfunction, with an ejection fraction <45%, fractional shortening <30%, and LV dilatation, although all four chambers may be dilated. Functional MR is present in about 43% of patients with PPCM, and LV thrombus is common in patients with LVEF <35%. Peripheral embolization to any part of the body, including the lower extremities, bowel, and brain, is possible, as is pulmonary embolism. Left ventricular hypertrophy (LVH) is often present on ECG, as are ST-T-wave abnormalities.

Treatment includes agents that reduce afterload and preload and increase contractility. **ACE inhibitors** are used in the postpartum patient, while hydralazine is used while the patient is still pregnant. **Beta blockers** are used to reduce heart rate, the incidence of arrhythmia and risk of sudden cardiac death, and are relatively safe. Beta-1–selective blockers (metoprolol and atenolol) are preferred, as this avoids beta-2 blockade, which results in peripheral vasodilation and uterine relaxation. **Digoxin** is also safe during pregnancy and should be used to augment contractility and rate control, although levels must be closely monitored in the pregnant patient. **Diuretics** are used for preload reduction and symptom relief. In those with thromboembolism, **heparin** is required, followed by warfarin (**Coumadin**) after delivery.

In general, the **prognosis** in PPCM is better than that seen with nonischemic cardiomyopathies. The extent of ventricular recovery at 6 months postdelivery predicts overall recovery, although continued improvement has been seen 2 to 3 years after diagnosis.

Subsequent pregnancies in patients with PPCM are associated with significant deterioration in LV function and can result in death. Family-planning counseling is essential after the diagnosis of PPCM is made, and women who do not recover LV function should be encouraged to consider forgoing future pregnancy.

Pregnancy and Congenital Heart Disease

Advances in medical and surgical therapy have helped more patients with congenital heart disease survive to reproductive age. With this increase in survival comes the challenge of managing the pregnant woman with congenital heart disease. There are risks to both the mother and the fetus, and a multidisciplinary approach with cardiology, obstetrics, and anesthesiology is needed to ensure a safe and successful pregnancy and delivery.

Maternal cardiovascular risks include **arrhythmia, stroke, HF, pulmonary edema, and death.** The risk of such an event is determined by a woman's ability to adapt to the physiologic stresses placed on her cardiovascular system during pregnancy. The risks associated with different congenital conditions (Table 28-1) are determined by the patient's anatomy, previous operations, and hemodynamic status.

TABLE 28-1 CONGENITAL HEART DISEASE IN PREGNANCY

Lesion	Potential Risks	Recommendations
Low risk		
Ventricular septal defects	Arrhythmia Endocarditis (if residual defect present)	Antibiotic prophylaxis if residual defect
Atrial septal defects	Arrhythmia Thromboembolic events	Thromboprophylaxis if on bed rest Consider low-dose aspirin
Repaired coarctation	Preeclampsia Aortic dissection Heart failure Endarteritis	Beta blockers for blood pressure control Elective C-section if aortic aneurysm or uncontrolled hypertension Antibiotic prophylaxis
Tetralogy of Fallot	Arrhythmia RV failure Endocarditis	Consider preterm delivery if RV failure Antibiotic prophylaxis
Moderate risk		
Mitral stenosis	Atrial fibrillation Thromboembolism Pulmonary edema	Beta blockers Low-dose aspirin Consider bed rest during third trimester with thromboprophylaxis Antibiotic prophylaxis
Aortic stenosis	Arrhythmia Angina Endocarditis LV failure	Bed rest during third trimester with thromboprophylaxis Consider balloon valvuloplasty for severe AS; cases of surgical AV replacement have also been reported in patients who are not candidates for balloon valvuloplasty Consider preterm delivery by C-section if cardiac decompensation Antibiotic prophylaxis
Systemic right ventricle (corrected transposition of the great arteries)	RV dysfunction Heart failure Arrhythmia Thromboembolism Endocarditis	Regularly monitor rhythm Cardioversion if atrial flutter Stop ACE inhibitors, consider beta blockers Low-dose aspirin Antibiotic prophylaxis
Cyanotic lesions (without pulmonary hypertension)	Hemorrhage Thromboembolism Worsening cyanosis Heart failure Endocarditis	Consider bed rest and supplemental oxygen Thromboprophylaxis Antibiotic prophylaxis

TABLE 28-1	CONGENITAL HEART DISEASE IN PREGNANCY (Continued)	
Lesion	Potential Risks	Recommendations
Fontan-type circulation	Heart Failure Arrhythmia Thromboembolism Endocarditis	Consider low-molecular-weight heparin and aspirin throughout pregnancy Maintain filling pressures during delivery Antibiotic prophylaxis
High risk		
Marfan syndrome with dilated aortic root	Dissection of ascending aorta	Beta blockers Elective C-section if aortic root >4.5 cm
Eisenmenger syndrome	30%–50% mortality related to pregnancy Arrhythmia Heart failure Endocarditis	Consider termination Close cardiovascular monitoring, early bed rest, pulmonary vasodilators and supplemental oxygen Monitor 10 days postpartum

ACE, angiotensin-converting enzyme; AS, aortic stenosis; AV, aortic valve.

Source: Adapted from Uebing A et al. Pregnancy and congenital heart disease. *BMJ* 2006; 332:401–406, with permission.

The risk of fetal adverse events is higher than that in the general population. These risks include intrauterine growth retardation, preterm birth, intracranial hemorrhage, and fetal loss. These risks are higher in women with poor functional class, cyanotic heart disease, and LV outflow tract obstruction (LVOT). In addition, there is a 3% to 12% risk that the congenital heart condition will recur in the fetus (compared with a baseline risk of 0.8% in the general population).

The level of care required during pregnancy depends on the severity of the patient's disease (Table 28-1). Low-risk patients can receive care locally. Moderate- to high-risk patients should be followed in a tertiary care facility, and those at highest risk may be hospitalized in the third trimester for bed rest, close monitoring, and oxygen if needed. Those at the highest risk—including women with Eisenmenger syndrome (or other forms of pulmonary hypertension [PH]), Marfan syndrome with an aortic root >4 cm in diameter, or severe LVOT obstruction—should be informed of the high risk of maternal morbidity and mortality and consider terminating the pregnancy.

Safety Profiles of Cardiac Drugs Commonly Used During Pregnancy

Reasonably Safe

- **Adenosine:** Rapid action and short half-life, rapid metabolism reduces amount crossing the placenta. First choice for SVT, no teratogenicity in second and third trimesters (unknown safety in first trimester). Fetal heart rate monitoring recommended if used to terminate maternal SVT.
- **Beta blockers:** Widely used in pregnancy to treat hypertension, hypertrophic cardiomyopathy, thyrotoxicosis, mitral stenosis, and fetal tachycardia. Use leads to

reduction in umbilical blood flow and increase in uterine contractility (beta-2). Beta-1–selective agents (atenolol, metoprolol) may be preferable, given peripheral vasodilation and uterine relaxation.

- **Calcium-channel blockers (CCBs):** Widely used to treat fetal SVT and to prevent preterm delivery and preeclampsia. Verapamil is preferred for maternal and fetal SVT (acute and chronic). No teratogenicity, but maternal/fetal hypotension, bradycardia, AV-nodal blockade, and decreased LV contractility reported. IV verapamil associated with maternal hypotension and decreased uterine blood flow. Excreted in breast milk.
- **Digoxin:** Widely used for maternal/fetal arrhythmias, safest antiarrhythmic agent at therapeutic doses. Freely crosses the placenta. Digoxin levels decrease by up to 50% due to increase in renal excretion. Digoxin toxicity associated with fetal loss.
- **Flecainide:** Not widely used, no evidence of teratogenicity or fetal adverse effects. Crosses placenta, but effective fetal renal excretion. Excreted in breast milk.
- **Heparin:** Used in atrial fibrillation/flutter for 3 weeks prior to cardioversion and 4 weeks postcardioversion; also in women with mechanical valves or thromboembolism. Unfractionated subcutaneous heparin better than low-molecular-weight heparin, as larger molecular weight decreases placental transfer.
- **Lidocaine:** Crosses placenta but not known to increase fetal malformations. Causes increase in myometrial tone, decrease in placental blow flow and fetal bradycardia. If fetus is acidotic, can result in neonatal cardiac and CNS toxicity. Small amounts excreted in breast milk.
- **Mexiletine:** Similar to lidocaine, crosses placenta; limited data.
- **Procainamide:** Used frequently, no reports of teratogenicity in first trimester. Limited data.
- **Quinidine:** Used in pregnancy since the 1930s, adverse events are uncommon but include mild uterine contractions, premature labor, neonatal thrombocytopenia. At toxic doses, miscarriage, cranial nerve VII injury. Low amounts in breast milk.

Cardiac Drugs NOT Safe for Use in Pregnancy

- **ACE inhibitors, ARBs:** Risk of neonatal renal failure, hypotension, renal tubular dysgenesis, intrauterine growth retardation, decreased skull ossification.
- **Amiodarone:** May be used in life-threatening conditions but carries risk of hypothyroidism and potential brain damage.
- **Phenytoin:** Carries risk of heart defects, intrauterine growth retardation, orofacial defects.
- **Spironolactone:** Defects in external genitalia seen in animal studies. Amiloride preferred if potassium-sparing diuretic needed.
- **Warfarin:** Risk of skeletal and CNS malformations, intracranial hemorrhage.

CARDIOVASCULAR ISSUES IN THE ELDERLY

Coronary Artery Disease

The elderly—those aged 75 years and older—are most rapidly growing population in the United States. The prevalence of CAD in the elderly is 21.7% in men and 12.9% in women. Thirty percent of in-hospital deaths due to MI and 20% of hospitalizations for MI are in patients ≥80 years old, despite the fact that this group makes up only 5% of the general population. Comorbid conditions—including diabetes, hypertension, chronic HF, and ST-segment abnormalities on ECG—are more common in the elderly than in younger patients, thus increasing the risk for cardiovascular events.

Many studies have shown an increased benefit of commonly prescribed cardiovascular medications and coronary revascularization in the elderly compared with younger patients, yet these therapies are underutilized in the elderly. At the individual level, these benefits include symptom improvement, prevention of death, prevention of recurrent vascular events (MI, stroke, arterial occlusive disease), improvement in quality of life, and prevention of disability. At the societal level, cardiovascular medications can reduce hospitalizations and institutionalizations, resulting in tremendous cost savings.

The following pages review the medications that provide cardiovascular benefits, their associated risks, and the nonpharmacologic treatment of CAD in this patient population.

Antiplatelet Agents

- **Aspirin:** Recommended for all patients at high risk for CAD, stroke, or vascular events. Studies have not focused specifically on the elderly, in whom there is increased risk of gastrointestinal bleeding and hemorrhagic stroke. The benefit of aspirin may be diminished when it is used in combination with ibuprofen.
- **Clopidogrel:** Alternative to aspirin in those with aspirin resistance or allergy. Well proven in the acute management of CAD, more expensive than aspirin for use in the chronic setting.

Lipid-Lowering Agents

- **HMG-CoA reductase inhibitors (statins):** Good data in older patients from both the Heart Protection Study and PROSPER. May offer the greatest morbidity and mortality benefits in both primary and secondary prevention of CAD. Despite the indisputable benefits of statins, they remain underutilized in the elderly. This is likely due to fear of adverse effects, the most serious of which is myopathy (especially in those over age 80). However trials have repeatedly shown statins to be remarkably safe in the elderly.
- **Fibrates:** Limited data in the elderly, although the Veterans Affairs High-Density Lipoprotein Intervention trial (VA-HIT), a secondary prevention study in men aged 73 years old and younger with low baseline serum HDL-C and normal LDL-C, demonstrated a lower combined endpoint of CAD and stroke. This risk reduction was greatest in those patients above 65 years of age.

ACE Inhibitors and Angiotensin II Receptor Blockers

ACE inhibitors and ARBs are indicated in the treatment of hypertension, acute MI, and HF. In addition, they have anti-inflammatory, antioxidant, antithrombotic, and plaque-stabilizing effects. Studies such as the Heart Outcomes Prevention Evaluation (HOPE) trial with ramipril and the Losartan Intervention for Endpoint (LIFE) trial with losartan have shown benefit in a subgroup of elderly patients. To date, however, the effects of ACE inhibitors and ARBs have not been studied specifically in the elderly.

Beta Blockers

Beta blockers are also underutilized in the elderly, despite proven benefits in patients post-MI as well as those with HF, arrhythmia, hypertension, and anginal symptoms. Side effects—including depressive symptoms, sexual dysfunction, and fatigue—were found to be only minimally increased in the elderly population.

Calcium-Channel Blockers

CCBs do not have the well-defined role that beta blockers and ACE inhibitors have for use in the elderly. There is little proven benefit and, in some cases, they have been shown to cause harm. They should be reserved for patients who continue to have anginal symptoms or refractory hypertension despite adequate treatment with beta blockers, ACE inhibitors, diuretics, and nitrates. If LV systolic function is normal, verapamil and diltiazem are acceptable; if LV function is depressed, amlodipine, felodipine, and nitrendipine are preferred.

Long-Acting Nitrates

Isosorbide has long been used to treat symptomatic ischemia. However, it is not indicated as monotherapy for angina and does not alter the prognosis in patients with stable coronary disease. Patients develop tolerance to nitrates over time, and it is possible that stable, asymptomatic patients may be taking these drugs unnecessarily.

Over-the-Counter Supplements and Vitamins

The elderly make up a large percentage of consumers who take vitamins and antioxidants, despite the lack of evidence for benefit in CAD. Two randomized trails failed to show a cardiovascular benefit for vitamin E alone or vitamin E plus vitamin C and beta carotene. Folic acid *may* be beneficial, as it is involved in homocysteine metabolism; it is inexpensive and probably safe, however, it has yet to be shown to have proven benefit in patients with CAD.

Early Invasive Strategy in Non–ST-Segment-Elevation Acute Coronary Syndromes

Historically, elderly patients have been less likely than younger patients to undergo coronary angiography and revascularization in the setting of non–ST-segment-elevation acute coronary syndromes (ACS).

A landmark study that investigated the benefit of early invasive versus conservative management of non–ST-segment elevation ACS in the elderly is the Treat Angina with Aggrastat and Determine Cost of Therapy with an Invasive or Conservative Strategy-Thrombolysis in Myocardial Infarction (TACTICS-TIMI) 18 trial. The trial included 2220 patients with non–ST-segment elevation MI (NSTEMI) and unstable angina, 43% of whom were 65 years of age or older. Several important conclusions were drawn from the study:

- Elderly patients with non–ST-segment elevation ACS have a marked increase in adverse ischemic outcomes, with a fourfold higher risk of death or nonfatal MI in patients 75 years of age and older compared with those <55 years of age.
- Early invasive management had an absolute risk reduction in nonfatal MI or death of 10.8% and a relative risk reduction of 56% compared with conservative management in those ≥75 years of age.
- The benefits of the early invasive strategy are greater in the elderly than in younger patients, and these benefits continue to increase with increasing age.
- The early invasive strategy is more cost-effective, as it prevents more deaths and recurrent MIs.
- There is no increase in stroke risk in the elderly with the early invasive strategy.
- There is a significant increase in bleeding risk with the early invasive strategy (16.6% vs. 6.5% with the conservative strategy). This increase in bleeding risk may be associated with use of glycoprotein IIb/IIIa inhibitors, arterial closure devices and newer antithrombin agents.

Heart Failure in the Elderly

HF is prevalent in the elderly and is the number one reason for hospitalization in those aged 65 and older. The incidence of HF increases with age, rising from 2% to 3% in patients aged 65 to over 10% in those over age 80.

The high prevalence of HF in the elderly can likely be accounted for by age-related changes in ventricular function and the increased prevalence of risk factors (hypertension, diabetes, dyslipidemia). Out of fear for adverse effects, these risk factors are often not aggressively treated in the elderly. In addition, the elderly commonly take medications that may exacerbate HF (i.e., nonsteroidal anti-inflammatory drugs [NSAIDs]).

Causes of HF in the elderly include ischemic heart disease, hypertensive heart disease, valvular heart disease, and nonischemic cardiomyopathy. Diastolic dysfunction with preserved systolic function is common in the elderly, and the elderly often present with atypical symptoms.

Making the diagnosis of HF begins with a comprehensive history and physical exam. The **history** should investigate the presence of previous MI, CAD, revascularization, risk factors, valvular disease, thyroid disease, medication noncompliance, infection, smoking status, functional capacity, and the presence of symptoms, including chest pain, exertional dyspnea and dyspnea at rest, orthopnea, paroxysmal nocturnal dyspnea, lower extremity swelling, weight gain, and increased abdominal girth.

The **physical exam** should include the patient's weight, blood pressure, and heart rate as well as an examination of the neck, lungs, heart, abdomen, and lower extremities. Ruling out reversible or treatable causes of HF in the history and correctly assessing level of congestion and volume overload on exam may help guide treatment and ultimately improve prognosis.

Initial diagnostic tests should include a chest x-ray, ECG, comprehensive metabolic panel, complete blood count, thyroid-stimulating hormone (especially in the setting of concomitant atrial fibrillation), and transthoracic echocardiography to assess LV function (both systolic and diastolic) and evaluate for valvular or structural heart disease.

There is no HF treatment regimen specific to the elderly population. In choosing a drug regimen, remember that the elderly have a narrow therapeutic range, may not respond as well to drugs as younger patients, and may be more prone to adverse drug effects.

The following are evidence-based recommendations for the management of HF in the elderly.

ACE Inhibitors

- Reduce new onset of symptomatic HF in those with asymptomatic LV dysfunction and reduce morbidity and mortality in those with LV dysfunction post-MI.
- Reduce morbidity, mortality, and symptoms and improve functional status in those who have symptomatic HF.
- Recent studies show benefit at lower doses.

Aldosterone Receptor Antagonists

- Spironolactone decreases risk of death from progressive HF and sudden cardiac death by 30% and is associated with a 35% decrease in hospitalization for worsening HF.
- Side effects include hyperkalemia, gynecomastia (less with use of eplerenone than of spironolactone).

Angiotensin II Receptor Blockers

- Reduce morbidity and mortality; improve clinical signs and symptoms of HF, LVEF, and functional class in both younger and older patients.
- May have additional benefit when given to patients who are already taking ACE inhibitors, although data are conflicting.

Beta Blockers

- Indicated for HF, asymptomatic LV dysfunction with EF <40%, NYHA functional class I–III unless there is a documented contraindication (e.g., bradycardia and decompensated HF).

- Reduce morbidity and mortality with benefit occurring as early as 3 months after initiation of drug; effects are similar in both elderly and younger patients.
- Similar 35% decreased risk of death in class IV HF regardless of age.

Calcium-Channel Blockers

- **Verapamil, nifedipine, and diltiazem are NOT indicated** in patients with HF and LVEF <40% because of an increased risk of pulmonary edema and cardiogenic shock in the short term treatment of HF and worsening HF and increased mortality in the chronic treatment of HF.
- **Amlodipine and felodipine** have not been shown to increase mortality, although their benefit is unclear.

Digoxin

- Does not reduce overall mortality but reduces hospitalization and worsening of symptomatic HF.
- Digoxin toxicity is common in elderly HF patients and can lead to significant morbity and mortality.
- Signs of digoxin toxicity include arrhythmia, confusion, nausea, anorexia, and visual disturbances.
- No evidence exists to support monitoring digoxin levels, but it is reasonable to obtain levels when digoxin toxicity is suspected.

Diuretics

- Reduce symptoms of dyspnea and edema.

Atrial Fibrillation in the Setting of HF in the Elderly

- **Anticoagulation** should be offered because elderly patients are at high risk of stroke and systemic embolization.
- If anticoagulation is contraindicated, the patient should be treated with aspirin, 75 to 325 mg/daily.

Device Therapy in the Elderly

Pacemakers

- 85% of patients who receive pacemakers are ≥65 years old.
- Dual-chamber pacemakers improve survival and quality of life in many elderly patients.
- The decision not to place a pacemaker when indicated may be appropriate if the patient is extremely sedentary or has a limited life expectancy.

Implantable Cardioverter-Defibrillators (ICDs)

- Ventricular arrhythmias occur in 70% to 80% of people ≥60 years old, although many are asymptomatic.
- Elderly patients with CAD, hypertensive or dilated cardiomyopathy, and valvular heart disease are at risk for sudden cardiac death (SCD).
- The pharmacologic therapy of ventricular arrhythmias is similar to that used in younger patients, but the physiology of aging—including decreases in renal and hepatic clearance of medications, volume of drug distribution, changes in body composition, and comorbidities—should be accounted for and doses adjusted when needed.
- ICDs confer similar or greater benefit in the elderly compared with younger patients in preventing SCD.
- Very elderly patients with poor functional capacity and multiple comorbidities and/or limited life expectancy may not be good candidates for ICDs.

CARDIOVASCULAR ISSUES IN MINORITIES

Over the last several decades, the population of the United States has become increasingly diverse. The percentage of non-Hispanic whites is declining and is now at 67%. Hispanics make up 14% to 15% of the population, African Americans 12%, and Asian and Native Americans the remaining 7%.

Studies have demonstrated a disparity between the levels of care that minorities receive compared with whites as well as a difference in outcomes. Minority populations are less likely to undergo percutaneous coronary intervention or coronary artery bypass grafting or to receive thrombolytic agents. Many factors contribute to the disparities in patient care, including the health care delivery system with its lack of cultural sensitivity, communication and financial barriers, patient choice, variations in disease presentation, and physician bias.

African Americans

The leading cause of death among African Americans is CVD, responsible for 36.3% of the such deaths in the United States each year. Compared with whites, African Americans have a higher prevalence of risk factors (hypertension, diabetes, obesity), receive less adequate care, and are more likely to die because of their CVD than the general population.

Hypertension (HTN) has a disproportionate effect on African Americans, affecting nearly 45% of African Americans living in the United States. African Americans develop HTN earlier in life, and it tends to be more severe. HTN contributes to a higher risk of stroke, CVD, death from CVD, left ventricular hypertrophy, HF, and end-stage renal disease. Despite these increased risks, HTN remains undertreated in this population, with only 45% of African Americans having well-controlled blood pressure, compared with 56% of whites.

For the uncomplicated African American patient with HTN, the initial drug of choice remains the thiazide diuretic. In view of the increased incidence of end-organ disease in African Americans, it is reasonable to consider such patients high risk and begin a multidrug regimen. There is evidence to support the use of ACE inhibitors, ARBs, and beta blockers, with benefits above and beyond their blood pressure–lowering effects.

The Antihypertensive and Lipid-Lowering Treatment to Prevent Heart Attack Trial (ALLHAT) demonstrated that lisinopril was a less effective antihypertensive agent than the thiazide diuretic chlorthalidone or the CCB amlodipine in African Americans and that thiazides were better than ACE inhibitors and CCBs in lowering risk of stroke, HF and CVD. Nevertheless, ACE inhibitors should still be included as part of a multidrug regimen for their renal and cardioprotective effects.

Different beta blockers may have different effects in African Americans. While bucindolol has not been seen to have a mortality benefit in African Americans, metoprolol, carvedilol, and propranolol have shown cardiovascular benefits, including decreased mortality and decreased hospitalizations. Beta blockers have also been shown to reduce arrhythmias and SCD in African Americans, particularly after a MI.

The African American Heart Failure trial (AHeFT) studied the use of fixed-dose combination isosorbide dinitrate/hydralazine along with standard HF therapy in black patients with NYHA functional class III or IV HF and found a 43% reduction in death from any cause, 33% relative risk reduction in hospitalization for HF, and improved quality of life.

Dyslipidemia is as common among African Americans as it is among whites; however, the lipid profile is different. African Americans tend to have lower mean LDL-C levels, lower small dense LDL-C, and higher HDL-C levels.

Hispanic Americans

CVD is the leading cause of death in the Hispanic population, accounting for 39.6% deaths. The National Health and Nutrition Examination survey (NHANES) has found that Hispanic women are disproportionately obese and have the highest incidence of the metabolic syndrome. Hispanic men have a high prevalence of CVD risk factors, including diabetes, HTN, and physical inactivity. In addition, HTN awareness among Hispanic Americans is lower, and it is less likely to be detected and treated in this population.

Interestingly, Hispanic Americans comprise only 3% of patients with acute decompensated HF despite the increased prevalence of risk factors in this population. Compared with whites, Hispanics have a worse outcome when they develop decompensated HF but a better outcome compared with African Americans.

Asian and Native Americans

Asian and Native Americans make up the smallest proportion of the general population, so they have been underrepresented in studies of CVD. What we know is the following:

- Heart disease is second to cancer as the leading cause of death among Asians and Pacific Islanders, accounting for 26% all deaths.
- Japanese men living in Hawaii have an increased risk of impaired glucose tolerance, and this is associated with a marked increase in thromboembolic and hemorrhagic stroke, CAD, SCD, and all-cause mortality.
- Asian Americans are less likely than white patients to undergo cardiac procedures.
- Response to antihypertensive agents is similar among South Asians and whites.
- The leading cause of death among Native Americans is heart disease.
- Native Americans have the least understood CVD profile. There is a great deal of heterogeneity among the >500 tribes in the United States.
- Mortality secondary to CVD among Native Americans is at least the same as or higher than that of the general population, and they have the highest rate of premature death from CVD.
- Native Americans have a particularly high prevalence of diabetes.

CARDIOVASCULAR ISSUES AMONG CANCER PATIENTS

This section reviews the issues of (1) the increased incidence of cardiomyopathy in the setting of chemotherapy and (2) that of late stent thrombosis.

Chemotherapy-Induced Cardiomyopathy

The development of cardiotoxicity is a key issue in cancer patients who receive many chemotherapeutic agents, including anthracyclines, high-dose cyclophosphamide, and trastuzumab, as well as those who receive mediastinal radiation.

Anthracyclines

Anthracyclines are among the most effective chemotherapeutic agents; however, they are associated with both early (within 1 year of treatment) and late (after 1 year following treatment) cardiotoxicity. Doxorubicin, epirubicin, idarubicin, and daunorubicin are the commonly used anthracyclines in the treatment of both solid and hematologic malignancies.

The reported **incidence** of HF related to anthracycline treatment ranges from 1.6% to 2.8%; however, up to 57% of long-term survivors have been found to have cardiac abnormalities, including both symptomatic and asymptomatic LV dysfunction.

Risk factors for the development of anthracycline-induced cardiomyopathy include age >50 years and treatment with >200 mg/m^2 doxorubicin. **Prior to initiating treatment**

with anthracyclines, patients should receive a baseline physical examination, ECG, and evaluation of resting LV function by radionuclide gated blood pool imaging. They require routine monitoring of LV function during and after treatment.

The **proposed mechanism** for anthracycline-induced cardiotoxicity involves myocyte damage from free radicals that form from ferrous complexes. Randomized trials have shown cardioprotection with the coadministration of **dexrazoxane**, an iron chelator; however, dexrazoxane may interfere with the efficacy of the anthracyclines in killing cancer cells, and its role remains unclear. In addition, a **liposomal encapsulated doxorubicin** has been formulated, in which the drug is sequestered from organs with tight capillary junctions like the heart; this may also offer some cardioprotection.

Treatment of chemotherapy-related cardiomyopathy is similar to that of HF due to other causes. It is unclear if cancer patients respond to treatment in the same manner as in the case of HF due to other causes, but chemotherapy-related HF may improve with proper management. Chemotherapy induced cardiomyopathy is associated with a high incidence of tachycardia; therefore beta blockers may play a greater role in this population.

Trastuzumab (Herceptin)

Trastuzumab is a humanized monoclonal antibody used either alone or in combination with anthracyclines for the treatment of HER-2–positive metastatic breast cancer. When added to traditional chemotherapy, it has been shown to increase median survival by 25% to 45%.

In the National Surgical Breast and Bowel Project (NSABP), trastuzumab in combination with anthracyclines plus cyclophosphamide plus paclitaxel (standard therapy) was found to be associated with a 4.1% incidence of cardiac events, CHF, and cardiac death compared with the 0.8% incidence seen when the latter agents were used without trastuzumab. In a pooled analysis of randomized trials of trastuzumab, the incidence of cardiotoxicity was found to be 10%, versus 2% in the standard therapy trials that did not include trastuzumab.

The mechanism of trastuzumab-related cardiomyopathy remains unclear. Unlike anthracycline-induced cardiotoxicity, it does not appear to be cumulative or dose-related. Risk factors for developing trastuzumab-related cardiomyopathy include older age, exposure to anthracyclines, previous cardiac disease, HF, LV dysfunction, and HTN.

Prior to receiving trastuzumab, patients should undergo evaluation of LV function, preferably by radionuclide imaging. It has been proposed that in patients with LVEF <40%, careful risk-benefit analysis should occur before initiating therapy with trastuzumab. EF should be monitored every 4 to 6 weeks during treatment. If the LVEF falls by more than 10% or to less than 40% or if symptoms of CHF develop, trastuzumab should be discontinued and resumed only if the EF improves to ≥40% and symptoms resolve.

Trastuzumab-induced cardiomyopathy appears to be more reversible than that seen with anthracyclines. Treatment is similar to that used in patients with HF due to other causes.

Stent Thrombosis in the Chemotherapy Patient

As endothelialization of the internal lumen of a coronary stent is necessary to protect against thrombotic stent occlusion, the possibility arises that patients who receive chemotherapy and require stent placement may have delayed neointimalization. This brings up multiple issues:

- When is it safe to discontinue taking antiplatelet agents if the neointimalization process is delayed by chemotherapy?
- A common side effect of chemotherapy is thrombocytopenia, and those who receive drug-eluting stents will require antiplatelet agents such as clopidogrel for at least a

year and aspirin indefinitely, exposing them to a greater increased risk of bleeding from both decreased number of platelets and decreased platelet function.

- Cancer is a risk factor for hypercoagulability and may further place patients at risk for subacute or late stent thrombosis.

These issues must be considered in treating the cancer patient who is diagnosed with CAD and requires percutaneous coronary revascularization.

CARDIOVASCULAR ISSUES IN THE PATIENT WITH HIV

Since the advent of highly active antiretroviral therapy (HAART) in the 1990s, survival of patients infected with the human immunodeficiency virus (HIV) has dramatically increased. In addition to the cardiovascular complications of the acquired immunodeficiency syndrome (AIDS)—including myocarditis, dilated cardiomyopathy, pericardial effusion, endocarditis, cardiac tumors, and pulmonary HTN—cardiologists are now faced with the increasing incidence of CAD in the HIV population. This section reviews the cardiovascular issues in the HIV patient and provide treatment recommendations where appropriate.

HIV and CAD

Studies evaluating the relative risk of CAD in the HIV patient have been conflicting. Overall, it seems that **there is a small increase in absolute risk of MI in HIV patients taking HAART, particularly protease inhibitors (PIs)**, compared with the general population. This risk increases with duration of treatment and is associated with the development of metabolic derangements, including dyslipidemia, insulin resistance, and central obesity.

The HIV virus itself causes atherosclerotic changes, including endothelial dysfunction, inflammation (with increased levels of C-reactive protein [CRP], tumor necrosis factor [TNF], and interferon gamma), increased platelet adhesion in the form of elevated von Willebrand factor, and hypercoagulability secondary to decreased levels of protein S.

The HIV patient with CAD tends to be younger (mean/median age 42–50 years), to smoke (>50% patients with HIV smoke), to have a very low HDL and a high triglyceride level, and more likely to have single-vessel disease. Up to one-third of HIV patients have HTN, and this is associated with HAART in some studies. There is a high rate of restenosis after PCI. While there are no studies yet reporting graft patency after coronary artery bypass grafting (CABG), the event-free survival is 81% at 3 years.

Lipodystrophy, or HIV-associated fat redistribution, occurs in 20% to 35% of patients 1 to 2 years after starting HAART. It manifests as a loss of fat from the face and extremities and accumulations of fat in the neck, abdomen, trunk, and dorsocervical region ("buffalo hump"). Lipodystrophy may be reduced by exercise training with or without metformin.

Although HAART increases the risk of CAD in the HIV patient, the benefits far outweigh the risk. **Treatment of CAD** in this population is similar to that in the general population with a few exceptions, mainly drug–drug interactions (Table 28-2). As with all CAD patients, HIV patients who smoke should be encouraged to quit. Reducing obesity should also be a target for lifestyle modifications.

Pericarditis/Myocarditis

Asymptomatic pericardial effusion is common in HIV patients, occurring in about 11% of HIV patients per year before the advent of HAART. Larger effusions leading to cardiac tamponade are uncommon. Since HAART, the incidence of pericardial effusions and pericarditis has declined. Up to one-third of cases are associated with myocarditis, which is associated with high mortality.

TABLE 28-2   DRUG INTERACTIONS IN THE HIV PATIENT

Drug	Mechanism/Adverse Reaction	Drugs to Avoid	Alternative Rx
Protease inhibitors (ritonavir, atazanavir, saquinavir)	Inhibit metabolism by cytochrome P450 system. Risk of myopathy, rhabdomyolysis	Statins-simvastatin and lovastatin	Pravastatin or fluvastatin (not metabolized by P450)
Protease inhibitors	Decrease concentrations of PI's	St. John's wort	Atorvastatin at reduced dose
Phosphodiesterase 5 inhibitors (sildenafil, tadalafil, vardenafil)	Increased side effects, including hypotension, vision changes, priapism	Protease inhibitors	
Atazanavir	Prolongs PR interval	Caution if conduction disease, avoid beta blockers, non-dihydropyridine CCBs, and digoxin	
Protease inhibitors (fosamprenavir, nelfinavir, ritonavir, saquinavir)	Inhibit CYP3A	Antiarrhythmic drugs (amiodarone, quinidine, flecainide, propafenone)	
Protease inhibitors	Increased risk of ergot toxicity, including peripheral vasospasm and limb ischemia	Ergots	

Most often, the pericardial effusions are **tuberculous**, although *Staphylococcus* and *Streptococcus* are also possible etiologies, as are lymphoma and Kaposi's sarcoma. **A specific cause of myocarditis is found in <20% of cases.** Rarely, infective myocarditis may be caused by toxoplasmosis, aspergillosis, histoplasmosis, tuberculosis, *Cryptococcus*, cytomegalovirus, herpes simplex virus, or even HIV itself.

Pericardiocentesis is essential for diagnosis and to guide therapy; it is certainly indicated in effusion causing hemodynamic compromise.

Treatment depends on the cause. Tuberculous pericarditis should be treated with antituberculous drugs, corticosteroids, and pericardial drainage if effusion is present.

HIV-Associated Cardiomyopathy

Before HAART, up to 15% of HIV patients were found to have global LV dysfunction by echocardiography and 2% of such patients developed CHF. Most were patients with the lowest CD4 cell counts, and the prognosis was very poor. Since HAART, the incidence of HIV-related cardiomyopathy and HF has declined.

The exact mechanism of HIV-induced cardiomyopathy remains unclear but may involve direct cardiotoxicity of the HIV virus itself, cardiotoxicity of HAART (particularly zidovudine through cardiac mitochondrial toxicity), increased cytokine activity, opportunistic infections, IV drug abuse, or nutritional deficiencies.

On echocardiography, these patients have biventricular dilatation. Biopsy shows both myocyte hypertrophy and evidence of myocarditis. Response to the treatment of HIV-induced cardiomyopathy may be complicated by the presence of opportunistic infections, autoimmune response to the HIV, and the cardiotoxic effects of HAART.

Cardiac Tumors

The cardiac tumors HIV patients most commonly develop are Kaposi's sarcoma and B-cell lymphoma.

Patients with **Kaposi's sarcoma** are usually asymptomatic and often have widespread mucocutaneous disease. Kaposi's can invade the pericardium, epicardium, and myocardium and an effusion may be present. Treatment may involve interferon alpha, which has been associated with reversible LV dysfunction.

The **B-cell lymphomas** are aggressive and may be primary or secondary cardiac tumors, usually located in the right atrium. Patients present with symptoms of HF, atrioventricular (AV) block, or other conduction abnormalities caused by myocardial infiltration, ventricular tachycardia, and pericardial effusion. Treatment involves chemotherapy to treat the lymphoma, but the patient should be monitored for arrhythmia caused by tumor necrosis.

Endocarditis in the HIV Patient

HIV by itself is not a risk factor for infective endocarditis (IE), but HIV is an independent risk factor for IE in IV drug abusers. IE also occurs in the setting of long-term indwelling central venous catheters in this population. The lower the CD4 cell count, the higher the risk for IE.

Staphylococcus aureus is the most common causative organism, although *Streptococcus viridans* is also common. **Prognosis** is better for right-sided IE, with a mortality of <5%, compared to 20% to 30% for left-sided lesions. Surgery reduces these mortalities to <2% for right-sided lesions and 15% to 20% for the left-sided lesions. Prognosis is the worst in IE caused by gram-negative bacteria or fungi. Mortality is higher in those with CD4 cell counts <200/μL or who have advanced to AIDS. AIDS patients require a maximum-duration antibiotic regimen.

HIV and Pulmonary Hypertension

The incidence of primary pulmonary HTN (PPH) is 0.5% in HIV patients compared with 1 to 2 per million in the general population.

No relation has been found between PPH and CD4 cell count or with the presence of RV dysfunction caused by opportunistic infections. One theory to explain the increased incidence of PPH in HIV patients implicates human herpesvirus 8 (HHV-8), the causative agent for Kaposi's sarcoma, but this remains to be proven. IV drug abusers commonly develop PPH, likely due to injection of foreign materials (i.e., talc), but this may be confounding.

Diagnosis is made via echocardiography and right heart catheterization. Histopathology reveals plexogenic arteriopathy similar to the PPH seen in non-HIV patients. **Treatment** is similar to the therapy used to treat PPH in the non-HIV population and includes CCBs, diuretics, anticoagulation, prostacyclin analogs, sildenafil, and the endothelin antagonist, bosentan. Prognosis is poor, and the effect of HAART on PPH is not known.

KEY POINTS TO REMEMBER

- CVD is the leading cause of death in women.
- Hormone replacement therapy should not be prescribed for the purpose of reducing CAD risk.
- Any arrhythmia can occur during pregnancy in women both with and without preexisting structural heart disease. Most antiarrhythmic drugs are safe, but all cross the placenta and should be used with caution.
- Peripartum cardiomyopathy is LV systolic dysfunction occurring in the last month of pregnancy or the first 5 months postpartum. The etiology is unclear. Treatment includes preload and afterload reduction, beta blockers, digoxin, diuretics, and anticoagulation.
- Maternal risk of pregnancy in women with congenital heart disease is determined by the patient's anatomy, previous operations, and hemodynamic status. Fetal risks are higher in women with poor functional class, cyanotic heart disease, and LV outflow obstruction. In those at highest risk, termination of pregnancy should be considered.
- CVD is common in the rapidly growing elderly population. Cardiovascular drug therapy and coronary revascularization have increased benefit in the elderly compared with younger patients but are often underutilized.
- HF is the number one reason for hospitalization in the elderly. Isolated diastolic dysfunction is common, and the elderly often present with atypical symptoms. Treatment should include ACE inhibitors, aldosterone receptor antagonists, ARBs, beta blockers, digoxin, diuretics, anticoagulation, and device therapy where indicated.
- CVD is the leading cause of death in African Americans and Hispanics and the second leading cause of death in Asians and Pacific Islanders, yet there are disparities in the level of health care minorities receive compared with whites.
- HTN has a disproportionate effect on African Americans, occurring earlier in life, with greater severity, and with increased incidence of end-organ damage. Treatment begins with thiazide diuretics, although most patients require a multidrug regimen including ACE inhibitors, ARBs, and beta blockers, with benefits above and beyond their blood pressure–lowering effects.
- Cancer patients who receive anthracycline, high-dose cyclophosphamide, and trastuzumab-based chemotherapy regimens are at risk for developing cardiomyopathy. Treatment of chemotherapy-related HF is similar to the treatment of HF due to other causes.
- Both the HIV virus and HAART result in an increased risk of CAD compared with the general population.
- Since the development of HAART, the incidence of HIV-associated cardiomyopathy has declined.
- Practitioners should be aware of drug interactions between HAART and commonly used cardiovascular drugs.

REFERENCES AND SUGGESTED READINGS

Alexander KP, Peterson ED. Medical and surgical management of coronary artery disease in women. *Am J Manag Care* 2001;7:951–956.

ALLHAT Officers and Coordinators for the ALLHAT Collaborative Research Group. Major outcomes in high risk hypertensive patients randomized to angiotensin converting enzyme inhibitor or calcium channel blocker vs diuretic. *JAMA* 2002;288(3):2981–2997.

Bach RG, Cannon CP, Weintraub WS, et al. The effect of routine, early invasive management on outcome for elderly patients with non–ST-segment elevation acute coronary syndromes. *Ann Intern Med* 2004;141:186–195.

Barrett-Connor E, Grady D. Hormone replacement therapy, heart disease, and other considerations. *Annu Rev Public Health* 1998;19:55–72.

Beta-Blocker Evaluation of Survival Trial Investigators. A trial of the beta-blocker bucindolol in patients with advanced chronic heart failure. *N Engl J Med* 2001;344:1659–1667.

Bonow RO, Carabello BA, Chatterjee K, et al. ACC/AHA 2006 Guidelines for the Management of Patients with Valvular Heart Disease. *JACC* 2006;48(3):1–148.

CDC/DHHS. *Heart Disease Facts and Statistics*. Available at http://www.cdc.gov/heartdisease/facts.htm

CDC/NCHS. *Heart Facts 2007*. Available at www.americanheart.org/downloadable/heart/1176927558476AllAmAfAm%20HeartFacts07_lores.pdf.

Cohn JN, Tognoni G. A randomized trial of the angiotensin receptor blocker valsartan in chronic heart failure. *N Engl J Med* 2001;345(23):1667–1675.

Daly C, Clemens F, Lopez Sendon JL, et al. Gender differences in the management and clinical outcome of stable angina. *Circulation* 2006;113:490–498.

Ferdinand KC. Coronary artery disease in minority racial and ethnic groups in the United States. *Am J Cardiol* 2006;97(2):12–19.

Ferrero S, Colombo BM, Ragni N. Maternal arrhythmias during pregnancy. *Arch Gynecol Obstet* 2004;269:244–253.

Fonarow GC. Quality indicators for the management of heart failure in vulnerable elders. *Ann Intern Med* 2001;135:694–702.

Garg R, Gorlin R, Smith T, et al. The effect of digoxin on mortality and morbidity in patients with heart failure. *N Engl J Med* 1997;336:525–533.

Gibbons RJ, Abrams J, Chatterjee K, Daley J, et al. ACC/AHA 2002 Guideline update for the management of patients with chronic stable angina. *J Am Coll Cardiol* 2003;91:159–168.

Grady D, Herrington D, Bittner V, et al. Cardiovascular disease outcomes during 6.8 years of hormone therapy. Heart and Estrogen/Progestin Replacement Study Follow-up (HERS II). *JAMA* 2002;288(1):49–57.

Gregoratos et al. ACC/AHA/NASPE 2002 Guideline update for implantation of cardiac pacemakers and antiarrhythmia devices. Available online at http://www.acc.org/clinical/guidelines/pacemaker/index.htm.

Hilfiker-Kleiner D, Kaminski K, Podewski E, et al. A Cathepsin D–cleaved 16 kDa form of prolactin mediates postpartum cardiomyopathy. *Cell* 2007;128:589–600.

Hsue P, Waters DD. What a cardiologist needs to know about patients with human immunodeficiency virus infection. *Circulation* 2005;112:3947–3957.

Hunt SA, Abraham WT, Chin MH, et al. ACC/AHA 2005 Guideline update for the diagnosis and management of chronic heart failure in the adult. *JACC* 2005;46:1–82.

James PR. A review of peripartum cardiomyopathy. *J Clin Pract* 2004;58(4):363–365.

Khan JM, Beevers DG. Management of hypertension in ethnic minorities. *Heart* 2005;91:1105–1109.

Kwok YS, Kim C, Segal M, et al. Exercise testing for coronary artery disease diagnosis in women: a meta-analysis. *Circulation* 1996;I-497:2916.

Limat S, Demesmay K, Voillat L, et al. Early cardiotoxicity of the CHOP regimen in aggressive non-Hodgkin's lymphoma. *Ann Oncol* 2003;14:277–281.

Manson LE, Hsia J, Johnson KC, et al. Women's Health Initiative Investigators: Estrogen plus progestin and risk of coronary heart disease. *N Engl J Med* 2003;349:523–534.

McMurray JJ, Ostergren J, Swedberg K, et al. Effects of candesartan in patients with chronic heart failure and reduced left ventricular systolic function takeing angiotensin-converting enzyme inhibitors: the CHARM-Added trial. *Lancet* 2003;362:767–771.

Mosca L, Banka CL, Benjamin EJ, et al. Evidence-based guidelines for cardiovascular disease prevention in women: 2007 update. *Circulation* 2007;115:1481–1501.

Ng R, Green MD. Managing cardiotoxicity in anthracycline-treated breast cancers. *Expert Opin Drug Saf* 2007;6(3):315–321.

Packer M, Coats AJS, Fowler MB, et al. Effect of carvedilol on survival in severe chronic heart failure. *N Engl J Med* 2001;344:1651–1658.

Panrath GS, Jain D. Trastuzumab-induced cardiac dysfunction. *Nucl Med Commun* 2007;28:69–73.

Patel H, Rosengren A, Ekman I. Symptoms in acute coronary syndromes, does sex make a difference? *Am Heart J* 2004;148(1):27–33.

Pilote L, Dasgupta K, Humphries KH, et al. A comprehensive view of sex-specific issues related to cardiovascular disease. *Can Med Assoc J* 2007;176(6):S1–S41.

Pitt B, Zannad F, Remme WJ, et al. The effect of spironolactone on morbidity and mortality in patients with severe heart failure. *N Engl J Med* 1999;341:709–717.

Polk DM, Naqvi TZ. Cardiovascular disease in women: sex differences in presentation, risk factors and evaluation. *Curr Cardiol Rep* 2005;7(3):166–172.

Redberg RF. Coronary artery disease in women: understanding the diagnostic and management pitfalls. *Medscape Gen Med* 1999. Available at http://www.medscape.com/viewarticle/408890.

Rodriguez BL, Curb JD, Burchfiel CM, et al. Impaired glucose tolerance, diabetes, and cardiovascular disease risk factor profiles in the elderly. The Honolulu Heart Program. *Diabetes Care* 1996;19:587–590.

Rosengren A, Wallentin L, Gitt AK, et al. Sex, age, and clinical presentation of acute coronary syndromes. *Eur Heart J* 2004;25:663–670.

Rossouw JE, Prentice Rl, Manson JE, et al. Postmenopausal hormone therapy and risk of cardiovascular disease by age and years since menopause. *JAMA* 2007;297(3):1465–1477.

Sliwa K, Fett J, Elkayam U. Peripartum cardiomyopathy. *Lancet* 2006;368:687–693.

Smith SC, Winters KW, Lasala JM. Stent thrombosis in a patient receiving chemotherapy. *Cathet Cardiovasc Diagn* 1997;40:383–386.

Strandberg TE, Pitkala KH, Tilvis RS. Benefits of optimising drug treatment in home-dwelling elderly patients with coronary artery disease. *Drugs Aging* 2003;20(8):585–595.

Sudano I, Spicker LE, Noll G, et al. Cardiovascular disease in HIV infection. *Am Heart J* 2006;151(6):1147–1155.

Taylor AL, Ziesche S, Yancy C, et al. combination of isosorbide dinitrate and hydralazine in blacks with heart failure. *N Engl J Med* 2004;351:2049–2057.

Trappe, HJ. Acute therapy of maternal and fetal arrhythmias during pregnancy. *J Intens Care Med* 2006;21(5):305–315.

Uebing A, Steer PJ, Yentis SM, et al. Pregnancy and congenital heart disease. *BMJ* 2006;332:401–406.

Yamasaki N, Kitaoka H, Matsumura Y, et al. Heart failure in the elderly. *Intern Med* 2003;42:283–288.

Yancy CW, Benjamin EJ, Fabunmi RP, et al. Discovering the full spectrum of cardiovascular disease: Minority Health Summit 2003 executive summary. *Circulation* 2005;111:1339–1349.

Yancy CW. Executive Summary of the African American Initiative. *Medscape Gen Med* 2007;9(1):28.

Yusif S, Sleight P, Pogue J, et al. Effects of an angiotensin-converting-enzyme inhibitor, ramipril, on cardiovascular events in high risk patients, the Heart Outcomes Prevention Evaluation Investigators. *N Engl J Med* 2000;342(3):145–153.

Zipes DP, Camm AJ, Borggrefe M, et al. ACC/AHA/ESC 2006 guidelines for management of patients with ventricular arrhythmias and prevention of sudden cardiac death. *JACC* 2006;48:247–346.

Diabetes and Cardiovascular Disease

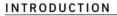

Kan Liu

INTRODUCTION

Diabetes mellitus affects more than 10% of the population of the United States, and its prevalence increases as the population ages and grows more obese. This disease claims a disproportionate fraction of the health-care budget, as the result not only of the costs involved in the care of diabetes itself but also of those involved in caring for the complications of this disease. Cardiovascular complications are the leading cause of diabetes-related morbidity and mortality. This chapter focuses on the pathogenesis, clinical manifestations, and management of various cardiovascular diseases including coronary heart disease (CHD) and congestive heart failure (CHF) as well as strategies for cardiac risk reduction in diabetic patients.

CORONARY HEART DISEASE IN DIABETES

Introduction

Compared with nondiabetics, diabetic patients have higher prevalence of CHD, higher rate of myocardial infarction (MI), greater ischemic burden, and poorer post-MI outcome and long-term survival. Cardiac risk in diabetic individuals is 2 to 4 times greater than that in nondiabetics. Diabetes is considered by the National Cholesterol Education Program/Adult Treatment Panel III (NCEP/ATPIII) guidelines to be a coronary artery disease (CAD) risk equivalent.

Causes

Pathophysiology

Multiple mechanisms have been proffered to account for the increased risk of CAD in the diabetic patient, including endothelial dysfunction and enhanced thrombosis development. Coronary atheromas from diabetic patients contains more lipid-rich tissue and macrophage infiltration, which increases the risk of plaque rupture and subsequent thrombosis development. There is also enhanced platelet aggregation and activation along with poor coronary collateral development.

Presentation

Clinical Presentation

The clinical severity of an acute MI in diabetics is often greater than that of nondiabetics even with similar infarct sizes and left ventricular ejection fraction (EF). Acute pulmonary edema due to CHF occurs more frequently in diabetic heart disease, as do arrhythmias due to regional heterogeneity in sympathetic innervation and myocardial electrical instability. Diabetic patients also have a higher risk of other noncardiac complications, such as renal failure.

Symptoms

Diabetics tend to have a blunted appreciation of ischemic pain, which may result in atypical angina symptoms, silent ischemia, or even silent infarction. Autonomic denervation due to diabetic neuropathy may be an underlying mechanism.

Management

Diagnosis

Current guidelines from the American College of Cardiology/American Heart Association (ACC/AHA) do not specifically address the diagnostic and prognostic utility of exercise electrocardiographic (ECG) testing among diabetic patients. The American Diabetes Association (ADA) advocates for stress testing in diabetic patients with:

- Typical or atypical cardiac symptoms
- Resting ECG suggestive of ischemia or infarction
- Peripheral or carotid occlusive arterial disease
- Sedentary lifestyle and age ≥35 years with plans to begin a vigorous exercise program
- Two or more of the following risk factors in addition to diabetes:
  - Total cholesterol ≥240 mg/dL
  - Low-density-lipoprotein cholesterol (LDL-C) ≥160 mg/dL
  - High-density-lipoprotein cholesterol (HDL-C) ≤35 mg/dL
  - Blood pressure ≥140/90 mm Hg
  - Smoking
  - Family history of premature CAD
  - Microalbuminuria

Diagnostic Testing

For a full description of diagnostic stress testing modalities, see Chapter 3. As applied to the diabetic patient, several points are worth mentioning:

- The diagnostic sensitivity and specificity of exercise ECG testing is similar for diabetic patients and nondiabetic patients.
- Myocardial perfusion imaging has higher sensitivity and specificity in this population compared with exercise ECG alone.
- **Diabetic patients with normal stress echocardiograms may have a greater risk for subsequent cardiovascular events than nondiabetic patients, particularly beyond 2 years.**
- More extensive coronary calcification in diabetics may interfere with the interpretation of coronary stenosis severity in computed tomography (CT) angiography.

Treatment of Acute Coronary Syndrome

- ST-segment elevation myocardial infarction (STEMI): As with nondiabetics, diabetic patients with STEMI should receive immediate coronary reperfusion with either primary percutaneous intervention (PCI) or thrombolytic therapy in the absence of a contraindication.
- Unstable angina (UA)/non-STEMI (NSTEMI): As with nondiabetics, diabetic patients with a UA/NSTEMI should be considered candidates for early invasive treatment followed by revascularization if appropriate.
- Medical therapy: Medical therapy in the setting of acute coronary syndrome (ACS) is similar to that of the nondiabetic (see Chapter 8). Like nondiabetics, diabetics should receive antiplatelet agents [aspirin (ASA), clopidogrel, and glycoprotein (GP) IIb/IIIa inhibitors], anticoagulation, as well as angiotensin converting enzyme

(ACE) inhibitors and angiotensin receptor blockers (ARBs). Notable points as applied to the diabetic patient are:

- Beta blockers were previously not favored because of the fear of masking hypoglycemic symptoms or worsening glycemic control. However, the overall benefit has been found to be at least equivalent to or greater than that seen in nondiabetics.
- Aldosterone antagonists have a class I indication for diabetic patients after an acute MI, in the setting of:
  - Left ventricular ejection fraction (LVEF) ≤40%
  - Receiving an ACE inhibitor
  - Serum creatinine ≤2.5 mg/dL (men) or ≤2.0 mg/dL (women)
  - Serum potassium ≤5.0 meq/L
- The goal of blood pressure control should be <130/80 for diabetic patients.
- The goal LDL-C is <70 mg/dL or 50% reduction from baseline.
- Glycemic control is very important. Both diabetics and nondiabetics who have had an acute MI or are critically ill benefit from tight blood glucose control. The 2004 ACC/AHA guidelines for glycemic control on STEMI (which should also be applicable to NSTEMI) are:
  - Class I recommendation: insulin infusion to normalize blood glucose in patients with a complicated course regardless of whether the patient has a diagnosis of diabetes.
  - Class IIa recommendation: insulin infusion in all MI patients with hyperglycemia.
  - Strict glycemic control should be maintained after discharge with a goal HbA1c of less than 7% (see **"Cardiac Risk-Factor Reduction,"** below).
- **For details regarding revascularization, see Chapters 8 and 9.**

Complications

Diabetic patients are more likely to experience complications associated with an MI, including postinfarct angina and heart failure.

Special Topics

Revascularization Therapy for Stable Angina in Diabetic Patients. Unlike diabetic patients with ACS, the revascularization strategies for diabetic patients with stable angina are controversial. In diabetic patients with stable CHD, is there a difference in outcomes between those who receive coronary revascularization and those who initially receive intensive medical management? The Bypass Angioplasty Revascularization Investigation 2 Diabetes (BARI 2D) is an ongoing clinical trial to address this issue. Based on BARI and ARTS I trials and subsequent meta-analysis, coronary artery bypass grafting (CABG) has traditionally been preferred to PCI in diabetic patients with multivessel disease. However, these recommendations were made before the availability of drug-eluting stents.

HEART FAILURE IN DIABETES

Introduction

Diabetes affects cardiac structure and function independent of blood pressure or CHD. More than 30 years ago, Rubler et al. introduced the term "diabetic cardiomyopathy," based on postmortem findings. The higher incidence of heart failure in diabetic patients has been ascribed to a preexisting subclinical impairment of left ventricular function.

In the presence of diabetes, the risk of heart failure is 2.4-fold higher in men and 5-fold higher in women. Diabetes predicts heart failure independent of coexisting hypertension or CHD. Each 1% increase in hemoglobin A1c is associated with an 8% increased risk of

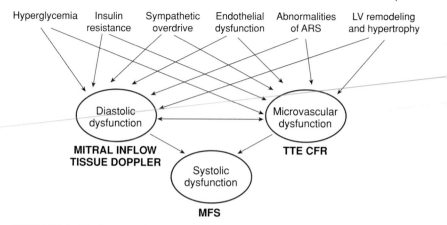

FIGURE 29-1. The hypothetical link of metabolic alterations to cardiac function in diabetes. Hyperglycemia, insulin resistance, sympathetic overdrive, endothelial dysfunction, abnormalities of the angiotensin-renin system (ARS), and LV remodeling/ hypertrophy may induce diastolic dysfunction (DD) and impairment of the coronary microcirculation. The LV systolic involvement appears subsequent to DD and/or coronary microvascular dysfunction. CFR, coronary flow reserve; MFS, midwall fractional shortening; TTE, transthoracic echocardiography. (From Galderisi M. Diastolic dysfunction and diabetic cardiomyopathy: evaluation by Doppler echocardiography. *J Am Coll Cardiol* 2006;48[8]:1548–1551, with permission.)

heart failure. The incidence of heart failure after revascularization with PCI or CABG is also greater in diabetics.

Causes

Pathophysiology

Grossly, diabetic hearts (Fig. 29-1) have increased left ventricular mass, wall thickness, and arterial stiffness. Microscopic pathologic changes include myocardial fibrosis, infiltration of the interstitium with periodic acid-Schiff–positive material, and alterations in the myocardial capillary basement membrane. In autopsy studies, myocardial catecholamine stores are depleted in diabetic patients, which could impair both systolic and diastolic cardiac function. Thus, autonomic neuropathy may partially contribute to the development of left ventricular dysfunction in the diabetic state. Insulin deficiency or resistance impairs glucose availability of cardiomyocytes, resulting in a shift from glucose to fatty acid metabolism. Coronary microcirculatory pathology plays a role in the development of diabetic cardiomyopathy. Impaired nitric oxide and vascular endothelial growth factor (VEGF) function contribute to this defect.

Presentation

Clinical Presentation

The clinical presentation of diabetic cardiomyopathy is similar to that of other kinds of cardiomyopathies. Clinical manifestations from either diastolic or systolic dysfunction can occur in patients with various stages of diabetes. Abnormal diastolic function has been noted in 27% to 70% of asymptomatic diabetic patients, based on various studies. Multiple studies indicate that the level of urine microalbuminuria is proportional to the degree of cardiac diastolic dysfunction in diabetic patients. In view of this, **the presence of urine microalbuminuria may warrant echocardiography with pulsed-wave Doppler evaluation, even in asymptomatic diabetic patients.**

Management

Treatment

Glycemic control is very important in diabetic patients to prevent advancement from early diastolic dysfunction to overt heart failure. **ACE-inhibitor therapy** should be prescribed regardless of the degree of left ventricular dysfunction to decrease left ventricular hypertrophy and myocardial fibrosis, prevent myocardial remodeling, improve endothelial function, and lower insulin resistance. If ACE inhibitors are not tolerated, an **ARB** can be used as an alternative treatment. **Beta blockers** should be utilized, since new diagnostic criteria consider the presence of diabetes as stage 1 heart failure. Beta blockers prevent the remodeling process and shift myocardial metabolism from fatty acid to glucose, which may reduce lipotoxicity on cardiomyocytes. **Thiazolidinediones** decrease myocardial fatty acid content and their toxic metabolites and also improve ventricular function. However, thiazolidinediones can cause fluid retention and are contraindicated in New York Heart Association (NYHA) functional class III or IV heart failure. Recent concerns over roziglitazone suggest caution when used in patients with significant CAD or CHF. **Aldosterone antagonists** have antifibrotic effects on the development of cardiomyopathy. However, no data are available specifically for their use in the treatment of diabetic cardiomyopathy. Diabetes has been considered a relative contraindication for **heart transplantation**. Patients with multiple diabetic comorbidities may have a better outcome treated with other therapies, such as mechanical assist devices. However, diabetics should not *a priori* be excluded from consideration for transplant, particularly if they are free of significant diabetic complications.

CARDIAC RISK-FACTOR REDUCTION IN DIABETES

Introduction

A number of modifiable risk factors for CHD and heart failure in the diabetic patient have been identified. These include obesity, hypertension, dyslipidemia, and smoking. There is considerable evidence indicating that a substantial reduction in cardiovascular mortality could be achieved by multifactorial cardiac risk reduction.

Management

Aspirin

Daily aspirin therapy is beneficial in diabetic patients with CHD. However, there is currently no randomized study available regarding aspirin for primary prevention in diabetes population.

Blood Pressure Control

The United Kingdom Prospective Diabetes Study (UKPDS) suggests that each 10 mm Hg reduction in mean systolic pressure is associated with a 12% reduction in the risk of diabetic complications. The blood pressure goal for diabetic patients is ≤130/80 mm Hg. Lower values may be beneficial in patients with diabetic nephropathy. Combination therapy with an ACE inhibitor/ARB and a beta blocker is often required for patients with hypertension and diabetes.

Serum Lipid Control

Screening for lipid disorders should be done at least annually in diabetic patients and more often if needed. Use of statins is recommended for secondary prevention in all diabetic patients with cardiovascular diseases, with a goal LDL-C of <70 mg/dL. The ADA recommends an LDL-C of <100 mg/dL as the primary goal for all diabetic patients even in the absence of known CHD. Statin therapy should be initiated in patients >40 years of age without overt cardiovascular disease to achieve a reduction in LDL-C of 30% to 40%, regardless of baseline LDL-C levels. Non–HDL-C appears to be a particularly strong predictor of CHD in both men and women with diabetes.

Glycemic Control

The progression of cardiovascular complications correlates not only with the duration of diabetes but also with the level of glucose control. Poor glucose control and onset of disease under the age of 20 years are often associated with progressive target-organ dysfunction, including coronary, cerebral, and peripheral vascular diseases. Strict glycemic control is recommended in both type 1 and type 2 diabetes because of demonstrated benefits in terms of microvascular disease. The importance of tight glycemic control for protection against cardiovascular disease has been established in type 1 diabetes. However, the similar association has not been established in type 2 diabetes. The current ADA recommendation is to achieve a hemoglobin A1c goal of <7%. More stringent goals can be considered in individual patients. Hemoglobin A1c should be checked at least twice yearly in patients with stable glycemic control and quarterly in patients with poor glycemic control.

Special Topics

CHD Before Diabetes. Diabetes may first be diagnosed in the setting of acute MI. Fasting plasma glucose and hemoglobin A1c should be routinely measured during hospitalization in nondiabetic patients with an acute MI. Values that are elevated but do not meet the criteria for diabetes (i.e., impaired fasting glucose or impaired glucose tolerance) must be repeated after discharge to identify those at increased risk. If the diagnosis is confirmed, glycemic therapy should be started as early as possible.

KEY POINTS TO REMEMBER

- Diabetes is considered a CAD risk equivalent.
- Diabetic patients have higher rate of MI, greater ischemic burden, more silent symptoms, and poorer post-MI outcome and long-term survival.
- CABG has traditionally been preferred to PCI in diabetic patients with multivessel disease, but this may change with the advent of drug-eluting stents and pending the results of ongoing clinical trials.
- Diabetes affects cardiac structure and function independent of blood pressure or CHD.
- Abnormal cardiac diastolic function often exists at a very early stage even in asymptomatic diabetic patients.
- Urine microalbuminuria is proportional to the degree of cardiac diastolic dysfunction in diabetic patients.
- In the absence of contraindications, ACE inhibitors or ARBs should be used in diabetic patients regardless of the degree of left ventricular dysfunction.
- The goal of blood pressure control in diabetics is ≤130/80 mm Hg and even lower in patients with diabetic nephropathy.
- The current goal for glycemic control is to achieve a hemoglobin A1c <7%. More stringent goals might be needed.
- Serum lipid control is extremely important in diabetic patients for cardiac risk reduction. The LDL-C goal for patients with CAD is <70 mg/dL.

REFERENCES AND SUGGESTED READINGS

Abaci A, Oguzhan A, Eryol NK, et al. Effect of diabetes mellitus on formation of coronary collateral vessels. *Circulation* 1999;100(22):2219–2223.

Adler AI, Stratton IM, Neil HA, et al. Association of systolic blood pressure with macrovascular and microvascular complications of type 2 diabetes (UKPDS 36): prospective observational study. *BMJ* 2000;321(7258):412–419.

Albers AR, Krichavsky MZ, Balady GJ. Stress testing in patients with diabetes mellitus: diagnostic and prognostic value. *Circulation* 2006;113(4):583–592.

Albers AR, Krichavsky MZ, Balady GJ. Stress testing in patients with diabetes mellitus: diagnostic and prognostic value. *Circulation* 2006;113(4):583–592.

Antiplatelet Trialists' Collaboration. Collaborative overview of randomised trials of antiplatelet therapy—I: Prevention of death, myocardial infarction, and stroke by prolonged antiplatelet therapy in various categories of patients. *BMJ* 1994;308(6921):81–106.

Bell DSH. Use of beta blockers in patients with diabetes. *Endocrinologist* 2003;13: 116–123.

Bypass Angioplasty Revascularization Investigation 2 Diabetes (BARI 2D) Trial Investigators. *Am J Cardiol* 2006;97(12A):9G–19G.

Camici PG, Crea F. Coronary microvascular dysfunction. *N Engl J Med* 2007;356(8): 830–840.

Galderisi M. Diastolic dysfunction and diabetic cardiomyopathy: evaluation by Doppler echocardiography *J Am Coll Cardiol* 2006;48(8):1548–1551.

Gundersen T, Kjekshus J. Timolol treatment after myocardial infarction in diabetic patients. *Diabetes Care* 1983;6(3):285–290.

Haffner SM, Lehto S, Ronnemaa T, et al. Mortality from coronary heart disease in subjects with type 2 diabetes and in nondiabetic subjects with and without prior myocardial infarction. *N Engl J Med* 1998;339(4):229–234.

Iribarren C, Karter AJ, Go AS, et al. Glycemic control and heart failure among adult patients with diabetes. *Circulation* 2001;103(22):2668–2673.

Kambara N, Holycross BJ, Wung P, et al. Combined effects of low-dose oral spironolactone and captopril therapy in a rat model of spontaneous hypertension and heart failure. *J Cardiovasc Pharmacol* 2003;41:830–837.

Kannel W, Hjortland M, Castelli W. Role of diabetes in congestive heart failure. The Framingham Study. *Am J Cardiol* 1974;34:29.

Lu W, Resnick HE, Jablonski KA, Jones KL, et al. Non–HDL cholesterol as a predictor of cardiovascular disease in type 2 diabetes: the strong heart study. *Diabetes Care* 2003;26(1):16–23.

Mak KH, Topol EJ. Emerging concepts in the management of acute myocardial infarction in patients with diabetes mellitus. *J Am Coll Cardiol* 2000;35(3):563–568.

Marso S. *The Handbook of Diabetes Mellitus and Cardiovascular Disease.* London: Remedica; 2003.

McQueen MJ, Gerstein HC, Pogue J, et al. Reevaluation by high-performance liquid chromatography: clinical significance of microalbuminuria in individuals at high risk of cardiovascular disease in the Heart Outcomes Prevention Evaluation (HOPE) Study. *Am J Kidney Dis* 2006;48(6):889–896.

Nathan DM, Cleary PA, Backlund JY, et al. Intensive diabetes treatment and cardiovascular disease in patients with type 1 diabetes. *N Engl J Med* 2005;353(25):2643–2653.

Porte D, Sherwin RS, Baron A, eds. *Ellenberg and Rifkin's Diabetes Mellitus,* 6th ed. New York: McGraw Hill; 2003.

Roffi M, Chew DP, Mukherjee D, et al. Platelet glycoprotein IIb/IIIa inhibitors reduce mortality in diabetic patients with non–ST-segment-elevation acute coronary syndromes. *Circulation* 2001;104(23):2767–2771.

Rubler S, Dlugash J, Yuceoglu YZ. New type of cardiomyopathy associated with diabetic glomerulosclerosis. *Am J Cardiol* 1972;30:595.

Russo MJ, Chen JM, Hong K, et al. Survival after heart transplantation is not diminished among recipients with uncomplicated diabetes mellitus: an analysis of the United Network of Organ Sharing database. *Circulation* 2006;114:2280–2287.

Sobel BE, Schneider DJ. *Medical Management of Diabetes and Heart Disease.* New York: Marcel Dekker; 2002.

Stevens MJ, Raffel DM, Allman KC, et al. Cardiac sympathetic dysinnervation in diabetes: implications for enhanced cardiovascular risk. *Circulation* 1998;98(10):961–968.

The Bypass Angioplasty Revascularization Investigation (BARI) Investigators. Comparison of coronary bypass surgery with angioplasty in patients with multivessel disease. *N Engl J Med* 1996;335(4):217–225.

Third Report of the National Cholesterol Education Program (NCEP) Expert Panel on Detection, Evaluation, and Treatment of High Blood Cholesterol in Adults (Adult Treatment Panel III) final report. *Circulation* 2002;106:3143.

Wackers FJ, Young LH, Inzucchi SE, et al. Detection of silent myocardial ischemia in asymptomatic diabetic subjects: the DIAD study. *Diabetes Care* 2004;27:1954–1961.

Yudkin JS. How can we best prolong life? Benefits of coronary risk factor reduction in non-diabetic and diabetic subjects. *BMJ* 1993;306(6888):1313–1318.

Zarich SW, Arbuckle BE, Cohen LR, et al. Diastolic abnormalities in young asymptomatic diabetic patients assessed by pulsed Doppler echocardiography. *J Am Coll Cardiol* 1988;12(1):114–120.

Zhou Y-T, Graburn P, Karim A, et al. Lipotoxic heart disease in obese rats: implications for human obesity. *Proc Natl Acad Sci USA* 2000;97:1784–1789.

Zuanetti G, Latini R, Maggioni AP, et al. Effect of the ACE inhibitor lisinopril on mortality in diabetic patients with acute myocardial infarction: data from the GISSI-3 study. *Circulation* 1997;96(12):4239–4245.

The Cardiac Patient Undergoing Noncardiac Surgery

30

Andrew M. Kates

O ne of the most common requests for consultation from both the internist and cardiologist is the evaluation of the patient with manifest or suspected cardiovascular disease undergoing noncardiac surgery. Recently, the American College of Cardiology (ACC) and the American Heart Association (AHA) published joint guidelines that provide updated recommendations for this purpose and are discussed in detail below. This publication and its Executive Summary provide an excellent framework for preoperative risk assessment.

The purpose of risk assessment is to identify the patient at risk for perioperative cardiac morbidity or mortality. Preoperative cardiac evaluation should be tailored to the circumstances that have prompted the evaluation and to the nature of the surgical illness. In the setting of a surgical emergency, preoperative evaluation may be limited to a rapid assessment including vital signs, volume status, hematocrit, electrolytes, renal function, and electrocardiogram (ECG). Only the most essential tests and interventions are appropriate until the acute surgical emergency is resolved. A more thorough evaluation can be conducted after surgery. Additionally, in patients in whom coronary revascularization is not an option, it is usually unnecessary to perform a noninvasive stress test. Under other, less urgent circumstances, the preoperative cardiac evaluation may lead to a variety of responses that may result in postponement or cancellation of an elective procedure. The algorithm for perioperative cardiac evaluation and care is shown in Figure 30-1.

Several points merit mention. The most recent guidelines have changed the previous "major clinical factors" to "active cardiac conditions." These conditions place the patient at significant risk for perioperative complications. As such, the presence of one or more of these conditions requires intensive management. It may be reasonable to delay or cancel surgery unless the surgery is emergent. These conditions include:

- Unstable coronary syndromes
- Unstable or severe angina
- Recent myocardial infarction
- Decompensated heart failure
- Significant arrhythmias
- Severe valvular disease

The intermediate-risk clinical risk factors have been changed to include those from the Revised Cardiac Risk Index. These clinical risk factors include:

- History of ischemic heart disease
- History of compensated or prior heart failure
- History of cerebrovascular disease
- Diabetes mellitus
- Renal insufficiency

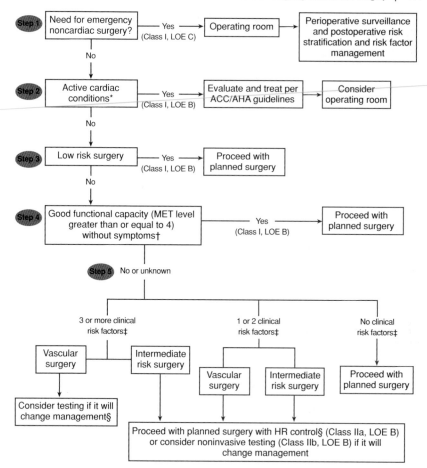

FIGURE 30-1. Algorithm for cardiac evaluation and management.

The level of risk with associated surgery has changed as well. Risk for specific surgeries is shown in Table 30-1.

Estimation of the patient's functional status is essential in this evaluation. Functional status based on different activities is shown in Table 30-2.

While there has been controversy recently regarding the benefits of beta-blocker therapy in the perioperative setting, it remains clear that aggressive beta-blocker therapy is beneficial for the high-risk patient. When possible, beta blockers should be started days to weeks before elective surgery. The dose should be titrated to achieve a resting heart rate of 60 bpm to increase the likelihood that the patient will receive the benefit of beta blockade. Rate control with beta blockers should continue during the intraoperative and postoperative periods to maintain a heart rate of 60 to 65 bpm. Specific recommendations are shown in Table 30-3.

The role of the consultant in this evaluation is to determine the stability of the patient's cardiovascular status and whether he or she is in optimal medical condition within

| TABLE 30-1 | RISK STRATIFICATION BASED ON TYPE OF SURGERY* |

Risk Stratification	Procedure Examples
Vascular (reported cardiac risk often >5%)	Aortic and other major vascular surgery Peripheral vascular surgery
Intermediate (reported cardiac risk generally 1%–5%)	Intraperitoneal and intrathoracic surgery Carotid endarterectomy Head and neck surgery Orthopedic surgery Prostate surgery
Low† (reported cardiac risk generally <1%)	Endoscopic procedures Superficial procedure Cataract surgery Breast surgery Ambulatory surgery

*Combined incidence of cardiac death and nonfatal myocardial infarction.
†These procedures do not generally require further preoperative cardiac testing.

| TABLE 30-2 | ESTIMATION OF FUNCTIONAL STATUS |

	Can you...		Can you...
1 MET	Take care of yourself?	4 METs	Climb a flight of stairs or walk up a hill?
	Eat, dress, or use the toilet?		Walk on level ground at 4 mph (6.4 kph)?
	Walk indoors around the house?		Run a short distance?
	Walk a block or 2 on level ground at 2–3 mph (3.2–4.8 kph)?		Do heavy work around the house like scrubbing floors or lifting or moving heavy furniture?
4 METs	Do light work around the house like dusting or washing dishes?		Participate in moderate recreational activities like golf, bowling, dancing, doubles tennis, or throwing a baseball or football?
		>10 METs	Participate in strenuous sports like swimming, singles tennis, football, basketball, or skiing?

kph, kilometers per hour; MET, metabolic equivalent; mph, miles per hour.
Fleisher LA, Beckman JA, Brown KA, et al. ACC/AHA 2007 guidelines on perioperative cardiovascular evaluation and care for noncardiac surgery: a report of the American College of Cardiology/American Heart Association Task Force on Practice Guidelines (Writing Committee to Revise the 2002 Guidelines on Perioperative Cardiovascular Evaluation for Noncardiac Surgery). *JACC* 2007;50(17): e159–241.

TABLE 30-3	INDICATIONS FOR BETA BLOCKER THERAPY			
Surgery	**No Clinical Risk Factors**	**1 or More Clinical Risk Factors**	**CHD or High Cardiac Risk**	**Patients Currently Taking Beta Blockers**
Vascular	Class IIb, Level of Evidence: B	Class IIa, Level of Evidence: B	Patients found to have myocardial ischemia on pre-operative testing: Class I, Level of Evidence: B Patients without ischemia or no previous test: Class IIa, Level of Evidence: B	Class I, Level of Evidence: B
Intermediate risk	...	Class IIb, Level of Evidence: C	Class IIa, Level of Evidence: B	Class I, Level of Evidence: C
Low risk	...	...	...	Class I, Level of Evidence: C

Fleisher LA, Beckman JA, Brown KA, et al. ACC/AHA 2007 guidelines on perioperative cardiovascular evaluation and care for noncardiac surgery: a report of the American College of Cardiology/American Heart Association Task Force on Practice Guidelines (Writing Committee to Revise the 2002 Guidelines on Perioperative Cardiovascular Evaluation for Noncardiac Surgery). *JACC* 2007;50(17): e159–241.

the context of the surgical illness. It is not the consultant's role to "clear" the patient, and use of this term is strongly discouraged. As stressed in the guidelines, preoperative tests should be recommended only if the information obtained will result in a change in the surgical procedure performed, a change in medical therapy or monitoring during or after surgery, or a postponement of surgery until the cardiac condition can be corrected or stabilized. Communication is a critical part of the preoperative evaluation. Discussions should be undertaken with the surgeon, anesthesiologist, and other physicians as well as with the patient and, if appropriate, the family, regarding the potential cardiac risks.

REFERENCES AND SUGGESTED READINGS

Fleisher LA, Beckman JA, Brown KA, et al. ACC/AHA 2007 guidelines on perioperative cardiovascular evaluation and care for noncardiac surgery: a report of the American College of Cardiology/American Heart Association Task Force on Practice Guidelines (Writing Committee to Revise the 2002 Guidelines on Perioperative Cardiovascular Evaluation for Noncardiac Surgery). *JACC* 2007;50(17):e159–241.

Appendix:
Cardiovascular Medications

ACKNOWLEDGMENT

The editors are indebted to James M. Hollands, PharmD, Clininal Pharmacist, Cardiac Intensive Care Unit at Barnes-Jewish Hospital for his considerate review of this appedix.

Abbreviations

ACLS: advanced cardiac life support
ACS: acute coronary syndrome
ACT: activated clotting time
ADP: adenosine diphosphate
AF: atrial fibrillation
AV: atrioventricular
BID: twice daily
CAD: coronary artery disease
CHF: congestive heart failure
CVA: cerebrovascular accident
CYP: cytochrome P-450 enzyme
ER: extended-release
g: gram
GI: gastrointestinal
GP: glycoprotein
h: hour
HDL: high-density lipoprotein
HIT: heparin-induced thrombocytopenia
HTN: hypertension
IHSS: idiopathic hypertrophic subaortic stenosis
ISA: intrinsic sympathomimetic activity
IV: intravenous
kg: kilogram
LDL: low-density lipoprotein
LV: left ventricle
μg: microgram

mg: milligram
min: minute
MI: myocardial infarction
PAD: peripheral arterial disease
PCI: percutaneous coronary intervention
PE: pulmonary embolism
PEA: pulseless electrical activity
PO: per os (by mouth)
PTT: partial thromboplastin time
q: every
QD: daily
QID: four times daily
RBC: red blood cell
SC: subcutaneous
SL: sublingual
STEMI: ST-segment elevation myocardial infarction
SVT: supraventricular tachycardia
TG: triglyceride
TID: three times daily
TTP: thrombotic thrombocytopenic purpura
U: units
VF: ventricular fibrillation
VT: ventricular tachycardia
VTE: venous thromboembolism

Angiotensin Converting Enzyme (ACE) Inhibitors

Generic Name	Trade Name	Tablet Size	Indications (Dosing Range)	Contraindications	Serious Reactions	Common Reactions	Metabolism (Half-life)	Unique Properties
Benazepril	Lotensin	5, 10, 20, 40 mg	HTN: 20–40 mg QD				Liver (10 h)	
Captopril	Capoten	12.5, 25, 50, 100 mg	HTN: 25–50 mg BID–TID CHF: 6.25–50 mg TID Nephropathy: 25 mg TID Post MI: 12.5–50 mg TID	**Black box warning: Pregnancy (fetal morbidity and mortality)**			Liver (<3 h)	
Enalapril	**Vasotec**	2.5, 5, 10, 20 mg IV dosing available	HTN: 2.5–40 mg QD CHF: 2.5–20 mg BID Post MI: 10 mg BID Nephropathy: 5–20 mg QD	Avoid in patients with prior angioedema due to ACE inhibitor or bilateral renal artery stenosis **Reduce Dose by 50% if Patient is Taking Diuretics**	Anaphylactoid reaction, **angioedema, hyperkalemia, renal failure,** agranulocytosis	**Cough,** hypotension, dizziness, hyperkalemia	Liver (11 h)	
Fosinopril	**Monopril**	10, 20, 40 mg	HTN: 10–80 mg QD CHF: 10–40 mg QD				Liver, GI tract (11.5 h)	

Generic	Brand	Forms	Dosing	Warnings	Side Effects	Metabolism (half-life)	Notes
Lisinopril	**Prinivil, Zestril**	2.5, 5, 10, 20, 40 mg	HTN: 10–40 mg QD CHF: 2.5–20 mg QD Post MI: 5–10 mg QD			None (12 h)	
Moexipril	**Univasc**	7.5, 15 mg	HTN: 7.5–30 mg QD			Liver (12 h)	Works at the tissue ACE level
Perindopril	**Aceon**	2, 4, 8 mg	HTN: 4–16 mg QD Stable CAD: 4–8 mg QD	**Black box warning: Pregnancy (fetal morbidity and mortality)**	Anaphylactoid reaction, **angioedema, hyperkalemia, renal failure,** agranulocytosis	Liver (1 h)	Works at the tissue ACE level
Quinapril	**Accupril**	5, 10, 20, 40 mg	HTN: 10–80 mg QD CHF: 5–20 mg BID	Avoid in patients with prior angioedema due to ACE inhibitor or bilateral renal artery stenosis		Liver, GI tract (1–2 h)	Works at the tissue ACE level
Ramipril	**Altace**	1.25, 2.5, 5, 10 mg capsules	HTN: 2.5–20 mg QD CHF, post-MI: 5 mg BID Cardiac risk reduction: 2.5–10 mg QD	**Reduce Dose by 50% if Patient is Taking Diuretics**	**Cough,** hypotension, dizziness, hyperkalemia	Liver (13–17 h)	Works at the tissue ACE level
Trandolapril	**Mavik**	1,2,4 mg	HTN: 2–4 mg QD CHF, post-MI: 4 mg QD			Liver (6 h)	Works at the tissue ACE level

Angiotensin Receptor Blockers (ARBs)

Generic Name	Trade Name	Tablet Size	Indications (Dosing Range)	Contraindications	Serious Reactions	Common Reactions	Metabolism, CYP (Half-life)
Candesartan	Atacand	4, 8, 16, 32 mg	HTN: 4–32 mg QD CHF: 32 mg QD				Liver (9 h)
Eprosartan	Teveten	400, 600 mg	HTN: 400–800 mg QD				Glucuronidation (5–9 h)
Irbesartan	Avapro	75, 150, 300 mg	HTN: 75–300 mg QD Nephropathy: 300 mg QD	**Black box warning: Pregnancy (fetal morbidity and mortality).**	**Hyperkalemia,** angioedema, renal failure, hypotension		Liver, 2C9 (11–15 h)
Losartan	Cozaar	25, 50, 100 mg	HTN: 25–100 mg QD Nephropathy: 50–100 mg QD	Bilateral renal artery stenosis		Dizziness, back pain, fatigue	Liver, 2C9, 3A4 (2–9 h)
Olmesartan	Benicar	5, 20, 40 mg	HTN: 10–40 mg QD				Minimal (13 h)
Telmisartan	Micardis	20, 40, 80 mg	HTN: 20–80 mg QD				Minimal (24 h)
Valsartan	Diovan	40, 80, 160, 320 mg	HTN: 80–320 mg QD CHF: 40–160 mg QD Post-MI: 20–160 mg QD				Liver, 2C9 (6 h)

Beta-Adrenergic Receptor Blockers

Generic Name	Trade Name	Tablet Size	Indications (Dosing Range)	Contraindications	Serious Reactions	Common Reactions	Metabolism (Half-life)	Unique Properties
Acebutolol	Sectral	200, 400 mg	HTN: 400–800 mg QD VT/VF: 600–1200 mg QD				Liver (3–4 h)	Beta-1 selective ISA
Atenolol	Tenormin	25, 50, 100 mg IV dosing available	HTN: 50–100 mg QD Angina: 50–200 mg QD Acute MI: 5mg IV X 2 doses, then 50 mg BID	**Black box warning (for select beta blockers): avoid abrupt cessation.**	**Bronchospasm, heart block,** bradycardia, Raynaud's phenomenon	**Fatigue, lethargy, constipation,** depression, cold extremities, vivid dreams	None (6–7 h)	Beta-1 selective
Betaxolol	Kerlone	10, 20 mg	HTN: 10–20 mg QD				Liver (14–22 h)	Beta-1 selective
Bisoprolol	Zebeta	5, 10 mg	HTN: 2.5–20 mg QD				Liver (9–12 h)	Beta-1 selective
Carvedilol	Coreg	3.125, 6.25, 12.5, 25 mg	CHF: 6.25–25 mg BID or 20–80 mg QD (ER)				Liver, 2D6 (6–10 h)	Blocks alpha-1, beta-1 and beta-2 receptors
	Coreg CR	10, 20, 40, 80 mg (ER)	HTN: 6.25–25 mg BID or 20–80 mg QD (ER) Post-MI LV dysfunction: 25 mg BID or 80 mg QD (ER)					

(continued)

Beta-Adrenergic Receptor Blockers

Generic Name	Trade Name	Tablet Size	Indications (Dosing Range)	Contraindications	Serious Reactions	Common Reactions	Metabolism (Half-life)	Unique Properties
Esmolol	**Brevibloc**	IV dosing only	SVT: 500 µg/kg load, then 50 µg/kg/min HTN: 80 mg load, then 150 µg/kg/min				RBCs (9 min)	Beta-1 selective Extremely short half-life
Labetalol	**Trandate**	100, 200, 300 mg IV dosing available	HTN: 200–400 mg BID HTN crisis: 40–80 mg IV q 10 min	**Black box warning (for select beta blockers): avoid abrupt cessation.**			Liver (5–8 h)	Blocks alpha-1, beta-1 and beta-2 receptors
Metoprolol	**Lopressor**	25, 50, 100 mg	HTN: 50–200 mg BID or 25–400 mg QD (ER)	Severe bradycardia, AV block, cardiogenic shock, decompensated heart failure	**Bronchospasm, heart block,** bradycardia, Raynaud's phenomenon	**Fatigue, lethargy, constipation,** depression, cold extremities, vivid dreams	Liver, 2D6 (3–7 h)	Beta-1 selective
	Toprol XL	25, 50, 100, 200 mg (ER) IV dosing available	Angina: 50–200 mg BID or 100–400 mg QD (ER) Acute MI: 5 mg IV q3 min, then 50 mg QID CHF: 12.5–200 mg QD (ER)					

Generic	Brand	Strengths	Dosing	Warnings	Side effects	Metabolism (half-life)	Notes
Nadolol	**Corgard**	20, 40, 80, 120, 160 mg	HTN: 40–80 mg QD Angina: 40–80 mg QD			None (20–24 h)	Nonselective beta blocker
Penbutalol	**Levatol**	20 mg	HTN: 20 mg QD			Liver (5 h)	Nonselective beta blocker ISA
Pindolol	**Visken**	5, 10 mg	HTN: 5–15 mg BID			Liver, 2D6 (3–4 h)	Nonselective beta blocker ISA
Propranolol	**Inderal**	10, 20, 40, 60, 80 mg	HTN: 80–240 mg BID Angina: 80–320 mg/day div BID–QID	**Black box warning (for select beta blockers): avoid abrupt cessation.** Severe bradycardia, AV block, cardiogenic shock, decompensated heart failure	**Bronchospasm, heart block,** bradycardia, Raynaud's phenomenon **Fatigue, lethargy, constipation,** depression, cold extremities, vivid dreams	Liver, 2D6 (3–5 h) (ER: 8–11 h)	Nonselective beta blocker
	Inderal LA InnoPran XL	60, 80, 120, 160 mg (ER) IV dosing available	MI: 180–240 mg/day div TID–QID AF: 10–30 mg PO TID–QID Migraine headache prophylaxis: 160–240 mg/day div BID–QID Essential tremor: 120 mg/day div BID–TID				IV dosing for SVT: 1–3 mg IV

(continued)

Beta-Adrenergic Receptor Blockers

Generic Name	Trade Name	Tablet Size	Indications (Dosing Range)	Contraindications	Serious Reactions	Common Reactions	Metabolism (Half-life)	Unique Properties
			IHSS: 20–40 mg TID-QID	**Black box warning (for select beta blockers): avoid abrupt cessation.**		**Fatigue, lethargy, constipation,**		
			Pheochromocytoma (adjunct): 60 mg/day div BID-QID		**Bronchospasm, heart block,** bradycardia, Raynaud's phenomenon	depression, cold extremities, vivid dreams		
Timolol	Blocadren	5, 10, 20 mg	HTN: 10–20 mg BID	Severe bradycardia, AV block, cardiogenic shock, decompensated heart failure			Liver, 2D6 (2–4 h)	Nonselective beta blocker
			MI: 10 mg BID					
			Migraine headache prophylaxis: 10-30 mg/day div QD-BID					

Calcium-Channel Blockers

Generic Name	Trade Name	Tablet Size	Indications (Dosing Range)	Contraindications	Serious Reactions	Common Reactions	Metabolism (Half-life), CYP	Unique Properties
Amlodipine	Norvasc	2.5, 5, 10 mg	HTN: 5–10 mg QD CAD: 5–10 mg QD				Liver, 3A4 (30–50 h)	Dihydropyridine
Diltiazem	Cardizem	30, 60, 90, 120 mg	HTN: 120–180 mg BID (12 h ER) Or 180–480 mg QD (24 h ER)	**Nondihydropyridines: avoid in patients with AV block, sick sinus syndrome, acute MI with pulmonary congestion, or with possible accessory AV bypass tract (WPW)**	**Dihydropyridines:** hypotension, syncope **Nondihydropyridines:** AV block, bradycardia, heart failure	**Dihydropyridines:** peripheral edema, headache, flushing, fatigue, gingival hyperplasia **Nondihydropyridines:** peripheral edeam, constipation	Liver, 3A4 (3–4 h)	Nondihydropyridine
	Cardizem CD Cardizem LA Cartia XT Dilacor XR Dilt-CD Diltia XT Taztia XT Tiazac	60, 90, 120 mg (12 h ER) 120, 180, 240, 300, 360, 420 mg (24 h ER) IV dosing available	Angina: 30–90 mg QID or 120–480 mg QD (24 h ER) AF: 0.25 mg/kg IV, may give 0.35 mg/kg IV after 15 min, then follow with 5–15 mg/h IV SVT: 0.25 mg/kg IV, may give 0.35 mg/kg IV after 15 min, then follow with 5–15 mg/h IV					
Felodipine	Plendil	2.5, 5, 10 mg	HTN: 2.5–10 mg QD				Liver, 3A4 (9 h)	Dihydropyridine

(continued)

423

Calcium-Channel Blockers

Generic Name	Trade Name	Tablet Size	Indications (Dosing Range)	Contraindications	Serious Reactions	Common Reactions	Metabolism (Half-life)	Unique Properties
Isradipine		2.5, 5 mg	HTN: 2.5–5 mg BID or 5 mg QD (ER)				Liver, 3A4 (8 h)	Dihydropyridine
	DynaCirc CR	5, 10 mg (ER)					Liver, 3A4 (8 h)	Dihydropyridine
Nicardipine	Cardene	20, 30 mg	HTN: 20–40 mg TID or 30–60 mg BID (ER) or 5 mg/h IV, titrate to BP					
	Cardene CR	30, 45, 60 (ER)				**Dihydropyridines:** peripheral edema, headache, flushing, fatigue, gingival hyperplasia		
		IV dosing available	Angina: 20–40 mg TID	**Nondihydropyridines: avoid in patients with AV block, sick sinus syndrome, acute MI with pulmonary congestion, or with possible accessory AV bypass tract (WPW)**	**Dihydropyridines:** hypotension, syncope **Nondihydropyridines:** AV block, bradycardia, heart failure			
Nifedipine	Procardia	10, 20 mg	Vasospasm: 10–20 mg TID or 30–90 mg QD (ER)				Liver, 3A4 (2 h) (ER, 7 h)	Dihydropyridine
	Procardia XL	30, 60, 90 mg (ER)	Angina: 10–20 mg TID or 30–90 mg QD (ER)			**Nondihydropyridines:** peripheral edeam, constipation		
	Adalat CC		HTN: 30–90 mg QD (ER) or 30–90 mg QD (ER)					
Nimodipine	Nimotop	30 mg	SAH: 60 mg q4h X 21 days				Liver, 3A4 (8–9 h)	Dihydropyridine
Nisoldipine	Sular	10, 20, 30, 40 mg	HTN: 20–40 mg QD				Liver, 3A4 (7–12 h)	Dihydropyridine

			Nondihydropyridines: avoid in patients with AV block, sick sinus syndrome, acute MI with pulmonary congestion, or with possible accessory AV bypass tract (WPW)	**Dihydropyridines:** hypotension, syncope **Nondihydropyridines:** AV block, bradycardia, heart failure	**Dihydropyridines:** peripheral edema, headache, flushing, fatigue, gingival hyperplasia **Nondihydropyridines:** peripheral edeam, constipation	Liver, 3A4 (6–10 h)	Nondihydropyridine
Verapamil	**Calan**	40, 80, 120 mg	Angina: 80–120 mg TID				
	Calan SR	120, 180, 240 mg (12 h ER)	HTN: 80–120 mg TID or 120–480 mg/day div BID (12 h ER) 120–480 mg QD (24 h AM) 100–400 mg QHS (24 h PM)				
	Verelan	120, 180, 240, 360 mg (24 h AM)	AF: 80–120 mg TID-QID or 2.5–10 mg IV				
	Verelan PM	100, 200, 300 mg (24 h PM) IV dosing available	SVT conversion: 2.5–10 mg IV SVT prevention: 80–120 mg TID-QID				

Cholesterol-Lowering Drugs

	Generic Name	Trade Name	Tablet Size	Contraindications	Serious Reactions	Common Reactions	Metabolism, CYP (Half-life)	Unique Properties
HMG-CoA Reductase Inhibitors	Atorvastatin	Lipitor	10, 20, 40, 80 mg				Liver, 3A4 (14–30 h)	**LDL: 39–60%** ↓ HDL: 5–9% ↑ TG: 19–37% ↓
	Fluvastatin	Lescol Lescol XL	20, 40 mg 80 mg (ER)	Unexplained elevated liver enzymes	**Myopathy and rhabdomyolysis, hepatitis, pancreatitis**	Constipation, diarrhea, dyspepsia	Liver, 2C9 (3 h, 9 h for ER)	**LDL: 33–38%** ↓ HDL: 3–11% ↑ TG: 19–25% ↓
	Lovastatin	Mevacor Altoprev	10, 20, 40 mg 10, 20, 40, 60 mg (ER)				Liver, 3A4 (3 h)	**LDL:21–42%** ↓ HDL: 2–10% ↑ TG: 6–27% ↓
	Pravastatin	Pravachol	10, 20, 40, 80 mg				Liver (77 h)	**LDL: 22–37%** ↓ HDL: 2–12% ↑ TG: 15–24% ↓
	Rosuvastatin	Crestor	5, 10, 20, 40 mg				Liver, 2C9 (19 h)	**LDL: 45–63%** ↓ HDL: 8–14% ↑ TG: 10–35% ↓
	Simvastatin	Zocor	5, 10, 20, 40, 80 mg				Liver, 3A4 (2 h)	**LDL: 26–47%** ↓ HDL: 8–16% ↑ TG: 12–34 % ↓

Fibrates	**Fenofibrate**	**TriCor**	48, 50, 54, 107, 145, 160 mg tablets; 43, 67, 130, 134, 200 mg capsules	Hepatitis, pancreatitis, **rhabdomyolysis, especially when prescribed with HMG-CoA reductase inhibitor**	Nausea, diarrhea, constipation, myopathy	Glucuronidation (16–20 h)	LDL: 20–30% ↓ HDL: 3–11% ↑ **TG: 23–54% ↓**
	Gemfibrozil	**Lopid**	600 mg			Liver, 2C9 (1.5 h)	LDL: 0–10% ↓ HDL: 10–20% ↑ **TG: 20–60% ↓**
Niacin	**Niacin**	**Niacor** **Niaspan**	500 mg 500, 750, 1000 mg (ER)	Hepatotoxicity	**Flushing,** pruritus, blurred vision	Liver (30 min)	LDL: 6–25% ↓ **HDL: 15–35%** **TG: 20–60% ↓**
Bowel Absorption	**Ezetimibe**	**Zetia**	10 mg	Anaphylaxis	Abdominal pain, diarrhea	GI tract and liver (22 h)	LDL: 18% ↓ HDL: 0–1% ↑ TG: 8% ↓
Bile Acid Resins	**Cholestyra-mine**	**Questran**	4-g packet	Constipation		None	LDL: 5–30% ↓ HDL: 0–5% ↑ TG: 0–10% ↑
	Colesevelam	**WelChol**	625 mg	**Fecal impaction**	**Constipation, flatulence**	None	LDL: 15–18% ↓ HDL: 3–5% ↑ TG: 0–10% ↑
	Colestipol	**Colestid**	1-g tablet 5-g packet			None	LDL: 15–30% ↓ HDL: 0–5% ↑ TG: 0–10% ↓

Nitrates

Generic Name	Trade Name	Tablet Size	Indications (Dosing Range)	Contraindications	Serious Reactions	Common Reactions	Metabolism (Half-life)	Unique Properties
Isosorbide dinitrate	Isordil Biovail Dilatrate-SR	2.5, 5, 10 mg (SL) 5, 10, 20, 30, 40 mg (ER)	Angina: 10–40 mg BID-TID Acute angina: 2.5–10 mg SL q2–3h				Liver, (1–5 h)	Onset (SL): 2–5 min Onset (ER): 60–90 min Duration (SL): 1–3 h Duration (ER): 12 h
Isosorbide mononitrate	Monoket Ismo Imdur	10, 20, 30, 60, 120 mg	Angina prevention: 20 mg BID or 30–60 mg QD				Liver, (5 h)	Onset: 30–60 min Duration: 5–12 h
Nitroglycerin ointment	Nitro-Bid	2% Ointment	Angina: ½ in. q6h	**Contraindicated with erectile dysfunction medications (phosphodiesterase-5 inhibitors, i.e. sildenafil, tadalafil, vardenafil)**	Severe hypotension, methemoglobinemia	**Hypotension, headache,** tachycardia, flushing	Liver, RBCs (1–3 min)	Onset: 30–60 min Duration: 8–12 h
Nitroglycerin transdermal	Nitro-Dur Minitran	0.1, 0.2, 0.3, 0.4, 0.6 mg/h patch	Angina: 0.2–0.4 mg/h patch QD				Liver, RBCs (1–3 min)	Onset: 30–60 min Duration: 3–5 h
Nitroglycerin translingual	NitroMist	0.4-mg metered spray	Angina: 1–2 sprays SL q3–5 min				Liver, RBCs (1–3 min)	Onset: 1-3 min Duration: 30–60 min
Nitroglycerin sublingual	NitroQuick NitroStat NitroTab	0.3, 0.4, 0.6 mg	Angina: 1 tab SL q3–5 min				Liver, RBCs (1–3 min)	Onset: 1-3 min Duration: 30–60 min
Nitroglycerin intravenous	Tridil	IV dosing	Unstable angina: 5 µg/min, titrate rapidly to effect; CHF with MI: 5 µg/min, titrate rapidly to effect				Liver, RBCs (1–3 min)	Onset: Immediate Duration: 3–5 min

Diuretics

	Generic Name	Trade Name	Tablet Size	Contraindications	Serious Reactions	Common Reactions	Metabolism, CYP (Half-life)
Loop	Bumetanide	Bumex	0.5, 1, 2 mg	**Caution with renal failure.** Use of diuretic requires frequent monitoring for renal function and electrolye abnormalities.	**Severe hypokalemia, volume depletion,** metabolic alkalosis, ototoxicity	**Urinary frequency,** hypokalemia, dizziness, **muscle cramps**	Liver, (1–2 h)
	Furosemide	Lasix	20, 40, 80 mg				Liver, (30–60 min)
	Torsemide	Demedex	5, 10, 20, 100 mg				Liver, 2C9 (3–4 h)
	Ethacrynic Acid	Edecrin	25 mg				Liver, (1 h)
Thiazide	Chlorothiazide	Diuril	250, 500 mg		**Severe hypokalemia, volume depletion,** metabolic alkalosis		None (1–2 h)
	Chlorthalidone	Hygroton	25, 50, 100 mg				None (40 h)
	Hydrochlorothiazide	Microzide	12.5, 25, 50, 100 mg				None (5–15 h)
	Indapamide	Lozol	1.25, 2.5 mg				Liver (26 h)
	Metolazone	Zaroxolyn	2.5, 5, 10 mg				None (14 h)
K-sparing	Amiloride	Midamor	5 mg	**Black box warning: Risk of severe hyperkalemia**	**Hyperkalemia,** renal failure, agranulocytosis, aplastic anemia	Headache, nausea, diarrhea, photosensitivity	None (6–9 h)
	Triamterene	Dyrenium	50, 100 mg				Liver (1–3 h)
	Spironolactone	Aldactone	25, 50, 100 mg	Monitor for hyperkalemia		Nausea, **gynecomastia, hirsutism,** rash, diarrhea	Liver (1–3 h)

Antiplatelets and Anticoagulants

Generic Name	Trade Name	Tablet Size	Indications (Dosing Range)	Contraindications	Serious Reactions	Common Reactions	Mechanism of Action	Metabolism CYP (Half-life)
Aspirin		81, 165, 325, 500, 650 mg	ACS: 162–325 mg X1 MI risk reduction: 81–325 mg QD	Aspirin-induced asthma, severe GI bleed	Anaphylaxis, bronchospasm, **GI bleed,** hepatotoxicity	Dyspepsia, tinnitus	Inhibits prostaglandin synthesis	Liver, plasma (2–6 h)
Cilostazol	**Pletal**	50, 100 mg	Claudication: 100 mg BID	**Black box warning: Contraindicated in CHF**	**Heart failure, agranulocytosis,** bleeding	Headache, diarrhea	Inhibits phosphodiesterase-3	Liver, 3A4 (11–13 h)
Clopidogrel	**Plavix**	75 mg	ACS: 300 mg X1, 75 mg QD Stent thrombosis prevention: 75 mg QD Recent MI, stroke, PAD: 75 mg QD	GI bleed, intracranial hemorrhage	Bleeding, TTP, angioedema	**Bleeding,** dyspepsia, bruising	Inhibits ADP receptor on platelets	Liver, 2C9 (8 h)
Ticlopidine	**Ticlid**	250 mg	Stroke prevention: 250 mg BID Stent thrombosis prevention: 250 mg BID	**Black box warning: Neutropenia, TTP, aplastic anemia**	Blood dyscrasia, TTP, bleeding			Liver, 2C19 (8–12 h)

Antiplatelet

Abciximab **Reopro**	IV dosing	PCI adjunct: bolus 0.25 µg/kg, then 0.125 µg/kg per min ACS: bolus 0.25 µg/kg, then 10 µg per min	Thrombocytopenia, bleeding	Thrombocytope-nia, bleeding, anaphylaxis	**Bleeding**, back pain, bradycardia, hematuria	Inhibits GP 2B-3A receptor on platelet	None (<30 min)	
Tirofiban **Aggrastat**	IV dosing	ACS: 0.4 µg/kg per min X 30 min, then 0.1 µg/kg per min	Bleeding	Bleeding, anaphylaxis			None (2 h)	
Eptifibatide **Integrilin**	IV dosing	PCI adjunct: 180 µg/kg bolus X 2 ten min apart, then 2 µg/kg per min ACS: 180 µg/kg bolus, then 2 µg/kg per min	Bleeding, thrombo-cytopenia, **renal failure**	Bleeding, thrombocy-topenia, ana-phylaxis			None (2.5 h)	

GP2B/3A Inhibitor

(continued)

Antiplatelets and Anticoagulants

Generic Name	Trade Name	Tablet Size	Indications (Dosing Range)	Contraindications	Serious Reactions	Common Reactions	Mechanism of Action	Metabolism CYP (Half-life)
Thrombolytics								
Urokinase	Abbokinase	IV dosing	PE: 4400 U/kg over 10 min, then 4400 U/kg per h × 12 h	**Bleeding, prior hemorrhagic stroke, any type of stroke within 1 year, known intracranial mass, severe uncontrolled HTN, trauma**	Bleeding, anaphylaxis, reperfusion arrhythmias	Bleeding	Converts plasminogen to plasmin, promoting fibrinolyis	Liver (12 min)
Alteplase	Activase		MI: weight-based; PE: 100 mg over 2 h					Liver (35 min)
			CVA: 0.9 mg/kg over 1 h (10% dose as bolus)					
Reteplase	Retavase		MI: 10 U IV X 2 (after 30 min)					Liver, kidney (15 min)
Tenecteplase	TNKase		MI: weight-based					Liver (2 h)
Direct Thrombin Inhibitors								
Argatroban	Argatroban	IV dosing	PCI adjunct: 350 µg/kg bolus, then adjust per activated clotting time; HIT: 2 µg/kg per min	Bleeding	Bleeding, cardiac arrest	Bleeding, False elevation of INR, hypotension	Direct thrombin inhibitor	Liver, 3A4 (45 min)
Bivalirudin	Angiomax		PCI adjunct: 0.75 mg/kg bolus, then adjust per activated clotting time	Bleeding	Bleeding, thrombocytopenia	Bleeding, back pain, anxiety		Kidney (25 min)
Lepirudin	Refludan		HIT: 0.4 mg/kg bolus, then 16.5 mg/h. Adjust for PTT	Bleeding	Bleeding, anaphylaxis	Bleeding, hematuria		Unknown (1.5 h)

Antithrombin Therapy

Drug	Route	Dosing				Mechanism	Metabolism (half-life)
Unfraction-ated heparin	IV, SC dosing	VTE prophylaxis: 5000 U SC BID-TID VTE treatment: 80 U/kg bolus, then 18 U/kg per h IV ACS: 60 U/kg bolus (max 4000 U) then 12 U/kg per hour (max 1000 U/h)	Bleeding, **thrombocytopenia, HIT**	Bleeding, thrombocytopenia, HIT	Bleeding	Inactivates thrombin and other clotting factors	Liver, (1.5 h)
Enoxaparin **Lovenox**	SC dosing	VTE prophylaxis: 30–40 mg QD-q12h VTE treatment: 1mg/kg q12h ACS: 1 mg/kg q12h STEMI: 30 mg IV + 1 mg/kg SC q12h	**Black box warning: epidural/spinal hematoma risk, renal failure, HIT**	Spinal hematoma, bleeding, thrombocytopenia, prosthetic heart valve thrombosis (Enoxaparin)	Injection site pain, bleeding, elevated LFTs	Low-molecular-weight heparin (LWMH), inhibits factor X > factor II	Liver, (4–7 h)
Dalteparin **Fragmin**		VTE prophylaxis: 5000 U SC QD VTE treatment: 200 U/kg SC QD ACS: 120 U/kg SC q12h					Liver, (3–5 h)
Tinzaparin **Innohep**		VTE treatment: 175 anti-Xa U/kg SC QD					Unknown (3–4 h)

(continued)

Antiplatelets and Anticoagulants

Generic Name	Trade Name	Tablet Size	Indications (Dosing Range)	Contraindications	Serious Reactions	Common Reactions	Mechanism of Action	Metabolism CYP (Half-life)
Fondaparinux	**Arixtra**		VTE prophylaxis: 2.5 mg SQ QD VTE treatment: 5, 7.5, or 10 mg SC QD based on weight				Selective factor X inhibitor	Unknown (17–21 h)
Warfarin	**Coumadin Jantoven**	1, 2, 2.5, 3, 4, 5, 6, 7.5, 10 mg	Anticoagulation: highly variable with genetic polymorphisms	**Black box warning: Fatal bleeding risk** Avoid in pregnancy	Bleeding, skin necrosis	Bruising, bleeding, GI upset, **many drug reastions**	Inhibits vitamin K–dependent coagulation factor synthesis	Liver, 2C9 + others (20–60 h)

Antithrombin Therapy

Antiarrhythmics

Generic Name	Trade Name	Tablet Size	Indications (Dosing Range)	Contraindications	Serious Reactions	Common Reactions	Metabolism (Half-life)	Mechanism of Action
Adenosine	**Adenocard**	IV dosing	ACLS, SVT: 6 mg IV X 1	Sick sinus syndrome (without a pacemaker)	Bradycardia, VF, VT	Transient asystole, flushing	RBCs, endothelium (<10 sec)	Slows AV node conduction
Isoproterenol	**Isuprel**	IV dosing	Bradycardia: 2–10 μg per min	Angina	Seizures, hypotension	Nervousness, restlessness, tremor	Liver, tissues (1–3 min)	Stimulates beta-receptors
1A Disopyramide	**Norpace**	100, 150 mg	VT/VF: 300 mg PO load, then 150 mg q6h or 300 mg PO q12h (ER)	**Black box warning: Increased mortality with recent MI, CAD**	Arrhythmia, CHF, blood dyscrasia	Hypotension, CHF, blurred vision, QRS prolongation	Liver, 3A4 (12 h)	Sodium channel blocker, causes slower conduction velocity and increased refractory periods
	Norpace CR	100, 150 mg (ER)						
1A Procainamide	**Pronestyl**	250, 375, 500 mg	VT/VF or AF: 15–17 mg/kg load IV over 30 minutes, then 1–6 mg/min IV. Load until QRS widens 50%, arrhythmia suppressed or max dose (1.5 g). Titrate infusion per procainamide levels	**Black Box Warning: Drug-induced lupus syndrome, proarrhythmic effects and blood dyscrasia**	Arrhythmia, asystole, seizures, blood dyscrasia, lupus syndrome	Hypotension, bradycardia, bitter taste, hallucinations, QRS prolongation	Liver (3–4 h)	
	Pronestyl-SR Procanbid	250, 500, 750 mg (ER) IV dosing available						

(continued)

Antiarrhythmics

Generic Name	Trade Name	Tablet Size	Indications (Dosing Range)	Contraindications	Serious Reactions	Common Reactions	Metabolism (Half-life)	Mechanism of Action
1A Quinidine	Quinidine gluconate Quinidine sulfate	324 mg (ER) 200, 300 mg 300 mg (ER)	AF or VT/VF: 324–648 mg or 300–600 mg q8–q12h. (ER) Titrate to therapeutic levels.	**Black box warning: Increased mortality if structural heart disease is present.**	QT prolongation, arrhythmia, AV block, TTP, lupus syndrome	Diarrhea, GI upset, altered color perception, nervousness, QRS prolongation	Liver, 3A4 (6–8 h)	Sodium channel blocker, decreases action potential duration and shortens refractory periods, but no effect on conduction velocity.
1B Mexiletine	Mexitil	150, 200, 250 mg	VT/VF: 200 mg q8h	**Black box warning: Increased mortality with recent MI, CAD.**	Arrhythmia	GI upset, tremor, dizziness	Liver, 2D6 (10–12h)	
1B Lidocaine	Xylocaine	IV dosing	ACLS, VT/VF: 1–1.5 mg/kg IV X 1 VT/VF: 1–4 mg/min		Seizures, bronchospasm, heart block	Tremor, confusion, vision changes, tinnitus	Liver, 3A4 (2 h)	Sodium channel blocker, markedly decreases conduction velocity but not refractory period.
1C Flecainide	Tambocor	50, 100, 150 mg	AF: 50–300 mg div BID–TID	**Black box warning: Increased mortality with recent MI, CAD.** Proarrhythmic effects	Arrhythmia, CHF, QT prolongation, blood dyscrasia	Dizziness, visual disturbance, nausea, tremor	Liver, 2D6 (20 h)	
1C Propafenone	Rythmol Rythmol SR	150, 225, 300 mg 225, 325, 425 mg (ER)	AF: 150 mg PO q8h or 225–425 mg q12h (ER)	**Black box warning: Increased mortality with recent MI, CAD.** Sick sinus syndrome without pacemaker, severe hypotension	Arrhythmia, QT prolongation, CHF	Dizziness, taste changes, anxiety, bradycardia	Liver, 2D6 (2–10 h)	

2,3	**Sotalol**	**Betapace** **Betapace AF**	80, 120, 160, 240 mg 80, 120, 160 mg	VT/VF: 80–160 mg q12h AF: 80–160 mg PO q12h	**Black box warning: Initiate with continuous ECG recording, calculate creatinine clearance prior to dosing.** Sinus bradycardia, long QT.	Arrhythmia, QT prolongation, heart block, bradycardia	Dyspnea, fatige, bradycardia	None (7–18 h)	Beta-receptor blocker and increases the action potential duration and therefore, refractory period.
3	**Amiodarone**	**Cordarone** **Pacerone**	100, 200, 400 mg IV dosing available	ACLS, VT/VF: 300 mg IV X1 VT/VF and AF: 200–600 mg PO QD (after several week oral loading at higher doses)	**Black box warning: Pulmonary, liver and proarrhythmic toxicities. Start medication in hospital and consider other agents first.** Sinus bradycardia	Pulmonary, liver, thyroid toxicity, severe bradycardia, arrhythmia	Corneal deposits, GI fatigue, blue skin discoloration, many drug reactions	Liver, 3A4 (58 days)	Increases the action potential duration and therefore, refractory period (K channel)
3	**Dofetilide**	**Tikosyn**	125, 250, 500 µg	AF: (877) 845–6796 for information	**Black box warning: Restricted to trained prescribers, hospitalize to monitor ECG and renal function.** Baseline QT prolongation, renal failure.	QT prolongation, arrhythmia	Headache, chest pain, dizziness	Liver, 3A4 (10 h)	Increases the action potential duration and therefore, refractory period (K channel)

(continued)

Antiarrhythmics

	Generic Name	Trade Name	Tablet Size	Indications (Dosing Range)	Contraindications	Serious Reactions	Common Reactions	Metabolism (Half-life)	Mechanism of Action
3	Ibutilide	Corvert	IV dosing	AF: 1 mg IV over 10 min	**Black box warning: Administer with continuous ECG monitoring by personnel trained in ventricular arrhythmia management.** Proarrhythmic. Do not use if class I or III antiarrhythmics have been given within 4 h	Arrhythmia	QT prolongation, NSVT, headache	Liver, (6 h)	Increases the action potential duration and therefore, refractory period (Na channel)
5	Digoxin	Lanoxin	0.125, 0.25 mg IV dosing available	CHF or AF: 0.75–1.25 mg PO loading dose, then 0.125–0.5 mg QD	IHSS, sick sinus syndrome	AV block, atrial and ventricular tachyarrhythmia, delirium	Dizziness, GI upset, headache, palpitations, many drug interactions	Liver (1.5–2 days)	Increases parasympathetic activity, which causes increased automaticity while decreasing AV node conduction

Vasopressors and Inotropes

Generic Name	Trade Name	Indications (Dosing Range)	Alpha Receptor (Vasoconstriction)	Beta Receptor (Cardiac Output)	Dopamine Receptor (Renal Vasodilation)
Atropine		ACLS, bradycardia/PEA:		(++++) via ACh receptor	
Epinephrine	Adrenalin	ACLS, PEA: 1 mg (1:10,000 sol) IV q3–5 min Anaphylaxis: 0.1–0.5 mg (1:1000 sol) SQ/IM	++++	+++	
Dobutamine	Dobutrex	Cardiogenic Shock: 2–20 µg/kg per min IV	+	++++	
Dopamine		ACLS, bradycardia: 2–10 µg/kg per min IV Hypotension: 1–50 µg/kg per min IV	[10–20 mg/kg per min]	[5–10 mg/kg per min]	[1–5 mg/kg per min]
Isoproterenol	Isuprel	Bradycardia: 2–10 µg/min		++++	
Norepinephrine	Levophed	Hypotension: 2–12 µg/min IV	+++	++	
Milrinone	Primacor	Cardiogenic Shock: 0.5 µg/kg per min IV		(++++) via PDE receptor	
Vasopressin	Pitressin	ACLS, PEA: 40 U IV X 1 Hypotension: 0.04 U/min	(+++) via V1 receptor		
Phenylephrine	Neo-Synephrine	Hypotension: 40–180 µg/min IV	++++		

Other Cardiovascular Agents

Generic Name	Trade Name	Tablet Size	Indications (Dosing Range)	Contraindications	Serious Reactions	Common Reactions	Metabolism (Half-life)
Clonidine	**Catapres** **Catapres TTS**	0.1, 0.2, 0.3 mg 0.1, 0.2, 0.3 mg/24 h patch	HTN: 0.1–0.3 mg BID or 1 patch/week		Rebound HTN	Dry mouth, sedation, bradycardia	Liver (12 h)
Eplerenone	Inspra	25, 50 mg	CHF, post-MI: 50 mg QD HTN: 50 mg QD–BID	**Hyperkalemia**, renal failure	Hyperkalemia, angina	Hyperkalemia, fatigue	Liver, 3A4 (4–6 h)
Hydralazine	Apresolone	10, 25, 50, 100 mg IV dosing available	HTN: 10–50 mg QID HTN crisis: 10–20 mg IV q2–4h CHF: 50–100 mg PO TID		MI, blood dyscrasia, lupus syndrome	Headache, tachycardia, angina	Liver, (3–7 h)
Hydralazine/ isosorbide dinitrate	BiDil	37.5/20 mg	CHF: 1 tab TID	Severe hypotension	Lupus syndrome, hypotension	Headache, dizziness, chest pain	
Methyldopa	Aldomet	125, 250, 500 mg	HTN: 250–500 mg BID	Liver failure	Liver failure, myocarditis, hemolytic anemia	Sedation, headache, weakness, black tongue	Neurons, liver (1.5 h)
Nesiritide	**Natrecor**	IV dosing	CHF, acute: 2 µg/kg bolus, then 0.01–0.03 µg/kg per min	Hypotension	**Hypotension, renal dysfunction**	Hypotension, renal dysfunction	Unknown (18 min)
Nitroprusside	**Nipride** **Nitropres**	IV dosing	HTN crisis: 3–4 µg/kg per min IV	**Black box warning: Rapid hypotension and cyanide toxicity risk**	Severe hypotension, methemaglobinemia, thiocyanate toxicity	Nausea, dizziness, GI upset, tachycardia	RBC, liver (2 min)
Ranolazine	Ranexa	500, 1000 mg	Angina: 500–1000 mg BID	Prolonged QT interval, liver or renal failure	QT prolongation, bradycardia	Constipation, dizziness, many drug interactions	Liver, GI tract, 3A4 (6–22 h)

Index